MAR 0 8 2019

D0450118

PRAISE FOR
DYING OF WHITENESS

"In this paradigm-shifting tour de force, Jonathan M. Metzl brilliantly illuminates the shocking ways that white supremacy, through backlash governance, kills white people too. Moving deftly between mountains of data and compelling storytelling, *Dying of Whiteness* makes a vital contribution to our national conversation about racism and its discontents. Metzl uncovers the contemporary paradox of whiteness: a struggle to preserve white privilege in the midst of the declining value of whiteness. This is a must-read if you want to understand how race and the color line operate in twenty-first-century America."

> —Dorian Warren, president, Community Change, and co-chair, Economic Security Project

"*Dying of Whiteness* brilliantly demonstrates the tremendous impediment that white racism and backlash politics pose to our society's wellbeing, at a time when many white Americans quite literally would rather die than support policies they see as benefiting people of color. Metzl issues an urgently needed call to acknowledge the deadly toll of investing in whiteness—and to work collectively toward a just society that would be healthier for everyone."

> —Dorothy Roberts, author of *Killing the Black Body*

"As a recent term-limited progressive Missouri state legislator, I applaud Jonathan M. Metzl's dive into policies and agendas which are destructive to those most in need. He is correct in that racial resentment is the primary reason Medicaid expansion was not allowed to be debated on the House floor the past eight years. He is also correct in exposing racism as a primary reason why my home state of Missouri has loosened gun restrictions even though suicides, accidental, and domestic shootings have skyrocketed in every zip code—including in predominantly white areas. Racial overtones also color healthcare and gun legislation debates in the Capitol, as well as many lobbying efforts. *Dying of Whiteness* boldly exposes the devastating consequences of these politics for everyone, and calls on us to push back against racial resentment for the benefit of all."

> —Hon. Stacey Newman, Missouri House of Representatives, 2010–2018

"Policy makers, scholars, and the public at large need to read Metzl's *Dying of Whiteness*. He forcefully but with empathy demonstrates how poor and working-class whites are literally killing themselves by supporting policies on guns, health care, and taxes framed as defending white authority but which, in truth, benefit the white elite."

> —Eduardo Bonilla-Silva, James B. Duke Professor of Sociology, Duke University

"Jonathan M. Metzl goes to Missouri, Tennessee, and Kansas to understand why people support gun, health, and school policies they will suffer from. An informative snapshot of how 'the other half' live and die."

> —Dr. Alfredo Morabia, editor-in-chief, *American Journal of Public Health*

DYING OF
WHITENESS

Also by Jonathan M. Metzl

The Protest Psychosis: How Schizophrenia Became a
Black Disease

Prozac on the Couch: Prescribing Gender in the Era of
Wonder Drugs

Against Health: How Health Became the New Morality

JONATHAN M. METZL

DYING OF WHITENESS

HOW THE POLITICS OF
RACIAL RESENTMENT IS KILLING
AMERICA'S HEARTLAND

BASIC
BOOKS
New York

Cover design Chin-Yee Lai
Cover image Michael Matthews/Alamy Stock Photo
Cover © 2019 Hachette Book Group, Inc.

Basic Books
Hachette Book Group
1290 Avenue of the Americas, New York, NY 10104
www.basicbooks.com

Printed in the United States of America

First Edition: March 2019

Published by Basic Books, an imprint of Perseus Books, LLC, a subsidiary of Hachette Book Group, Inc.

The publisher is not responsible for websites (or their content) that are not owned by the publisher.

Print book interior design by Amy Quinn.

The Library of Congress has cataloged the hardcover edition as follows:

Names: Metzl, Jonathan, 1964– author.
Title: Dying of whiteness : how the politics of racial resentment is killing
    America's heartland / Jonathan M. Metzl.
Description: First edition. | New York : Basic Books, March 2019. | Includes
    bibliographical references and index.
Identifiers: LCCN 2018040108 (print) | LCCN 2018041118 (ebook) | ISBN
    9781541644960 (ebook) | ISBN 9781541644984 (hardcover)
Subjects: | MESH: Health Status | Healthcare Disparities | Health Services
    Accessibility | Socioeconomic Factors | Politics | Racism | Missouri |
    Tennessee | Kansas
Classification: LCC RA563.M56 (ebook) | LCC RA563.M56 (print) | NLM WA 300
    AM8 | DDC 362.1089—dc23
LC record available at https://lccn.loc.gov/2018040108

ISBNs: 978-1-5416-4498-4 (hardcover), 978-1-5416-4496-0 (ebook)

LSC-C

10 9 8 7 6 5 4 3 2 1

To the Metzl families, who persist, and in persisting, flourish. And to Anna and Clara, our future.

CONTENTS

INTRODUCTION

DYING OF WHITENESS

BEFORE DONALD TRUMP could implement his agenda—in some cases, before he even took the oath of office—reporters and pundits were already tallying the negative implications of his proposals for many Americans. This isn't surprising; changes in government policy inevitably create winners and losers. The twist here was that Trump's plans would hurt the working-class white populations who formed the core of his own base.

"Trump Voters Stand to Suffer Most from Obamacare Repeal and a Trade War" announced an NBC.com piece soon after the 2016 presidential election, quoting George Washington University economist Michael O. Moore. "I think you're going to get a disproportionate impact on people who supported Donald Trump but maybe don't realize that his policies may end up hurting them instead of helping them," Moore claimed. *Salon* echoed Moore's assessment: "Donald Trump is about to victimize his own voters." Meanwhile, a lead editorial in the *New York Times* announced that "Trumpcare Is Already Hurting Trump Country."[1]

Trump didn't bother denying any of it. During an interview on Fox News in March 2017, Tucker Carlson told the president that "counties that voted for you, middle-class and working-class counties, would do far less well" under the proposed repeal of the Affordable Care Act (ACA). "Yeah. Oh, I know that. It's very preliminary," Trump replied.[2]

As promised, the new administration soon pushed a steady stream of cuts to health care delivery systems, financial regulations, environmental

1

protections, job and child support programs, and drug treatment initiatives, all of which imperiled communities and locales where government functions were weak to begin with.[3]

Of course, voters endorsing politicians whose policies seem likely to hurt them is nothing new. Many Southern and midwestern states boast long histories of leaders who enact laws that disadvantage their own constituents and constituents who nonetheless repeatedly vote for these same politicians. As I show in the following chapters, that dynamic took on particular urgency in the decades leading up to the Trump presidency, when an emerging American conservatism promised to make white America "great" in ways that directly harmed lower- and middle-income white voters who supported conservative politics and policies in the first place.

This book details a seeming contradiction that I observed with increasing frequency during six years of research across the midwestern and Southern United States. Between 2013 and 2018, I traveled to places like Franklin, Tennessee; Olathe, Kansas; and Cape Girardeau, Missouri—in Sarah Palin's once controversial words, the "real America"—and asked people about urgent and contested political issues facing the American electorate, including health care, guns, taxes, education, and the scope of government. I wanted to learn how people balanced anti-government or pro-gun attitudes while at the same time navigating lives impacted by poor health care, widening gun-related morbidity, and underfunded public infrastructures and institutions.

I uncovered a diversity of complex opinions. Many people with whom I spoke longed for a middle ground in an increasingly polarized political climate and remained surprisingly open to compromise even under an endless drone of Twitter feeds and news reports that suggested America was in the midst of civil Armageddon. Grieving white mothers of gun suicide victims in Missouri told me that guns and the NRA represented "our way of life," while at the same time lamenting that local governments did not mandate background checks, gun safes, and trigger locks. African American men in Tennessee voiced support for Obamacare because they believed that expanded health insurance benefited low-income black, white, and Hispanic populations alike and in ways that could help everyone. Kansas parents who identified as Republicans and Tea Party supporters wished that their lawmakers would raise state taxes to bolster the public school system. These and other persons, whose voices appear frequently throughout this book, suggest how on-the-ground reality is far more complicated than are the polarized positions we are frequently fed—positions that benefit politicians, donors, foreign governments, or corporations by convincing different groups of Americans that they have nothing in common with each other. At many points along the way, I became convinced that reasonable people of vastly divergent, pro-this or anti-that backgrounds might find middle ground if left to their own devices.

But just as frequently, when I met with middle- and lower-income white Americans across various locales, I found support for a set of political positions that directly harmed their own health and well-being or the health and well-being of their own families. For instance, in early 2016, I spoke with Trevor (most identifying details are changed throughout this book, unless otherwise noted), a forty-one-year-old uninsured Tennessean who drove a cab for twenty years until worsening pain in the upper-right part of his abdomen forced him to see a physician. Trevor learned that the pain resulted from an inflamed liver, the consequence of "years of hard partying" and the damaging effects of the hepatitis C virus. When I met him at a low-income housing facility outside Nashville, Trevor appeared yellow with jaundice and ambled with the help of an aluminum walker to alleviate the pain he felt in his stomach and legs.

As it turned out, debates raged in Tennessee around the same time about the state's participation in the Affordable Care Act and the related expansion of Medicaid coverage. Had Trevor lived a simple thirty-nine-minute drive away in neighboring Kentucky, he might have topped the list of candidates for expensive medications called polymerase inhibitors, a lifesaving liver transplant, or other forms of treatment and support. Kentucky adopted the ACA and began the expansion in 2013, while Tennessee's legislature repeatedly blocked Obama-era health care reforms.

Even on death's doorstep, Trevor wasn't angry. In fact, he staunchly supported the stance promoted by his elected officials. "Ain't no way I would ever support Obamacare or sign up for it," he told me. "I would rather die." When I asked him why he felt this way even as he faced severe illness, he explained, "We don't need any more government in our lives. And in any case, no way I want my tax dollars paying for Mexicans or welfare queens."

Trevor's attitude points to an existential question at the center of my explorations: Of what was Trevor dying? At the most basic level, he died of the toxic effects of liver damage caused by hepatitis C. When the liver becomes inflamed, it fails to filter toxins from the blood and loses the ability to produce vital compounds such as bile and albumin. Without treatment, death comes by systematic deterioration. Jaundice gives way to ascites, which then gives way to hepatic encephalopathy and coma. It's an exceedingly slow, painful way to go out.

Yet I could not help but think that Trevor's deteriorating condition resulted also from the toxic effects of dogma. Dogma that told him that governmental assistance in any form was evil and not to be trusted, even when the assistance came in the form of federal contracts with private health insurance or pharmaceutical companies, or from expanded communal safety nets. Dogma that, as he made abundantly clear, aligned with beliefs about a racial hierarchy that overtly and implicitly aimed to keep white Americans hovering above Mexicans, welfare queens, and other nonwhite others. Dogma suggesting to Trevor that minority groups received lavish benefits from the state, even though he himself lived and died on a low-income budget with state assistance. Trevor voiced a literal willingness to die for his place in this hierarchy, rather than participate in a system that might put him on the same plane as immigrants or racial minorities.[4]

Trevor also slowly died because the dogmas and hierarchies he supported reflected the agendas of politicians who clamored that health care reform and Medicaid expansion represented everything from government overreach to evil incarnate. Anti-ACA invective found particular champions in GOP lawmakers in Tennessee, a once centrist state that turned hard right. These politicians repeatedly made sure that Tennessee did not create its own Obamacare exchange, expand Medicaid, or embrace the health care law in any way.

Thus, routine screenings, filled prescriptions, visits to doctors' offices, and many other factors linked to better health outcomes rose steadily in Kentucky in the four years after that state expanded Medicaid. Such trends lifted the overall well-being of many Kentuckians and particularly helped people who suffered from what are oddly called *preexisting conditions* like hepatitis C—oddly, in my opinion, because "preexisting" assumes that a person's existence begins at the consummation of health insurance coverage. Meanwhile, preventive care and proper treatment remained unattainable for many lower-income Tennessee citizens, in large part because of their state's political choices.

As a physician, I had some sense of the complex medical and psychological explanations for Trevor's symptoms. I worked in an intensive care
unit during my internship, where I saw firsthand the devastating effects of
organ failure. I then trained in psychiatry, where I came to appreciate how
people's deep defense mechanisms and projected insecurities can lead
them to act in ways that seem at odds with their own longevity.

Yet the more I spoke with Trevor, the more I realized how his experience of illness, and indeed his particular form of white identity, resulted
not just from his own thoughts and actions but from his politics. Local and
national politics that claimed to make America great again—and, tacitly,
white again—on the backs and organs of working-class people of all races
and ethnicities, including white supporters. Politics that made vague mention of strategies for governance but ultimately shredded safety nets and
provided massive tax cuts that benefited only the very wealthiest persons
and corporations. Politics that, all too often, gained traction by playing
to anxieties about white victimhood in relation to imagined threats posed
by "Mexicans and welfare queens." Dying for a cause then amounted to a
modern-day form of kamikaze. But in this case, death wasn't announced
with headlines of a flaming plane flown into a battleship. Instead, this form
of death was slow, excruciating, and invisible.[5]

I met many people like Trevor over the course of my research. People
who were dying in various overt or invisible ways as a result of political
beliefs or systems linked to the defense of white "ways of life" or concerns
about minorities or poor people hoarding resources. People like Trevor
who put their own bodies on the line, rather than imagining scenarios in
which diversity or equity might better the flourishing of everyone. The stories these people told me became jumping-off points for a more sustained
investigation of how particular American notions of *whiteness*—notions
shaped by politics and policies as well as by institutions, history, media,
economics, and personal identities—threaten white well-being.

My narrative highlights a reality that liberal Americans were often
slow to realize: Trump supporters were willing to put their own lives on
the line in support of their political beliefs. As a result, when viewed more
broadly, actions that may have seemed from the outside to be crazy, uninformed, or self-defeating served larger political aims. Had Southerners
like Trevor embraced the Affordable Care Act and come to depend on its
many benefits, it would have been much harder for politicians like Trump

to block or overturn healthcare reform. Similar arguments hold true for a number of the topics I analyze in the pages that follow, where on-the-ground white Americans make tradeoffs that negatively affect their lives and livelihoods in support of larger prejudices or ideals. By design, vulnerable immigrant and minority populations suffered the consequences in the most dire and urgent ways. Yet the tradeoffs made by people like Trevor frequently and materially benefitted persons and corporations far higher up the socioeconomic food chain—whose agendas and capital gains depended on the invisible sacrifices of lower income whites.

I track the full extent to which these political acts of self-sabotage came at mortal cost to the health and longevity of lower- and, in many instances, middle-income white GOP supporters—and ultimately, to the well-being of everyone else. The white body that refuses treatment rather than supporting a system that might benefit everyone then becomes a metaphor for, and parable of, the threatened decline of the larger nation. Rather than landing a man on the moon, curing polio, inventing the internet, or promoting structures of world peace, a dominant strain of the electorate voted in politicians whose platforms of American greatness were built on embodied forms of demise.

DYING OF WHITENESS explores the effects of what became central GOP policy issues—loosening gun laws, repealing the Affordable Care Act, or enacting massive tax cuts that largely benefited wealthy persons and corporations—on white population-level health. Over the course of my research for this book, I studied the intersecting histories of race and health in Southern and midwestern states. I collected any number of published reports detailing injuries and deaths among white Americans, even when the injured or deceased appeared to have no obvious connection to racism or politics. I also tracked the health effects of what various authors have called anti-government, anti-tax, pro-gun, and oft-Republican forms of "white backlash conservatism"—a dynamic illustrated by Trevor's rejection of the ACA because of concerns about nonwhite minorities taking away his resources. I repeatedly found examples of policies, politics, or products that claimed to restore white authority but silently delivered lethality. An example that I discuss at length below: pro-gun legislators, the NRA, and gun advertisements touted the abilities of semiautomatic weapons to restore white men's "privilege" and the "balance of power" in an ever-more-diverse world, even as firearms emerged as leading causes of white, male suicide. I then took deep dives into data from a number of scientific and medical databases in order to track systematically the health and mortality consequences that followed political decisions like Tennessee's refusal to expand Medicaid or Missouri's choice to ease regulations governing the purchase and carry of firearms.[6]

These inquiries unearthed trends that inform the book's central arguments. First, a host of conservative political movements emerged (or reemerged) in Southern and midwestern states over the later twentieth and early twenty-first centuries that brought into mainstream US politics once fringe agendas, such as starving government of funding, dismantling social programs, or allowing free flow of most types of firearms. These movements—ranging from the Tea Party to iterations of libertarianism funded by the Koch brothers, to the Freedom Caucus, to the so-called alt-right given voice through outlets such as *Breitbart*—arose from vastly different agendas and points of origin. However, their interests grew ever-more aligned as they came to power in Southern and midwestern states in ways that shaped state agendas, national GOP platforms, and, ultimately, policies of the Trump administration. As this played out, theories of backlash conservatism gave way to something even more powerful: practices of *backlash governance*.

Second, these increasingly unified forms of conservatism advanced politically through overt or implicit appeals to what has been called *white racial resentment*. In other words, these agendas gained support by trumpeting connections to unspoken or overt claims that particular policies, issues, or decisions served also to defend or restore white privilege or quell threats to idealized notions of white authority represented by demographic or cultural shifts. This was both a top-down process (politicians used racial resentment as a tool for class exploitation) and a bottom-up one (the language of white resentment became an increasingly accepted way of talking about whiteness more broadly).[7]

To be sure, groups like the Tea Party rose to prominence for a wide array of cultural, economic, and religious reasons, many of which had relatively little to do with whiteness or race. Lower-income communities left behind by globalizing economies, disenchantment with Democrats, and the growing influence of corporate lobbies and megarich donors on party politics unquestionably played major roles. A number of people with whom I spoke, when I explained the thesis of my book, told me that positions that appeared to reflect racism instead reflected a larger, color-blind "hatred of the poor."

Yet a major part of these movements' appeals lay in rallying cries that tapped into emotionally and historically charged notions that white Americans should remain atop other racial or ethnic groups in the US social hierarchy, or that white "status" was at risk. This is not to say that any one specific person was expressly racist. Rather, frameworks of white racial resentment shaped debates about, and attitudes toward, various public policies and acts of legislation. Sometimes, the racial agendas of these calls to arms were overt and obvious. For instance, posters of then president Obama photoshopped as an African witch doctor with a feather headdress and a bone through his nose began to appear at anti-ACA Tea Party rallies. In 2016, former Missouri Republican Party director Ed Martin told a cheering Tea Party for Trump rally in Festus, Missouri, that "Donald Trump is for Americans first. . . . You're not racist if you don't like Mexicans." (That same year, the Tea Party Patriots funded Asia-bashing advertisements featuring fictional Chinese executives in suits speaking Mandarin and laughing about how they were able to buy thousands of acres of Missouri farmland.) At other times, the racial underpinnings of the agendas appeared all but invisible to people on the ground, as with decisions to rally around issues such as guns, health insurance, or public schools—issues whose racially charged histories had been obscured by the passage of time.[8]

Third, the policies that took shape when these once fringe forms of conservatism entered the mainstream GOP and assumed legislative power often negatively affected the health of middle- and lower-income populations. While some of these policies and actions directly affected health care, others not expressly linked to health, such as the proliferation of civilian-owned firearms, nonetheless carried profound medical implications. White backlash politics gave certain white populations the sensation of winning, particularly by upending the gains of minorities and liberals; yet the victories came at a steep cost. When white backlash policies became laws, as in cutting away health care programs and infrastructure spending, blocking expansion of health care delivery systems, defunding opiate-addiction centers, spewing toxins into the air, or enabling guns in public spaces, the result was—and I say this with the support of statistics detailed in the chapters that follow—increasing rates of death.

Fourth, a wide array of middle- and lower-income people experienced negative health consequences from these policy decisions—again, largely because the policies involved elaborate strategies for tearing down community structures for middle- and lower-income Americans but hardly any blueprints for building them back up. Minority and immigrant communities, often the targets of backlash's ire, suffered greatly and needlessly. But the data I track in this book reveals the shocking extent to which the health and well-being of white Americans suffered from the health effects of these policies as well. Such effects played out in public ways—such as when white concertgoers died in high-profile mass shootings linked to gun policies (or lack thereof) enacted by conservative white politicians. Other effects were far less obvious—such as the long-term implications of blocking health care reform or defunding schools and infrastructure.[9]

Finally, as with Trevor, many lower- and middle-income white Americans continued to support these policies and ideologies—with their inherent links to narratives of imagined victimhood and domination—even after their negative effects became apparent and promises made by politicians such as Trump unraveled. Indeed, for a variety of reasons, white Americans in parts of the United States saw unprecedented drops in life expectancy over the time of my study. But instead of scrapping these state-level policies as examples of historically bad governance, they became the foundations for legislation at the national level, in the form of Trump-era tax bills, gun policies, health care strategies, and other ill-fated initiatives. All the while, the issues themselves—such as guns, health care, or taxes—accrued larger symbolic or moral meanings in ways that rendered conversations about the effects of specific policies ever-more difficult.[10]

The confluence of these trajectories led to a perilous state of affairs that I analyze in the sections that follow. Succinctly put: a host of complex anxieties prompt increasing numbers of white Americans like Trevor to support right-wing politicians and policies, even when these policies actually harm white Americans at growing rates. As these policy agendas spread from Southern and midwestern legislatures into the halls of Congress and the White House, ever-more white Americans are then, literally, *dying of whiteness*. This is because white America's investment in maintaining an imagined place atop a racial hierarchy—that is, an investment in a sense of whiteness—ironically harms the aggregate well-being of US whites as a demographic group, thereby making whiteness itself a negative health indicator.

Claims about lower- and middle-income people who vote against their self-interests often use frameworks based in economics. Scholars and writers have long argued that the Republican Party rose to influence in the US South by taking advantage of white backlash against integration and civil rights to cajole white working-class people to vote against their own financial self-interests. Thomas Frank, in his modern classic *What's the Matter with Kansas?*, writes that backlash conservatism rests on the foundation that "ignoring one's economic self-interest may seem like a suicidal move to you and me, but viewed differently it is an act of noble self-denial; a sacrifice for a holier cause." In her thoughtful study *Strangers in Their Own Land*, Arlie Hochschild poses the paradoxical question: "Why, with so many problems [in poor white communities], was there so much disdain for federal money to alleviate them?"[11]

My research measures just how deeply modern-day American backlash conservatism demands that lower- and middle-class white Americans vote against their own *biological* self-interests as well as their own economic priorities. Over the course of the narrative, I meet with white Americans who continue to support GOP policies, even as these same policies negatively affect their own health in measurable ways. The ways that these persons literally bet their lives and livelihoods on such policies and politicians forced me to recognize, time and again, the depths of their investments in GOP policy issues.

To be very clear, it is in no way my intention to expose anyone with whom I spoke as being duped or uninformed. Many of the people I met were trying to get by as best they could under deeply challenging circumstances. I tried to be transparent with people about the aims of this book, which led to honest conversations that challenged my own core beliefs. As the following chapters make clear, many people I spoke with were not exactly thrilled with their own political leaders and fought for reform in unexpected ways. I uncovered numerous other examples of working-class white resentment directed at other white people. As essayist Sarah Smarsh puts it, "Most struggling whites I know live lives of quiet desperation mad at their white bosses, not resentment of their co-workers or neighbors of color." Moreover, health is just one of the many factors people take into account when making decisions that affect their lives—and writing this book has made me think repeatedly about choices I make in my own life that might negatively impact my own longevity.[12]

Perhaps most important, I myself am a white American who grew up in the Midwest. Any approach I might adopt that suggests *them*, conservatives, versus *us*, enlightened liberals, is tempered by the fact that I, too, receive the benefit of the doubt when I walk down the street and that I am neither profiled by police nor subject to arrest and incarceration by ICE agents. I have no doubt that many of the conversations I recount in this book reflect commonalities between myself and the people I interview. It seems to me a lost opportunity to address Southern forms of whiteness as existing only in another "country," rather than as exaggerations of systems of privilege that surround North and South, liberal, progressive, and conservative, interviewee and interviewer both. It's too easy to blame the rise of white nationalism on politicians like Trump, Jeff Sessions, or Steve Bannon and far harder to address how the ideologies these politicians support benefit white populations more broadly. In this sense, the larger conversation about the effects of whiteness is the one we, white Americans, badly need to have.

Coming from the Midwest and writing about my home states—I grew up in Kansas and Missouri and now live in Tennessee—also made me keenly aware of just how much the politics of backlash upended the ground-level conciliatory work done since slavery, Jim Crow, segregation, and other vestiges of a shameful past. This work at least tried to rectify inequality through policies that promoted principles of diversity and social justice, but were rendered impossible by political agendas that defunded supporting governmental programs and agencies. All the while, politics fueled by racial resentment eroded faith in hallmark American democratic institutions more broadly.[13]

I kept thinking that at some point, the drive for self-preservation might trump political ideology. Why would someone reject their own health care, or keep guns unlocked when their children were home? Yet because of the frames cast around these and other issues hued with historically charged assumptions about privilege, it became ever-more difficult for many people with whom I spoke to imagine alternate realities or to empathize with groups other than their own. Compromise, in many ways, coded as treason.

THE HEART OF the book delves into three state-level narratives that illustrate how politics that claimed on face value to bolster white America ended up making even white lives sicker, harder, and shorter. I begin in Missouri, where pro–National Rifle Association (NRA) conservative lawmakers passed pro-gun laws that allowed citizens to carry concealed handguns at schools, annulled most city and regional gun restrictions, and allowed just about anyone over the age of eighteen to carry a concealed weapon. Though framed as universal expressions of Second Amendment rights, racial tensions lurked around every corner of these legislative decisions. Corporate-gun-lobby-backed politicians, commentators, and advertisements openly touted loosened gun laws as ways for white citizens to protect themselves against dark intruders, while white open-carry advocates paraded through largely African American sections of downtown St. Louis brandishing semiautomatic handguns and long guns. Meanwhile, black men who attempted to demonstrate their own open-carry rights were attacked and jailed rather than lauded as freedom-loving patriots.

When I began to sift through the statistics for gun injury and death in Missouri, I quickly realized that the primary victims of gun mortality were not criminals or inner-city gang members, as the NRA and some politicians implied. Rather, as gun laws were liberalized, gun deaths spiked . . . among white people. This was because white Missourians dominated injuries and deaths via gun-related suicides, partner violence, and accidental shootings—and in ways that outpaced African American gun deaths from homicides. Gun regulation is such a politically sensitive question in the United States that there has long been a congressional ban on funding for research on the health impact of firearms. Through a back door into data on mortality, I detail how legislation that substantially deregulated gun purchases set Missouri on a path toward becoming a top state for gun suicide, even among other pro-gun states, and that the primary victims of these trends were white Missourians, particularly white men living in rural areas. As I show, lax gun laws ultimately cost the state roughly $273 million in lost work between 2008 and 2015 and ultimately led to the loss of over *10,506 years* of productive white male life.

We next travel to Tennessee, where the conservative Republican establishment blocked the state's participation in the Affordable Care Act and Medicaid expansion at every turn. I talk to white men like Trevor, who vigorously resent government intrusion into their lives and fear that their tax dollars will go toward lazy minorities—even as they themselves suffer the consequences of restricted access to health care. These types of attitudes complicate attempts to sell health care reform in rural America and might doom progressive calls for "Medicare for all"—since attempts to promote expanded health care rarely address the racial anxieties surrounding government health care in places like Tennessee. As I show, social programs such as Medicare and Medicaid carry particular racial histories and as a result convey intonations about networks that connect the well-being of white Americans with the actions and contributions of persons from other racial or ethnic groups. Here as well, racial anxiety comes at a cost. Looking closely at the data on health outcomes between Tennessee and neighboring Kentucky uncovers how, when averaged across the population, Tennessee's refusal to expand Medicaid cost *every single* white resident of the state *14.1 days of life.*

The book's final section takes us to Kansas, where citizens struggle with the aftermath of a Tea Party–fueled economic "experiment" led by controversial Governor Sam Brownback, in which the largest income tax cut in state history turned the state budget surplus into a substantial deficit. Parents and school administrators describe how politicians often framed the resultant cuts to Kansas public schools as ways to punish "wasteful" minority districts who supposedly splurged on "party busses" instead of classrooms. And indeed, early budget cuts overwhelmingly impacted schools in low-income minority districts. But these initial cuts were not enough to fill the gaping holes in state budgets. Soon, as a thoughtful Kansas state legislator told me, "the fire that we set in the fields burned all the way up to the home." Popular resistance began to form only when cuts began to affect suburban white schools, but then it was often too late. When the data began to roll in, it turned out that white student populations saw flatlining test scores and rising high school dropout rates—trends that correlate directly with poor health later in life. As but one example, 688 additional white students dropped out of Kansas public high schools in the first four years of budget cuts than would have done so otherwise. On average, in the United States, dropping out of high school correlates with nine years of lost life expectancy. When calculated against average life expectancy, the cuts correlated by conservative estimates with *6,195.51 lost white life years.*

Guns, health care systems, and the impacts of tax cuts on schools are decidedly different issues, and the health effects that arise from these issues manifest in divergent ways. Getting shot leads to one form of mortality; not going to the doctor when you get sick or dropping out of high school leads to another. It's sometimes a matter of speed versus slow decay. As such, the narratives I tell in the three parts of the book differ in important ways. For instance, gun and health insurance policies affect health and mortality rates far more directly than do taxation and education spending policies.

Yet these issues overlap, not just because of their centrality to present-day GOP political platforms but because of connections to particular histories of race and place in America. For nearly two centuries, gun ownership was a privilege afforded mainly to white citizens in states such as Missouri, and guns became particular symbols as a result. Health insurance similarly represented a privilege afforded only to whites in many Southern states: through the antebellum period, insurers covered black bodies as property. Kansas became a national flashpoint for the limits of "separate but equal" public education, leading to the landmark *Brown v. Board of Education of Topeka* Supreme Court decision in 1954.

These histories imbue debates about guns, health care systems, taxes, and schools with larger meanings about race in America and about American whiteness. The history of race in America also helps explain why these topics cut to the heart of present-day debates about what it means to provide resources, protections, and opportunities for everyone in a diverse society versus providing securities and opportunities for a select few. Debates over firearm rights in Missouri revolve around questions of "Whose lives are worth protecting?"; over health care coverage in Tennessee around similar questions of "Whose lives are worth insuring?"; and over schools in Kansas around questions of "Whose lives are worth funding and educating?"

At the same time, prior to the emergence of the Tea Party and other far-right movements, so-called purple states also represented centrist examples where people with differing ideologies worked together to try to find common, if often unstable solutions to polarizing societal problems. Missouri claimed a long history of gun rights but also enforced some of the strictest handgun laws in the nation. Bipartisan groups of Tennessee lawmakers aimed to create a Southern oasis of health care in which every citizen of the state had health insurance. Kansas boasted some of America's best public schools. Then, polarization took over, and things changed.

MY FOCUS ON the health risks of American backlash politics for white Americans is in no way meant to minimize the larger effects of racism in the United States. It should be taken as a matter of fact, but all too often is not, that systems in which race correlates with privilege have devastating consequences for minority and immigrant populations. Cuts to health delivery networks, communal safety nets, schools, and social services, alongside policies that enable the proliferation of guns, often impact minority populations first and most severely. Racism itself can also have profoundly negative health consequences. Epidemiologist Yvette Cozier and her colleagues have uncovered associations between frequent experiences of racism—such as receiving poor service in restaurants and stores or feeling unfairly treated on the job or by the police—and higher risks of illness and obesity among African American women. Sleep researcher Michael Grandner has found links between perceived racism and sleep disturbances. And public health scholar Mario Sims found that lifetime discrimination was associated with greater rates of hypertension among adult African Americans.[14]

Increasingly, we now hear that people with racist attitudes fare poorly as well. Racist views make people "sick" and "unhealthy," neuroscientists claim, because the psychological effort of discrimination can raise blood pressure or cortisol levels and heighten risk for heart attacks or strokes. "Harboring prejudice may be bad for your health," neuropsychologist Elizabeth Page-Gould writes, because racially prejudiced people experience such "biological reactions . . . even during benign social interactions with people of different races."[15]

My findings in this book suggest that we make a wrong turn when we try to address racism mainly as a disorder of people's brains or attitudes, or try to "fix" the problem simply by attempting to sensitize people or change their minds. On an aggregate level, people's individual racial attitudes have relatively little correlation to their health. Yes, in extreme cases like that of Trevor, racial animus can lead to medical disaster. Yet this correlation rarely holds true at the level of population health. Racial animosity rarely makes a person sick in and of itself—otherwise, there would be many more sick people of all backgrounds in the world. Research suggests that certain racist policies might be medically advantageous for white people. For instance, sociologists Mark Beaulieu and Tracey Continelli have studied the "benefits of segregation for white communities."[16]

Instead, racism matters most to health when its underlying resentments and anxieties shape larger politics and policies and then affect public health. I say this in part because many of the middle- and lower-income white Americans I met in my research were not expressly or even implicitly racist. Race does not even come up in many of our conversations. Yet racism remained an issue, not because of their attitudes but because they lived in states whose elected officials passed overly permissive gun policies, rejected health care reform, undercut social safety net programs, and a host of other actions. In these and other instances, racism and racial resentment functioned at structural levels and in ways that had far broader effects than the kinds of racism that functions in people's minds.

Addressing racism structurally allows me to raise what became the most troubling findings of my research: I found that, when tracked over time, racially driven policies in Missouri, Tennessee, and Kansas functioned as mortal risk factors for all people who live in these states. This is because illness and death patterns that followed actions such as expanding gun proliferation or massive tax cuts mimicked those once seen in relation to other man-made pathogens, such as water pollution, secondhand smoke, or not wearing seat belts in cars, or during certain disease outbreaks. Society mobilized to reduce risk and improve health when toxins dumped into the water, cigarettes, or faulty automobiles led to declining health. But when the pathogens were policies and ideologies, they instead laid the foundations for politics furthered at the national level by the GOP, the NRA, and the Trump administration.[17] In these ways, stories like Trevor's come to embody larger problems of an electorate that, in its worst moments, votes to sink the whole ship (except for a few privileged passengers who get lifeboats) even when they are on it, rather than investing in communal systems that might rise all tides. Anti-blackness, in a biological sense, then produces its own anti-whiteness. An illness of the mind, weaponized onto the body of the nation.

Finally, I realize that "whiteness" is a highly sensitive and contested term, one that ties deeply to identity. In this book, I do not mean white as a biological classification or a skin color but as a political and economic system. I do so because of historical precedent: throughout American history, supporters of pretty much all American political backgrounds and parties have risen to defend the economic and political privileges built around "whiteness" when these privileges seem under "attack." For instance, the defense of whiteness proved a powerful tool for politicians aiming to rally forces against perceived threats to white privilege posed by desegregation during the American civil rights era of the 1960s. In 1964, then Democratic senator Strom Thurmond of South Carolina warned that the Civil Rights Act of that year would lead to "upheaval of social patterns and customs that are more than a century old" in many Southern white communities and that "to force people to change their pattern of living overnight . . . creates a potentially dangerous situation." Similar opposition resulted when the Johnson administration introduced Medicare and Medicaid in 1965, based on widespread concerns among white Southerners that new laws would require previously segregated hospitals to integrate in order to receive federal funding.[18]

Paying attention to "whiteness" as a political and economic system is also important because, according to the work of historians and race theorists, the seeming benefits afforded by such systems of privilege can blind working-class white populations to these system's negative effects, opening the door for potential manipulation. In his seminal work on Reconstruction, historian W. E .B. Du Bois famously argued that whiteness served as a "public and psychological wage," delivering to poor whites a valuable social status derived from their classification as "not-black." "Whiteness" thereby provided "compensation" for citizens otherwise exploited by the organization of capitalism—while at the same time preventing working-class white Southerners from forming a common cause with working-class black populations in their shared suffering at the bottom of the social ladder. In his classic text *The Wages of Whiteness*, historian David Roediger shows how "racial folklore" fuels racial ideologies in ways that open white working-class communities to "economic exploitation" by ruling-class whites. More recently, writer Toni Morrison states the inherent conflict of American whiteness bluntly: to "restore whiteness to its former status as a marker of national identity, a number of white Americans are sacrificing themselves." And in his elegiac *Tears We Cannot Stop: A Sermon to White America*, sociologist and pastor Michael Eric Dyson laments the "the politics of whiteness . . . it's killing us, and, quiet as it's kept, it's killing you too."[19]

Again, the health risks that Dyson describes go along with substantial real-world *benefits*, such as not being disproportionally shot by police, deported, or mass incarcerated. Yet present-day social scientists now catalog the trade-offs that many white Americans make to maintain a system that appears set up for their advantage. As a team of researchers led by sociologist Jennifer Malat writes, white Americans increasingly represent a "paradox" of privilege, access, and social rewards on one hand and relatively poor health outcomes on the other. For Malat, this paradox helps explain why "whites in the USA . . . rank poorly in international health comparisons."[20]

History also teaches us that it's best to avoid knee-jerk assumptions that more government, money, or health care are automatically good or that either end of the political spectrum corners the market on problematic racial assumptions. I've spent enough time working in hospital systems such as the United States Department of Veterans Affairs to realize that more investment in health care does not automatically result in better health outcomes. Indeed, sometimes a person is well advised to avoid seeing a doctor altogether. There are also far too many examples of ostensibly liberal or Democratic initiatives that result in poor health for minority and low-income populations—indeed, Democrats sustained segregation in the US South for decades prior to the 1960s. Liberals and progressives have at times used disdain for conservatives, or a sense of superiority over them, as ways to mask their own ways of promoting inequity.

Yet the Tea Party, the alt-right, and the populism of Donald Trump seem to signal a marked shift in the course of American history and hasten the downfall of what remains of white conservative political traditions of compromise. In the words of writer Ta-Nehisi Coates, Trump then became "the first white President" as a result. The results are potentially catastrophic. I've come to believe, and argue in this book, that playing to white anxieties has implications beyond "whipping up the base" against immigrants, liberals, and minorities. When politics demands that people resist available health care, amass arsenals, cut funding for schools that their own kids attend, or make other decisions that might feel emotionally correct but are biologically perilous, these politics are literally asking people to die for their whiteness. Living in a state or a county or a nation dominated by a politics of racial resentment then becomes a diagnosable, quantifiable, and increasingly mortal preexisting condition.[21]

I've written this book because, as a physician, I've become increasingly concerned about population-level policies constructed with disregard for population-level health. And as a researcher, I began to realize that the overarching negative health effects of these policies resulted not from people's deep biases or fear of minorities lodged deep in their brains but from specific electoral, economic, and policy decisions made at particular moments in time. Brains, genetics, feelings, and attitudes make racial hierarchy feel impossible to address because they suggest that people are and will always be the same. But decisions are communally made and can thus be communally unmade and remade in better ways.

Couching politics in racial mistrust also makes it harder for white America to see how we—and I include myself as a white American here—would benefit self and country far more by emphasizing economic, legislative, and everyday cooperation rather than by chasing the false promise of supremacy. Investing in communal health care solutions, workers' rights, better roads and bridges, research into climate change and opiate addiction, common-sense gun laws, or expanded social safety nets benefit everyone, not just the immigrant and minority populations or "liberals" that red- and purple-state white Americans have been taught to doubt or see as taking more than their fair share of entitlements. In the book's conclusion, I argue that the way forward requires a white America that strives to collaborate rather than dominate, with a mind-set of openness and interconnectedness that we have all-too-frequently neglected.

This is not to suggest that everyone become a Democrat—far from it. Rather, our nation urgently needs to recognize how the systems of inequality we build and sustain aren't benefiting anyone. Forms of white disconnect emerging today—and not coincidentally, at the very moment when US white populations begin to imagine an end to demographic dominance—instead encourage a host of anxieties and decisions that threaten the well-being of a great many people. Political fissures that the GOP, wealthy interest groups, and even foreign nations manipulate seemingly at every turn then further balkanize a country whose power derives from putting aside differences in the common cause of a greater, united confederation of states. Compromise then grows ever-less possible to imagine—under Trump, researchers at the Centers for Disease Control and Prevention (CDC) now even limit use of the word *diversity* in budget requests. All the while, we move closer to a system that benefits the very few at the expense of the many.[22]

Writing this book has led me to believe that understanding why conservative white Americans vote in ways that might negatively affect their own lives involves far more than pointing out ways that these voters may have been conned or deceived, as headlines like the ones with which I began this introduction tend to do. The particular issues about which Trump supporters appear to have been "duped" also tap into larger histories, myths, and ideologies. These histories, myths, and ideologies go a long way toward explaining the complex tension between promises of restored "greatness" on one hand and practices of self-sabotage on the other. Better awareness of this paradoxical tension might allow us to better promote an alternative investment in collaboration and equality—in many instances, by addressing ideologies of whiteness head-on rather than by proxy.[23]

However, at this writing at least, the electorate has chosen a regime whose policies come cloaked in the promise of restored privilege, enacted through mechanisms of polarization and divisiveness. As a result, we talk about eliminating financial safety nets and social support programs, allowing ever-more guns, defunding roads and bridges while at the same time enacting tariffs and building walls. Such talk, and the policies that flow from it, often signify protection, preservation, or continued supremacy. But in many instances, they ultimately serve to hemorrhage our collective abilities to solve problems or help people in times of need.[24]

The recent histories of Missouri, Tennessee, and Kansas thus serve as object lessons and cautionary tales that suggest how the racial system of America fails everyone. The health trajectories of people in these states also offer dire warnings against emulating gun policies like Missouri's, health care systems like Tennessee's, and tax cuts like those inflicted on Kansas across the entire United States. Ultimately, the three states we visit in this book show ways that, when white voters are asked to defend whiteness, whiteness often fails to defend, honor, or restore them.

PART 1

MISSOURI

THE CAPE

THE SUPPORT GROUP meets in a room off the main stacks at the public library of Cape Girardeau, Missouri, and provides community for people who have lost loved ones to suicide. It's December, and red-and-green Christmas decorations adorn a table in the center of the room. Next to the holiday decor sit small piles of pamphlets, DVDs, and refrigerator magnets that offer resources, uplifting phrases, or action plans. *Coping with Your Grief* is the title of one pamphlet, *With Help Comes Hope* of another.

The room is warm and brightly lit, in sharp contrast to the freezing conditions outside. Wind blows against the windows. Through the windows, one sees only darkness, save for the light illuminating the gate to the county cemetery that abuts the library grounds.

Eleven people in various stages of grief sit in a circle. At one end of the grief spectrum is Billie, a talkative woman in her late forties whose mother died by suicide nineteen years ago. At the other end is Kim, thirty-nine, whose father called her and then killed himself while they were still on the phone—it's been less than six months now. For Kim, getting through each day is a struggle.

December is a particularly hard time for everyone. Christmas conjures family memories and portends happy gatherings, but it also highlights the absence of the departed. The holidays also mark agonizing anniversaries for those in the room whose husbands, wives, siblings, parents, or other loved ones ended their lives during the season of joy.

Pain and empathy reverberate through the early parts of the meeting as the participants tell their stories. *I feel uniquely abandoned and alone,* each person says in one way or another. *We have been there and understand what you are going through*, replies the group. Together the members of this monthly meeting work to make sense of the nonsensical, the unthinkable, and to process the persistent existential questions at the core of their survivorship: *How could I have not seen? What could I have done differently? Could I have prevented this?*

I came to Missouri to better understand the real-world consequences of gun suicide and gun death, in large part because the state often serves as ground zero for gun violence prevention researchers. Located at the junction of the South and the Midwest, Missouri boasts a long history of gun use for hunting, warfare, and dueling. At the same time, through the early 1990s, Missouri's handgun laws were among the strictest in the nation, including a requirement that handgun buyers undergo background checks in person at sheriffs' offices before obtaining permits.[1]

However, in the past twenty years, an increasingly conservative and pro-gun legislature and citizenry had relaxed limitations governing practically every aspect of buying, owning, and carrying firearms in the state. In the six years prior to my 2016 visit to Cape Girardeau, the Missouri legislature ended prohibitions on the concealed and open carry of firearms in public spaces, lowered the legal age to carry a concealed gun from twenty-one to nineteen, and repealed many of the requirements for comprehensive background checks and purchase permits. In 2014, Missouri voters approved Amendment 5 to the state constitution, which established the "unalienable right of citizens to keep and bear arms, ammunition and accessories associated with the normal functioning of such arms, for the purpose of defense of one's person, family, home and property," and effectively negated the rights of cities or towns to enact practically any form of gun control.[2]

And in 2016, Missouri lawmakers overrode their governor's veto to enact Senate Bill 656, the so-called guns everywhere bill. Among other stipulations, SB 656 eliminated requirements for training, education, background checks, and permits needed to carry concealed weapons in Missouri. Bill 656 also annulled most city and regional gun restrictions, vastly expanded so-called Castle Doctrine coverage—the notion that "a man's home is his castle and he has a right to defend it . . . free from legal prosecution for the consequences of the force used"—and extended "stand-your-ground" protections for people who took lethal action against perceived dangers outside the home as well.[3]

The *New York Times* described what followed as a "natural experiment" in whether more guns led to more safety and less crime. Gun advocates hailed the legislative moves as boosting public security. The National Rifle Association (NRA), a not particularly silent partner in all of this, lauded the ultimate passage of SB 656 as "a great day for freedom in Missouri" and for "the constitutional rights of law-abiding citizens." State GOP legislators such as state senator Brian Munzlinger argued that Castle Doctrine laws enhanced the rights of "law-abiding citizens to protect themselves and their families." *Guns and Ammo* magazine cited Missouri as "ahead of the curve when it comes to gun rights" and a "top state for gun owners."[4]

At the same time, research suggested that gun injuries and deaths rose after it became easier for people to buy and carry firearms. For instance, a team of investigators led by Daniel Webster, director of the Johns Hopkins Center for Gun Policy and Research, analyzed crime data from Missouri and found that the state's 2007 repeal of its permit-to-purchase (PTP) handgun law "was associated with a 25 percent increase in firearm homicides rates." Between 2008 and 2014, the Missouri gun homicide rate rose to 47 percent higher than the national average. Rates of gun death by suicide, partner violence, and accidental shooting soared as well. In 2014, gun deaths topped deaths by motor vehicle accident for the first time in the state. News outlets referred to Missouri as the "Shoot Me State."[5]

I traveled through Missouri over the summer, fall, and winter of 2016 to learn about people's experiences, beneath the numbers and the data, of living in an increasingly armed society. I conducted structured interviews, met with groups, and talked to people I met along the way, all against the backdrop of the 2016 US presidential election that presented voters with starkly differing approaches to gun rights and gun violence prevention. Donald Trump earned the endorsement of the NRA through full-throated promotion of gun rights, promising to end restrictions on legal gun owners. Trump ultimately garnered the support of most counties in the increasingly red state of Missouri. Meanwhile, Hillary Clinton ran on a platform that included banning assault weapons, closing background-check and gun show loopholes, and limiting gun access for persons deemed at risk of violence.[6]

I spoke with people in small towns like Cape Girardeau as well as larger cities like Kansas City, St. Louis, Columbia, and Jefferson City about ways that the proliferation of guns may have changed how they interacted with people or lived their daily lives. The terrain was far from unfamiliar to me; I was born on a military base, and my parents settled our family in Kansas City after my father's service ended. I stayed in Missouri through college and medical school. My work as a doctor and a professor took me elsewhere, but I return to Missouri several times each year.

The Missouri I recalled was a Show Me State marked by attempted compromise. Leaders came from various ranks of society and represented a wide array of constituencies. As recently as 2000, when the election handed the state senate an even number of Democrats and Republicans with neither side holding a majority, party leaders arranged for a unique power-sharing agreement that split power among them. Under the agreement, the state senate had two co–presidents pro tem, one Republican and one Democrat, who rotated between days as to whom exercised the chamber powers, and selected committee cochairs appointed from each party.[7]

Over the course of the early twenty-first century, rightist agendas came to dominate the state legislature in ways that loosened gun laws, slashed public spending, blocked health care reform, and undercut social safety net programs. Meanwhile, racial tensions came to full boil in November 2014, after Darren Wilson, a twenty-eight-year-old white police officer in Ferguson, shot and killed an unarmed African American teenager named Michael Brown. A US Department of Justice report later revealed that the shooting happened within the context of a state where minority populations were subject to "unconstitutional policing," systemic bias, and law enforcement practices shaped more by a "focus on revenue rather than by public safety needs." With each visit over recent years, I could not help but notice that the tenor of the state became increasingly tense, polarized, and ever-more-heavily armed.[8]

Many of the people I met saw the increasing availability of firearms as a positive development. Tom, who wore a holstered gun while shopping for toiletries at a Walmart in Independence, told me that he appreciated the ability to protect himself against possible threats at all times. An advertising consultant from Columbia named John told me that he liked being able to carry a concealed firearm when he visited printing factories and other work sites. "The thought that I can bring a gun just makes me feel safer," he explained. Eleanor, owner of Smokin' Guns BBQ in North Kansas City, said that she welcomed customers who carried concealed weapons into her restaurant and that she was bothered much more by "intrusive government regulations about the food we serve."

Conversely, numerous Missourians described anxieties about guns and armed civilians in public spaces. "I've seen people with guns in their belts at the supermarket," a Columbia parent named Megan told me. "It makes me reconsider bringing my kid on shopping trips." A Democratic Missouri state representative worried that lawmakers and their staff carried concealed weapons during heated debates on the House floor. "With new laws, capital security can no longer ask lawmakers to check their firearms at the door," she explained. "And I often find it quite unnerving that the people I'm working with or arguing against might well be carrying secret guns during our legislative sessions."

Any number of African American citizens voiced concern about the charged implications of white citizens brandishing guns in mixed-race settings. In Kansas City, I met a Vietnam veteran named John, who told me that he now thinks twice about shopping at Sam's Club. John used to stop by the wholesale megastore on his way home from his job as a home health care provider. That was before he saw armed white men strolling through the aisles. For John, the result was often intimidation. "I see white guys and their sons walking around Sam's Club, Walmart, and other places where we shop, strolling with guns on their hips like it's the Wild West," he told me. "They're trying to be all macho, like they have power because of their guns, walking down the aisles. It just makes me . . . stay away."

For Cassandra, an African American pastor in St. Louis, situations such as the ones described by John illustrated a double standard through which society coded white gun owners as "protectors" and black gun owners as "threats." Her church hosted an intense debate among congregants after the horrific church shooting in Charleston, South Carolina, in June 2015 that yielded a decision to ban guns in their house of worship. Cassandra supported the decision: "Even though I want us to be protected, I can't escape the fact that these are the same guns that are oppressing communities of color in our state."

Cape Girardeau, in the southeastern part of Missouri, proved in many ways the most complex stop on my tour. The city of 78,000 is named after Jean Baptiste de Girardot, a French soldier who established a temporary trading post in the area in the early eighteenth century. The "Cape" refers to a rock promontory overlooking the Mississippi River that was later destroyed by railroad construction. The city's official website describes Cape Girardeau as a "regional destination for healthcare, education, shopping, and employment." But the city and the surrounding region recovered slowly from the recession of 2008, and stability remained elusive for many people and small businesses. Opioid and heroin abuse also became growing problems in the 2010s. In 2015, the average per capita income was $24,479, and 16 percent of people lived below the poverty line.[9]

Like much of southern Missouri, "Cape," as locals call it, is overwhelmingly white and Republican. The Quick Facts from the US Census listed 88.3 percent of residents as white in 2015, and the region went heavily for Trump in 2016.[10] Well-known native sons include conservative commentators David and Rush Limbaugh.

I flew into Cape Girardeau in December 2016, via a tiny propeller plane not much bigger than a crop duster. Before boarding in St. Louis, the pilot asked me and the four other passengers to weigh ourselves and our belongings, and he then seated us accordingly. He placed my carry-on in a small compartment in the nose of the plane, as if my change of clothing, running shoes, books, and computer might keep us on course. The flight from St. Louis took just under an hour, most of which we spent at low altitude over a flat farmland so vast and open that a bullet could travel for miles and not hit anything.

The centrality of gun culture to people's daily lives in Cape Girardeau struck me immediately on my arrival to town—in fact, it was hard to miss. Practically everyone waiting or working in the small airport wore some sort of camouflage. Middle-aged men sported camo jackets and pants, often accompanied by baseball caps bearing the logos of gun companies or hunting clubs. I saw a teenage girl wearing a camouflage T-shirt pushing an elderly man in a wheelchair, and the man wore a camo hat and cradled a camo lunchbox on his lap. Even the dogs bore camouflage—a woman in a camo jacket led a guide dog decked out in a camouflage bandanna. Were we in the woods on a fall day, these people would likely have been invisible. But because we were in a small regional one-room airport, they simply blended in with one another.[11]

I called a cab from the regional dispatch, and fifteen minutes later, the driver, Jim, arrived wearing camouflage pants and carrying a not-very-concealed weapon on his belt. We drove out of the airport and immediately passed a business called Shooters Gun Shop Inc., soon followed by a series of billboards for gun ranges, gun shops, and gun shows. I asked Jim about the ubiquity of firearms and camo, and he gave a thoughtful reply. "I'm sure it must seem strange coming in from the outside," he said, "but for us, it's what we've grown up with." I asked him what guns meant to him, and he immediately responded, "Freedom. Liberty. Patriotism. That's why we just voted Trump. No way we were going to let 'Crooked Hillary' take those things away from us."

Guns also feature prominently in the stories people tell at the support group and in the lengthy one-on-one interviews I conducted with group members and other people from Cape in the days and weeks following the gathering at the library. For pretty much everyone I speak with, the language of patriotism and protection collides with memories of extraordinary trauma and pain.

"We've been holding this meeting for five years," Billie, the coleader, announces to the group about halfway through the hour-and-a-half session. "And I would guess that tonight, yet again, over 90 percent of us are here because of a suicide by gun." Billie says this in part for my benefit—she reached out and invited me to observe a meeting after I posted an essay about my research on a Missouri listserv. Billie also raises the specter of firearms because doing so gives permission for people to share some of the more excruciating remembrances of their losses.

"I guess I'll go first," a man named Rick replies after a heavy moment of silence. Rick, in his early fifties, attends the meeting with his wife, June. The couple lost their son to suicide by gun four years earlier. Up to that point in the meeting, Rick often smiled and offered encouragement to others. But now he grows sullen.

"There's nothing prepares you for being first on the scene, finding your son after he's shot his self," he begins. "That memory's seared into my mind and will always be. It was like . . . he'd exploded. It was just . . . everywhere."

Rick later tells me more about his son, Kyle, who he describes as a sensitive soul trapped inside the body of a linebacker. Kyle was good with his hands and found work restoring old cars at a local body shop. Like many young people in southern Missouri, Kyle also struggled with opiate addiction but seemed to have kicked the habit, only to fall into heavy drinking.

Rick reveals only a small part of the story to the group, but his words have a profound effect on everyone. He then falls silent, and June speaks up. "We are grieving parents," she says. "But Rick has another level of trauma that I can't even imagine what he's going through, having found Kyle's body. How can you prepare for that? How can you ever forget it?"

"And don't forget the funeral," Rick adds.

"The funeral?" asks Billie.

"Where we come from, you say goodbye with an open casket. That's how it's done," Rick answers. "But Kyle was . . . gone. There was nothing left that looked like our son. I worked so hard with the undertakers, there was hardly anything left." He begins to weep. "We got the left arm. In the end, we got the left arm."

"They did a good job getting the left arm to a place where it looked like part of Kyle," June says stoically. "We held . . . they, they covered what was left of the body, but we held an open casket showing the left arm. It felt like enough. We got to say goodbye to him."

The metonymy of the arm for the son hangs in the air. People look down at their hands.

Kim speaks next. "It was pretty much the same for me. My dad never needed guns when we was growing up. An' then he got worried about protection, security, you know, and terrorism and intruders. I have no idea why; maybe that's what everyone was saying." She, too, begins to cry. "So my ex and I . . . we took him out and taught him to shoot. I had no idea that he would ever . . . he called me in the middle of the night, told me it was all my fault. Did it right then. And why? It's the same thing, when someone shoots himself in the head; all you can do is cremate them. You're searching for . . . memories."

"We've had four suicides in our family—no, wait, five if you count my cousin," adds Kelly, a woman in her late twenties who came late to the meeting after getting off work in a local nail salon. "All done by gun."

"I've only just now learned to relax at the holidays," a man named James says. "My uncle shot himself on Christmas Eve."

At this point in the conversation, I imagine, for a fleeting moment, a different kind of support group, where people who suffer excruciating loss by means other than gun suicide voice anger or despair at the commercial or societal forces that enabled their tragedies. *Why do they make it so easy to buy cigarettes when we know they are addictive?* families in a lung-cancer victims group might say. If this were a group mourning those killed by drunk driving, I might hear how bars, car companies, and beer sellers must do more to stop people who have been drinking from getting behind the wheel.

But that's not how survivors sound in Missouri when guns are the common bond. To be sure, the group reaches a point in the conversation in which outpourings of pain and despair turn to strategies for moving forward and helping others. "I would do anything to help other people so that their families don't have to go through this nightmare," June says at one point in the conversation. "What can we do to prevent more suicides?" Dawn, Billie's coleader, asks.

Grief is, by its very nature, immensely personal and isolating. Anne Lamott describes living with grief as akin to "having a broken leg that never heals perfectly—that still hurts when the weather gets cold, but you learn to dance with the limp." For C. S. Lewis, grief felt "so like fear." But grief can also produce community. Toni Morrison once said that in times of grief, instead of words or wishes, "I think you should just hug people and mop their floor."

So it was with this group. "With help comes hope," Dawn, a trained social worker, explains while expanding on one of the pamphlets on the table. "It's important to recognize warning signs and reach out to loved ones in despair when we notice that they're feeling hopeless or withdrawing from friends and family, or showing mood swings. Drinking alcohol makes it worse. Antidepressant medications can be of great help."

"We hope you all can join us when we do an *Out of the Darkness* walk in the spring," Billie adds. "It means so much to the community."

I want to be as respectful as I possibly can about people's experiences and about their ways of coping and moving forward. Indeed, as I sit in the room, I feel exceedingly grateful that the group allows me in and shares their stories with me.

At the same time, I cannot help but notice that, unlike my imagined lung cancer or impaired driving meetings, not one person makes a critical comment about guns, bullets, gun manufacturers, or gun laws. No one suggests that rethinking the role of guns in personal and public life might impact suicide. The comments that people make focus entirely on individual-level stressors, warning signs, and plans of action, never on larger societal ones.

I strive to know more about this gap in individual and collective narrative. So, toward the end of the meeting, I ask, "Have your experiences in any way changed the ways that you might think about the role of guns in everyday life?" I try my best to avoid any friction in my choice of words, and not sound like I'm asking a political question, or a gun-control question, or a seize-your-gun question. I am not here to change anyone's mind—I honestly want to understand.

The room responds in much the same way as had many of my prior and subsequent interview subjects when I ask any type of question that contained words such as *firearm* or *gun*: they circle the wagons.

"I don't think any of us blame the gun," Billie replies without a hint of defensiveness. "It's not the gun's fault. I still own many guns. Guns are important to us and to our liberties. Heck, I'm teaching my nieces to shoot in case they need to protect themselves."

"Lot of us come from military or come up with hunting," says June. "Guns are a way of life."

"We pass down guns in our family, strong NRA," James adds.

These replies are not surprising. Guns are a part of the culture in white rural Missouri, and often proudly so. Guns mean protection, self-preservation, and patriotism, as my cab driver Jim told me. And perhaps phrasing the question in the way I do, and the fact of my being an outsider, implies on some level that I ascribe culpability to the culture itself and to its inhabitants, even though this is not my intention. Perhaps as someone who grew up without guns, it's impossible for me to even ask this question in the right way.

And perhaps for this reason, the same guns that the NRA, Amendment 5, and SB 656 define as "weapons of defense and attack" become objects in need of communal protection. Protection even within a circle of people in pain, a circle defined by a radius in which fateful bullets forever changed, altered, and ended futures and lives. Guns, like life, are a way of life. Guns are connective tissue, or forms of interstitium. And as such, guns themselves, within the trajectory of the narratives in the room, remain, like whiteness, assumed, unexamined, invisible. They are a part of us that helps us identify each other when we are all dressed in camouflage, seeking to blend in.

"I'm totally pro-gun, always will be," a sixty-three-year-old Cape Girardeau grandmother named Sally who was not at the group tells me in an interview the following day when I ask about the role of guns in the suicide of her fourteen-year-old grandson. "You know you're in gun country now, right?"

The meeting ends. We gather our belongings, wrap ourselves in winter gear, and prepare to head back into the cold. Billie, Dawn, and I will go to Starbucks afterward to process, but before we head off, the two leaders swap holiday gifts and cheer with Rick, June, Kelly, and others.

I walk toward the lobby to wait, but Kim stops me as I head toward the door. "Thank you so much for coming and listening to us," she says. "And just wanted you to know that what she said is right. We don't blame the gun. It's never the gun—it's the person. Besides, if they say it's the gun's fault—well, they might come take away our guns, too."

RISK

I N SO MANY ways, the pain shared in a room in the Cape Girardeau Public Library defied categorization. Each person told his or her own unique narrative. Each narrative joined unimaginable suffering from losing an irreplaceable person with almost inconceivable trauma brought about by coming to terms with what happened in an attempt to move on. The singularity of each life, and each death, was its own complete story.

Yet I was in the room not as a participant but as a researcher—a researcher whose purpose involved understanding the larger frameworks that encompass rooms such as these in order to better address the tensions, trends, politics, experiences, and blind spots surrounding American gun mortality. From this perspective, the initial framework that became apparent, as I stepped back and began to process what I saw and heard, was neither whiteness nor race per se—I will get to these topics shortly and in detail. Rather, I thought first about the contested politics of *risk*.

Risk is generally the first and greatest focus for suicide researchers. This makes sense when you think about it. A main goal of suicide research is to anticipate which persons are most likely to harm themselves in order to then prevent their self-destructive actions. Prediction is particularly important because suicide is often a solitary, individual act. As Émile Durkheim wrote in his seminal work on the subject, "Each victim of suicide gives his act a personal stamp which expresses his temperament, the special conditions in which he is involved." We must intervene before because intervening during or after is rarely an option. Identifying risk is of little solace in retrospect.[1]

In pretty much all other forms of suicide except suicide by firearm, researching risk appears rather straightforward. Researchers develop hypotheses based on their areas of expertise, apply for research funding, and map trends. For instance, researchers in psychiatry map suicide patterns using frameworks of psychiatric diagnosis. *Are people with major depressive disorder more likely to try to harm themselves?* a researcher might ask, or, *Do anomalies in the brains of persons with post-traumatic stress disorder (PTSD) predict suicidal acts?* Dr. Lisa Pan and colleagues did one such study, funded by the National Institutes of Health, which found surprising metabolite abnormalities in the spinal fluids of depressed people who attempted suicide multiple times. Dr. Nigel Bush and colleagues used a grant from the Military Suicide Research Consortium to analyze the impact of the Virtual Hope Box, a smartphone app designed to improve stress-coping skills and perceived reasons for living among veterans at elevated risk of self-harm.[2]

Substance abuse experts assess the impacts of drugs, alcohol, or prescription medications on suicidal behaviors. *Does drinking increase the risk of suicide?* a researcher might ask, or *What are the impacts of illicit or prescription drugs?* For instance, in an important study funded by the National Institute of Mental Health, Dr. W. Vaughn McCall and colleagues found that people who take prescription sleep aids for insomnia may be at increased risk for suicidal thoughts.[3]

Public-health scholars and health-policy experts study the best methods for intervention when people are potentially suicidal. Looking over demographic data, they might ask, *What kinds of targeted suicide-prevention strategies work with what kinds of people?* For example, with funding from the National Institute of General Medical Sciences and the Indian Health Service, Dr. Mary Cwik and colleagues discovered that a comprehensive community-surveillance suicide-prevention program helped reduce teen suicide rates among the White Mountain Apache population of Arizona.[4]

These scientific approaches help society create lists of warning signs, events out of the ordinary, pre-event triggers, and other changes to the norm that help people better understand and assess suicide risk. Research also forms the foundation for activism in suicide-prevention communities. Mental health advocacy groups distill key findings and promote them via websites, brochures, and public-information campaigns. For example, the American Foundation for Suicide Prevention's public-information website lists expert knowledge about "Risk Factors and Warning Signs": "Something to look out for when concerned that a person may be suicidal is a change in behavior or the presence of entirely new behaviors . . . (such as) acting recklessly, withdrawing from activities, isolating from family and friends." The National Alliance on Mental Illness (NAMI) similarly promotes a "Risk of Suicide" page on its website that warns: "Someone experiencing suicidal thoughts should seek immediate assistance from a health or mental health care provider." And the Missouri Suicide Prevention Resource Center provides refrigerator magnets—indeed, the very same magnets handed out to participants at the Cape Girardeau meeting—listing crisis hotlines and two columns of suicide warning signs for which people should be on the lookout:[5]

- Threatening or talking about wanting to hurt or kill oneself
- Feeling hopeless
- No reason for living, no sense of purpose in life
- Withdrawal from friends, family, and society
- Increased alcohol or drug use

Support and survivor networks save lives by spreading vital information culled from research. Such efforts are particularly needed at the current moment because American suicide rates are on the rise. "U.S. Suicide Rate Surges to a 30-Year High," read an August 2016 *New York Times* headline, above an article that detailed how "suicide in the United States has surged to the highest levels in nearly 30 years . . . the increases were so widespread that they lifted the nation's suicide rate to 13 per 100,000 people, the highest since 1986." Subsequent research suggested that rates were particularly high in rural areas of the United States.[6]

Research also shifts the discourse about suicide from shame and blame to empathy and community. Suicide was long considered an offense toward God or a crime when approached through religion or the law. Christian dogma in seventeenth-century Europe promoted the notion that suicide was a sin. People actually dragged the bodies of suicide victims facedown through the streets before throwing them onto garbage heaps. In nineteenth-century England, the state deemed suicide victims criminals, buried them at night, and confiscated their estates and belongings. By 2015, however, surveys suggested that nearly 90 percent of Americans associated

suicide with mental illness, and 94 percent of Americans believed that suicide was "at least sometimes preventable" and would want to "do something" if someone close to them was considering harming themselves.[7]

Yet there is a crack in this enlightenment narrative. What if suicide
researchers are barred by their own government from obtaining federal
funding to research or compile data about the leading method of lethal
suicide in the United States? The method of suicide that kills more Americans than all other intentional means combined, including hanging, poisoning, overdosing, jumping, suffocating, or cutting? The method that kills
more Americans than all of the murderers, robbers, terrorists, and attack-
ers put together as well?[8]

This is not a what-if scenario—it was a reality in the United States
for much of the early parts of the twenty-first century. In 1996, Congress
passed a ban on federally funded gun research. Legislators—lobbied heavily by the National Rifle Association—added a rider to the federal budget.
That rider is known as the Dickey Amendment, and it stripped the Centers
for Disease Control (CDC) of funding for gun violence prevention research
and stipulated that "none of the funds made available for injury prevention
and control at the Centers for Disease Control and Prevention may be used
to advocate or promote gun control." *Prevention* is a particularly important word in this sentence because it means that researchers must climb
an immensely high wall if they wish to conduct federally funded research
about guns—unlike pretty much every other kind of risk and pretty much
every other kind of disease known to mankind. Congress renewed the ban
continually since 1996 until the time of writing of this book and extended
similar restrictions to other federal agencies, including the National Institutes of Health and the National Institute of Mental Health. Researchers
must then scramble to obtain funding from a number of private foundations
or, in some instances, reframe their research or hide its purpose in order to
receive baseline amounts of funding.[9]

Supporters of the ban—generally Republicans—assert that the restrictions are needed to block a "public health bias" or "tainted public
health model" that inexorably pushes for gun control. Similar arguments
often take aim at homicide and domestic violence studies as well—and
arose in the aftermath of CDC-funded research suggesting that having
guns in the home sharply increases the risk of fatal violence.[10]

Conversely, many of the nation's leading public health organizations and medical groups have now come out against the research ban. After decades of relative silence on the matter, the membership of the American Medical Association (AMA) in 2016 voted to take a stand. "An epidemiological analysis of gun violence is vital so physicians and other health providers, law enforcement, and society at large may be able to prevent injury, death, and other harms to society resulting from firearms," AMA president Steven J. Stack said at the time. That same year, a group called Doctors for America led a coalition of 141 medical organizations that sent a letter and petitioned senior members of the House and Senate appropriations committees, urging restoration of funding for gun violence research. Alice Chen, executive director of the group, explained that "we have heard from doctors everywhere who have talked about patients they've cared for who have been affected by gun violence. They've been shot, their family members have been shot, they're living with the consequences 20 years later. And research is an obvious thing that needs to be done in order to help everybody figure out the right solution."[11]

Even traditionally nonpolitical medical journals join in. A landmark editorial penned in 2017 by the editors of the *Journal of the American Medical Association* (*JAMA*) argued that Dickey represented an ongoing "attempt to suppress research into gun violence."[12]

Of course, no profession is without bias, and many disciplines by nature tend to privilege particular political points of view. I know all too well from my earlier research that, despite an overall focus on healing, biomedicine has been used to promote problematic ideologies and agendas. Indeed, part of why we need oversight bodies like the CDC in the first place is to continually assess research objectivity and promote gold-standard research methods.[13]

Yet Dickey potentially pushed gun violence prevention researchers into the trap of needing to prove basic or obvious hypotheses at the expense of more nuanced ones. For instance, it would hardly seem shocking from a population-level perspective that more people get shot in places where there are more guns, or that locales with basic restrictions on the purchase and carry of firearms see better health outcomes than locales that have none. These are the types of fundamental claims that gun researchers have been forced to continually validate and defend against the headwinds of a congressional ban and a well-funded corporate lobby that counters research with provocation rather than with counterbalanced research.

More to the point here, the debate over the research ban also often focuses on research regarding gun homicide, while giving secondhand status to the implications for suicide. Yet part of the initial impetus for the Dickey Amendment resulted from the outcry from the gun lobby about a 1992 study in the *New England Journal of Medicine* (*NEJM*) titled "Suicide in the Home in Relation to Gun Ownership," which tested the hypothesis that "limiting access to firearms could prevent many suicides." After an extensive analysis of nearly a thousand cases, the authors found evidence supporting the notion that "the ready availability of guns increases the risk of suicide in the home" and advised that "people who own firearms should carefully weigh their reasons for keeping a gun in the home against the possibility that it may someday be used in a suicide."[14]

This seemingly straightforward suggestion raised the ire of pro-gun lobbyists and politicians and eventually led to the ongoing deep freeze on funding for research on all forms of gun violence prevention, including gun-suicide prevention. In the fifteen years after the ban went into effect, federal funding for firearm injury prevention fell 96 percent, and peer-reviewed academic publishing on firearm violence fell by over 60 percent. Scholars who depended on federal funding and publication to advance professionally were often advised to stay away from researching gun violence prevention because of the potentially harmful effects on their careers. A 2017 analysis published in the *JAMA* found that gun violence was the least researched major cause of death in the United States as measured by the number of papers published, and the second-least-funded cause of death related to its death toll. It was as if someone placed a silencer on knowledge.[15]

As a researcher, it's hard not to get frustrated about this foolish and misguided ban and the censorship it produces when you sit in a meeting of people who have lost family members to suicide. The frustration is not because you are pro-gun, or anti-gun, or whatever—most people, for the most part, are both depending on the context (myself included), and this binary of pro- or anti- feels forced and oversimplified in relation to the real world in any case.

Rather, the frustration arises because it will be increasingly difficult for researchers to study what balanced suicide prevention might look like in parts of the country like Cape Girardeau, where there are so many guns in people's daily lives. Because of the ban and its downstream effects, researchers rarely study why a small number of gun owners chose to turn their guns on themselves while many others do not. They cannot determine the most effective points of intervention to prevent deaths among lawful gun owners or within particular social networks. They cannot compare various safe-storage methods in rural communities to find out whether gun lockers, trigger locks, or smart-gun technologies work best in households with guns and children. They cannot even receive a grant to study the potential psychological benefits of owning a gun.

In other words, the federal ban on funding gun research and the polarization it produces makes it harder to create common knowledge about some of the issues that most affected the people in the room in the Cape library, and the communities in which they strive, work, and try to survive. These were the red-state, pro-gun communities whose Second Amendment rights were never in doubt, but who lived in armed petri dishes with the lights turned out when it came to identifying risk factors and promoting strategies for suicide prevention. They were the communities in which the most lethal means to a self-inflicted end often lay, armed and loaded, beneath people's pillows or under their beds. Everyday people who most needed guidance even as they lived with, and often fell in line with, the politics and agendas that promoted the ban in the first place. In other words, the people who stood to benefit the most from the very research that their politics and politicians prohibited.

In most all other kinds of illness and injury-prevention research, federal funds help create large multisource databases of what is called morbidity and mortality, or illness, injury, and death, from which researchers can then track trends over time. For instance, an influenza researcher might access a large database to track how many people got sick from the flu over a ten-year period in a certain county and cross-check that with data that detailed how many people received the flu vaccine. Yet gun violence prevention researchers have had no such luxury. Without access to federally supported databases devoted specifically to gun-related injuries or interventions, researchers are often left to rely on backdoor strategies to answer even the most basic questions about gun-related patterns in the United States. One back door, morbidly, involves death—in the form of federally compiled databases that track causes of mortality in the United

States. This end around exists because firearms are listed as an option in the extensive "cause of death checklists" compiled by coroners and reported to local and federal health officials, who then assemble data on death trends. Researchers can use the resulting databases to compare death trends by region, age, race, gender, or other indicators. This system is far from perfect, but at present, death represents the best available metric to study one potential outcome of gun possession without actually doing a study on guns.

From the perspective of death data, there is relatively little debate that more gun suicides occur in homes, cars, garages, schools, and yards where there are more guns than in homes, cars, garages, schools, and yards where there are fewer guns. The controversial 1992 *NEJM* study foretold an emerging consensus. Quietly, beneath the radar of public outcry, researchers used death data to uncover associations between guns in people's homes and increased risk of gun suicide. For example, a 2013 aggregation of survey data by the Harvard Injury Control Research Center found strong statistical correlation between gun ownership and gun suicide "after controlling for other factors." And a 2018 *JAMA* study performed an extensive cross-sectional analysis of death data from 3,108 counties in the 48 contiguous states of the United States and found that states with strong gun laws had lower firearm suicide rates.[16]

Simply knowing a person's cause of death, however, does not answer the questions asked in the room at the Cape Girardeau Public Library or the questions I wanted to pursue after hearing the stories. Questions not just about how to stop or prevent this awful trend but about how to empathically understand relationships among guns, families, and communities without casting blame. Questions that explored the potential distinctiveness of gun suicide in red states where even the cab drivers roll up armed, just in case. Questions not about death but life among guns in gun country.

For instance, I wanted to know whether the risk factors printed on the refrigerator magnet were the right ones for predicting gun suicide in places like southern Missouri. Undoubtedly, many of the departed suffered from feelings of loneliness, hopelessness, and despair. It also seems possible that the magnet risk factors read like a guide for identifying ways that researchers thought about suicidality when they thought only of the despair of Sylvia Plath, Kurt Cobain, Robin Williams, or other people who suffered long histories of mental anguish and previous suicide attempts and psychiatric hospitalizations leading up to final, fateful acts. A suicidality that people call a cry for help, and for which, as the NAMI "Risk of Suicide" web page claims, "mental health professionals are trained to help a person understand their feelings . . . and can improve mental wellness and resiliency." Resiliency is important because the vast majority of people who try suicide by means other than firearm survive their initial attempts. For instance, drug overdose, the most common method in suicide attempts in the United States, is fatal in less than 3 percent of cases.[17]

But gun suicide often has its own temperament, its own pace, its own urgent, mercurial linearity. Turning a firearm on oneself (or a loved one in some cases of armed domestic murder-suicide) can fall into a category that experts call "impulsive"—a spontaneous response to immediate stressors, such as a romantic breakup, job loss, fight, or rejection. One landmark study of impulsive suicide attempts in Texas found that 24 percent of young people spent less than five minutes between the decision to commit suicide and the actual attempt, that 70 percent took less than an hour, and that "male sex" and a history of having been in a physical fight—but *not* depression—were found to be risk factors for these impulsive suicide victims.[18]

Firearms also represent especially lethal conduits between suicidal intentions and tragic ends. Roughly 85 percent of firearm suicide attempts result in death. For this reason, firearms rank at the top of what researchers call "case-fatality charts" that list the percentages of people who die from the different methods of suicide. As suicidologists describe it, guns top the list because of their "inherent deadliness," "ease of use," and "accessibility"—in other words, because of many of the same qualities that draw people to guns in the first place.[19]

Given the quick interval between thought and action and the lethality of firearms, scholars often argue that the use of a gun shifts the discourse on suicide from *why* to *how*. As the Harvard public health research report describes it, gun suicide often represents "an irreversible solution to what is often a passing crisis." How do you make a refrigerator magnet for that?[20]

As a researcher, you can't help but wonder: How many passing crises or cries for help end up entombed in the death data? How many people just wanted to make a statement, only to become a number in the column for completed firearm suicide? In what ways does the distinction between a cry for help, an accident, and an intended act matter when the outcome is often the same? What would it even look like to intervene beforehand

on a five-minute, armed impulse not linked to depression? It would stand
to reason that risk factors for the five-minute, armed group might look different from how they might for a person with a long history of severe depression, like Sylvia Plath. In other words, how do you make a refrigerator
magnet for that?

As I thought more about it, the ban on federally funded research made
less and less sense. While the block on gun research funding might in its
conception be aimed at scholars who are ostensibly (and for the most part
incorrectly) identified as diehard liberals or anti-gun zealots, its real-world
effects were most profoundly felt in the rooms, towns, and communities
with the most firearms and the most pressing needs to promote best practices for gun safety and gun suicide prevention. The places that needed the
most research and knowledge were the places, like Cape Girardeau, that
had the most guns.

This doesn't mean that research inherently promotes any one agenda
or automatically aims to take away anyone's gun. The best research respects the culture and the traditions it studies and should feel grateful
to be let in. Yet, in the Cape at least, it seemed clear to me that better
research and a more robust knowledge base could have lessened the blame
and guilt that survivors felt for missing so-called warning signs, especially
if the signs they were told to monitor were not wholly relevant in their particular cases. Research could have developed better models for recognizing risk. To put it very simply, better research could have helped the group
to have better refrigerator magnets.

THEN THERE WERE the hovering demographic questions regarding *race*. I am
a white American who sat in a room with other white Americans in a town
that is overwhelmingly white, non-Hispanic, and American. Highlighting
another, oft-unspoken distinctive factor about gun suicide is its connection
to whiteness in general and white maleness in particular.

A skew toward death by suicide for any one race or ethnicity seems
somewhat confounding. From what we know, thoughts of suicide probably affect all demographics of people. Freud defined drives toward death
and self-destruction (*todestriebe*) as central aspects of human development.
More to the point, present-day studies suggest little variability among
ethnic groups regarding what is called *suicidal ideation*—or thoughts of
self-harm.[21]

Perhaps as a result, non-gun suicide *attempts* are diversely distributed among races and genders, with particular demographic groups showing particular trends. For instance, women of all ethnic and racial backgrounds are far more apt than men to overdose on pills; African American men are at high risk after release from incarceration; Hispanic and American Indian and Alaska Native young adults skew toward suffocation/hanging at startling rates; and Asians/Pacific Islanders have shown relatively high rates of suicide attempt–related hospitalization. Women, Native Americans, and Hispanic-origin Americans show particularly worrisome trends of suicide attempts among teens. In other words, diverse conditions of helplessness and despair often mirror the gendered, ethnic, and socioeconomic diversity of the United States.[22]

But white Americans dominate death-per-suicide-attempt categories for one main reason: they remain dramatically overrepresented in civilian death data about firearm suicides. According to the most frequently used database of morbidity and mortality in the United States—the Web-based Injury Statistics Query and Reporting System (WISQARS)—gun suicides between 2009 and 2015 looked like this:

- 2009: Non-Hispanic white gun suicides = 16,351; total gun suicides = 17,172
- 2010: Non-Hispanic white gun suicides = 16,928; total gun suicides = 18,365
- 2011: Non-Hispanic white gun suicides = 17,536; total gun suicides = 18,984
- 2012: Non-Hispanic white gun suicides = 18,022; total gun suicides = 19,572
- 2013: Non-Hispanic white gun suicides = 18,561; total gun suicides = 20,087
- 2014: Non-Hispanic white gun suicides = 18,619; total gun suicides = 20,152
- 2015: Non-Hispanic white gun suicides = 19,161; total gun suicides = 20,779

(As defined by the Census Bureau, Non-Hispanic whites are people in the United States who are considered racially white and are not of Hispanic or Latino origin/ethnicity.)

Put another way, 92 percent of gun suicides in the United States were committed by non-Hispanic white persons. These percentages were dramatically higher than those seen in other "race" groups in the census database—such as gun suicides committed by persons categorized as black, Asian, or Native Americas. Put into graph form, the numbers by race appeared as follows:

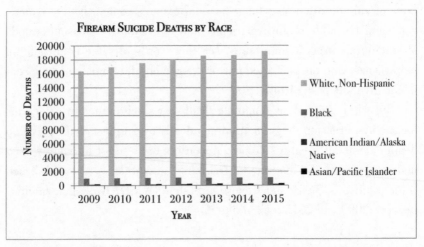

Source: WISQARS Fatal Injury Data via the National Vital Statistics System, organized by the Centers for Disease Control and Prevention, retrieved from https://www.cdc.gov/injury /wisqars/index.html.

Of course someone might think, *Doesn't this data simply reflect how the majority of people in the United States self-identify as white?* While this statement is true, these shocking trends held even when the numbers were sifted through what statisticians call age-adjusted and crude rate calculations, which balance out the numbers of suicides in relation to total populations. It's also important to consider that the percentage of non-Hispanic whites in the United States *declined* over the latter twentieth and early twenty-first centuries. Non-Hispanic white persons comprised 80 percent of the US population in 1980 but only 69 percent of the population in 2000. According to the US census, the percentage of non-Hispanic white people in the United States hit an all-time low of 62 percent in 2013 and kept falling every year after that. And yet over this same time period, 2009–2015, white populations consistently committed 92 percent of all gun suicides.[23]

As we can see in more detail below, the death numbers effectively represented gun suicides committed by white, non-Hispanic *men*. Women attempted suicide three times more often than did men but typically opted for pills or poisons, which are significantly less lethal on average. By contrast, the WISQARS data for completed gun suicide shows the following relationships between white men and everyone else in the United States:

- 2009: Non-Hispanic white male gun suicides = 14,168; total gun suicides = 17,1725
- 2010: Non-Hispanic white male gun suicides = 14,762; total gun suicides = 18,365
- 2011: Non-Hispanic white male gun suicides = 15,132; total gun suicides = 18,984
- 2012: Non-Hispanic white male gun suicides = 15,588; total gun suicides = 19,572
- 2013: Non-Hispanic white male gun suicides = 15,921; total gun suicides = 20,087
- 2014: Non-Hispanic white male gun suicides = 15,925; total gun suicides = 20,152
- 2015: Non-Hispanic white male gun suicides = 16,397; total gun suicides = 20,779

From 2009 to 2015, non-Hispanic white men accounted for nearly 80 percent of all gun suicides in the United States, despite representing less than 35 percent of the total population.[24]

Of course, it's important to be at least somewhat skeptical about these kinds of numbers. US census race and ethnicity categories are frequently critiqued as oversimplified and in any case represent people's self-reports rather than underlying biological realities. Race categories also frequently represent social and political biases—until relatively recently, for instance, American society did not consider Jews and Italians to be "white."[25]

Moreover, race factors a great deal in other categories of US gun death—inasmuch as there are deep racial differences in the means by which Americans die by gunshot. For instance, African Americans are far more likely than other Americans to die by gunshot in cases of homicide, assault, and in encounters with police. A far-ranging 2013 report by the Pew Research Center used US death certificate data to detail how "blacks were 55% of shooting homicide victims in 2010, but 13% of the population." By contrast, whites were 25 percent of the victims of gun homicide in 2010, but 65 percent of the population.[26]

Similarly, a 2015 Brookings Institution report relied on data from the National Center for Injury Prevention and Control (NCIPC) database to show a remarkable segregation whereby the vast majority (77 percent) of white gun deaths were suicides, while "less than one in five (19 percent) is a homicide." These figures were nearly opposite in black populations, where "only 14 percent of gun deaths are suicides but 82 percent are homicides." Broadly put, a white person in the United States is five times as likely to die by suicide using a gun as to be shot with a gun; for each African American who uses a gun to commit suicide, five are killed by other people with guns.[27]

Statistically speaking, then, white Americans die by gun suicide more than they should and die by gun homicide and police shootings less than other groups of people. For African Americans, it's the exact opposite. But here as well, the patterns are more complicated than they might seem. This is because the trends of white suicide and black homicide followed opposite trajectories over past decades (and indeed over the same decades when many US states loosened their gun laws). While white gun suicides skyrocketed between the late 1990s and the mid-2010s, this same period saw one of the more dramatic drops in firearm homicide rates in modern memory. Once again, from an extensive Pew research report:

> Compared with 1993, the peak of U.S. gun homicides, the firearm homicide rate was 49% lower in 2010, and there were fewer deaths, even though the nation's population grew. The victimization rate for other violent crimes with a firearm—assaults, robberies and sex crimes—was 75% lower in 2011 than in 1993. Violent non-fatal crime victimization overall (with or without a firearm) also is down markedly (72%) over two decades.[28]

According to the data from Pew, gun suicides rose even as rates of gun homicide and other forms of gun crime fell. By 2015, even *Breitbart News* reported that gun suicides accounted for two-thirds of firearm deaths in the country. And because white Americans, and for the most part white men, comprised the majority of gun suicide victims, this meant that white men increasingly drove the overall data on US gun deaths.[29]

These startling racial and gender trends in death were frequently marked by their invisibility. Surveys of US public opinion suggest that many Americans remain largely unaware of the prevalence of white gun suicide—or of the links between gun ownership and gun suicide at all. A 2017 survey found that "fewer than 10% of gun owners with children (or gun owners who had received firearm training) agreed that household fire-arms increase suicide risk."[30]

Public discourse about gun death instead focuses on violence toward others and homicides and relies more on racial and media stereotypes and anxieties about black criminals than on-the-ground realities. A widely cited opinion study published in the journal *PLOS ONE* found that "at-titudes towards guns in many US whites appear to be influenced . . . by illogical racial biases" related to the "fear of black violence and crime." Meanwhile, as the Pew report put it, the dramatic drop in gun homicide rates was not just invisible—most Americans believed the opposite to be true:

> Despite national attention to the issue of firearm violence, most Americans are unaware that gun crime is lower today than it was two decades ago. According to a new Pew Research Center survey, today 56% of Americans believe gun crime is higher than 20 years ago and only 12% think it is lower.[31]

THESE RACIAL DISPARITIES between white suicide and black homicide did not exist in a vacuum. Rather, they are in many ways reflective of ways that Americans talk about race, violence, and mortality more broadly. I say this because, all too often, when questions of aggression or violence involve blackness, many observers are quick to look for clues based in "biology" or "culture." Straight-faced scientists ask whether "blacks" express so-called warrior genes, leading "them" to attack "us" more frequently. They shamelessly suggest that the overrepresentation of African Americans in the criminal justice system results from underlying biological differences that cause "blacks" to commit more crimes, or demonstrate more psychopathic personalities, or act more impulsively or with less cultural regard for long-term consequences than do everyone else. Most scientists and scholars would rightly call this kind of research what it is—namely, racist. But the implicit frame whereby "black" minds or bodies or cultures function as causal categories of analysis in violence research remains too often in place.[32]

Here's a thought experiment: try posing the same kinds of questions about self-directed, mainstream, and predominantly white gun violence. To even ask a question such as whether "whites" are biologically, genetically, or culturally prone to gun suicide (not a position that I in any way endorse but that nonetheless would seem the correlate of a question about whether "blacks" are more biologically prone to gun homicide) seems innately counterintuitive. Ask this question to leading research search engines such as PubMed or AJP Online. Ask search engines like Google. Ask a stranger on the street. The answer will more than likely be confusion, silence, or the reply that we should give to all questions about the biology of violence—that violence is social and structural and that "white" in any case is not a true biological grouping but a social one. Or, as we will see, that politics shape outcomes much more than do genes. The point being that the implicit binary of black aggressors toward others and white victims of themselves should itself be the problem we should aim to critique and change rather than justify and support.[33]

Ultimately, the complex interactions of race, gender, and violence lead back to risk. Risk helps people identify the possibility of peril in their loved ones and is something that we all want to avoid in our own lives. Risk implies peril, hazard, and the possibility of loss. Risk, as anthropologist Lochlann Jain puts it, is a form of American autobiography—inasmuch as it reveals a great deal about our relationships with cars, machines, and other objects and technologies. As a doctor or as a researcher, I believe that a life with less risk is a life that is often longer, happier, and more secure. Risk is something that we should want to study, identify, and, ultimately, prevent.[34]

Yet risk feels *particularly* complicated in the context of the stories of white firearm suicide. Lessons seem hard to cull when the support groups are comprised only of grieving loved ones because the primary victims do not survive long enough to tell you what was going through their minds. Knowledge about best practices is fleeting because Congress effectively

blocks federally funded research on gun-related risk, leading to a knowledge vacuum unlike anything ever seen for every other leading cause of
injury and death. Ultimately, risk is embodied not in the imagined intruder
but in the person who already lives in the house. Risk then becomes at
once prevalent and invisible. Risk is an ellipsis, an evanescent void.

All too often, the language of "crisis" is used to fill the void provided
by this lack of research, knowledge, and common sense. Assumptions
about "whiteness in crisis" often drive coverage, not just about white gun
suicide but also about the identity of the American plurality in the age of
globalization and economic change. "Behind 2016's Turmoil, a Crisis of
White Identity," read a *New York Times* headline published days before
Trump's shocking victory, above an article that detailed how "whiteness
means being part of the group whose appearance, traditions, religion and
even food are the default norm" and in which experts saw "a crisis of white
identity" leading to Brexit and the rise of Trump.[35]

This kind of language often rightly reflects the painful everyday experiences and emotions that emerge when modes of production change,
companies leave town, and good, hardworking people and communities are
left holding the bag. In the 1890s, Durkheim, the sociologist, introduced
the concept of *anomie* to describe a crisis of disconnect that emerged between personal lives and social structures. Durkheim wrote in an era of
mass industrialization, a time when workers and collective guild labor
found themselves left behind by evolving economies. *Anomic suicide*, as
he called it, results when people lose a sense of usefulness and of where
they fit in within their societies, leading to feelings of "derangement" and
"insatiable will."[36]

Anomie seems an apt description for the experiences of working-class
white communities in places like Missouri during the latter twentieth and
early twenty-first centuries. The value of many goods and services these
communities produced diminished in the global economy. There was always someone somewhere else who could do the work faster and cheaper.
Pills, addictions, and even guns became modes of coping, ways of filling
the void. Studies charted the anomic crisis that emerged as a result. Research conducted by economists Anne Case and Angus Deaton detailed
"a marked increase in the all-cause mortality of middle-aged white non-
Hispanic men and women in the United States between 1999 and 2013,"
and suggested that not only were white bodies dying off at higher rates—so,

too, were the skills, structures, and hierarchies that gave American whiteness its valences in the first place.[37]

Here as well, however, we must be wary of making automatic assumptions without thinking them through. The working definition of a "crisis" often assumes an upheaval felt by a dominant group in the face of a threat or change that leaves previous power structures upended. We often hear, for instance, of a crisis of masculinity brought about by women's suffrage, or the women's movement, or women's entry into the workforce, or the #MeToo movement, or any number of other social changes in which strivings for equality by women are met by uncertainty in men. For instance, in 2015, Cardinal Raymond Burke blamed "radical feminism" for causing a "man crisis" in the Roman Catholic Church, which left men feeling "marginalized." Cardinal Burke insisted that feminism forced the church to constantly address women's issues at the expense of "critical issues important to men; the importance of the father . . . the importance of a father to children . . . the critical impact of a manly character; the emphasis on the particular gifts that God gives to men for the good of the whole society."[38]

Burke is only the latest to make such an argument—in the 1940s and '50s, authors such as Philip Wylie and David Reisman described crises in patriarchal authority brought about when corporate cultures and suburban lifestyles forced middle-class men to take on qualities and skills traditionally identified with women. In fact, the durability of these arguments led contemporary authors as far ranging as Susan Faludi, Ina Zweiniger-Bargielowska, and James Gilbert to explore crisis as a perpetual component of Western masculinity.[39]

Of course, masculinity crises likely felt very real from the perspectives of men who experienced them. Somewhere, sometime, some men woke up one morning to learn that the hierarchies on which they built their picket fences and senses of accomplishment appeared threatened or already overturned. Instead of the automatic authority they accrued by simply showing up, these men found themselves in a world in which they faced more competition and enjoyed less prestige. Maybe they even had to make their own dinners or type their own memos. According to evolutionary biology, these men responded in predictable ways—by smoking, fighting, drinking, pumping iron, driving too fast, or other modes of chest-beating that restored a sensation of order but also increased their blood pressures and shortened their collective life spans.[40]

The ways we define crisis allow us to attach the language of calamity to whiteness, men, or other seemingly dominant groups, while at the same time making it harder to see the suffering of women, immigrants, people of color, and other persons who do merit a "crisis of authority"—because they are supposedly built for it, or because they have lived with crisis all along. This logic suggests that men need to be on top because they embody no skills for acting otherwise; and everyone else, to paraphrase an important book about women-of-color feminism, are born with bridges called their backs.[41]

Such framing of crisis is also often based more in an imagined sense of nostalgia than in any lived reality, inasmuch as many men fought to maintain what they held to be their natural authority even though every man was not a king, a boss, a plantation owner, or a CEO. By definition, the majority of men needed to be underlings for the system to survive.

If there is any correlation between crisis masculinity and white male gun-suicide trends in the United States, then perhaps attempts to link guns to mortality should more fully consider the meanings of guns in relation to the myths of "decline" and "fall from grace" that play out when certain white Americans talk about their guns. This is the approach taken by emerging sociologists such as Jennifer Carlson and Angela Stroud, who study what Carlson calls the "everyday politics of guns in an age of decline." Both researchers study not how guns kill but why guns are deemed worth living and dying for. Stroud, for instance, extensively interviews white, permit-holding, "good guys with guns" and finds that these men carry firearms "because a white person with a gun is not presumed to be a criminal, he or she can navigate the world with some confidence that other people, most notably the police, will not presume they are bad guys." White privilege allows these men to "distinguish themselves not only from bad guys but also from versions of masculinity that do not measure up to the [armed, white, good-guy] ideal."[42]

Further, these sociological approaches suggest that placing a biomedical frame around gun mortality data and calling the loss of life a threat to public health, as medical researchers like myself are admittedly liable to do, can overlook how guns came to convey particular forms of authority or power in the first place.

As subsequent chapters will reveal, a traditional public health approach overlooks how, from the perspective of white men, guns became not only lethal but sublime. And how relying just on databases and mortality statistics cannot explain how firearms emerged in defense of particular notions of authority or supremacy, as sanctioned by pro-gun legislation and public policy and manipulated by industry, popular culture, and politicians. And, ultimately, how the armed defense of this notion of white male authority itself became a potent form of risk.[43]

I CAN'T JUST MAKE IT GO AWAY

Interview excerpts, December 15, 2016, Sikeston. Speaker 2: white male, 47, father.

Speaker 2: At the time we lost Connor, he was about three months past his twenty-sixth birthday. He was by all accounts, I thought, a very happy person. Laughed and joked all the time. He was a very giving person. If someone needed a favor, he would do it. If they needed a ride somewhere, he would take them. It didn't matter if that meant he was burning the last gallon of gas he had. He would loan money. He would do whatever. . . .

He was a very passionate person about things that he was interested in, and he would research them to get all the facts and information. He was just a joy to us and to our family. Of course, I guess everybody feels that way about their loved one that they've lost, but that's kind of who he was. He wasn't a perfect person. He made mistakes just like everybody else, but he was . . . my pride and joy. . . .

I knew that he was going to go out with someone female the night that we lost him, and that trip didn't turn out well.

I talked to him about 9:30 that night, and he told me kind of how things had gone. She'd really hurt his feelings, so we'd talked a little bit. We talked about doing the job the next morning and going out to eat, and everything seemed fine. At about 2:00 in the morning, I got a call, woke me up. . . .

I got up and got dressed and went over to his place; he lived down the street from us. At 2:00 in the morning, you're asleep. I really was half out of it. When I walked in, there he sat. He had taken a rifle. Our family's all hunters. He had taken a rifle and then he put it in his mouth and pulled the trigger. . . .

I had no idea that that had happened, so I just opened the door and stepped into the room and, you know, there it was. You're left dealing with a mountain of blood and . . . everything else. For me as a parent, guilt is huge, to go back and you look at their life as you raised them, and you wonder what you may have done wrong, what you should have done better. Connor was a happy child. He had friends growing up. Did really well in school.

JMM: What is your understanding of what took place?

Speaker 2: Those two had been dating for a while, at least that's how he saw it, I think. She had asked him to take her into town, and so he did thinking that they were going to, you know, hang out or whatever.

But actually, there was another guy. And she wanted to go see him, and she wanted to be with him. She wouldn't come back home with Connor. . . . Of course he was upset, but she said, "I do need one favor before you leave," and he said, "What's that?" She said, "He's hungry. Will you go across the street and get us something to eat?" He did and took it back to them—that's how he was—and then he drove home. He stopped on the way home and bought a couple bottles of whiskey, and he had drank most of a fifth of whiskey, whenever he did this. . . .

Of course, I didn't realize that he was probably dealing with depression at the time. He hid it well. Alcohol is a depressant and it lowers your inhibitions, so I think that may have had a lot to do with that decision, but we didn't see any signs of it before. He had never talked about it before, and we were talking on the phone and making plans for the next day, you know, and like five hours later he was gone. . . .

In that moment and with alcohol involved and a lot of, my understanding is a lot of deaths with firearms, alcohol is involved a lot of times. It was instantaneous. He didn't have to wonder how long it would last before it was over. The way that he did it, it was over in a fraction of a second.

JMM: Before he had time to think. . . . Then you're then left with such impossible questions.

Speaker 2: You go back, even back to . . . I'll sometimes go back to even when he was younger, and decisions that I made so far as discipline or things like that. Did I choose the wrong thing? Did I do that correctly? As far as the last day that I was with him and we were together, how did I not see that this was going on when I talked to him? How did I not hear it in his voice? How did I not know? I'm his father. How could I not know? Why didn't I pay closer attention? That type of thing. There are things that you go back and say, and as a parent sometimes, you have to use tough love because you feel like it's better for your child. Sometimes you tell them things—"You should do this," or "You should do that," or "You really shouldn't have done that."

What you're trying to do is guide them and help them learn, but you look back at those instances, which would normally, in the normal course of life, just be a learning moment for them or for you. You look back and they feel almost tragic because you feel like, I wish I hadn't have said that, or I wish I hadn't have used that tone of voice, or I wish . . . I've still got receipts where he stopped at 7-Eleven and got a soda and a pack of cigarettes that day. I know that stuff didn't mean anything to him. If he was here, he would probably tell me, "Throw that junk away."

JMM: We were talking before about guns, and I'm wondering, given what you and your family have been through, if you feel there might be anything distinctive about firearm suicide or the trauma it creates in survivors?

Speaker 2: I think, and of course suicide is horrible regardless. I think with gun suicide and especially in my case because of the way that things happened . . . because of what I found, I think it has made it difficult for me to, because people will say, "You know, remember happy times, remember him laughing and smiling, remember . . . " And I have many, many pictures of that, but you know the last memory I have of my son is sitting on a couch in the condition that he was in. I don't know if he had taken pills or if he had died by another means that it would not have been as graphic, if that would have been different for me. If that would have changed the way that I cope with it or deal with it.

   I think in that respect, death by suicide with a firearm is different than the others maybe in that respect, especially if you find them. Other people that I've talked to that didn't actually find their loved one, having to have read reports that were very graphic or they in their mind conjure up images of what they must have looked like. I think that visual is very, very hard to deal with. Well, it is for me. It's hard for me to deal with and hard for me to just make go away. I can't just make it go away. . . .

   It doesn't come to me as often as it did in the beginning. In the beginning, it was like just constantly. Every time I closed my eyes, that's what I saw. Then I think the other aspect with suicide by firearm . . . that has to be cleaned up and taken care of. It was a massive amount of cleanup. . . . The room and the floor was basically covered with his blood, parts of him. . . .

   I just keep thinking, you know, you're twenty-six years old and you're so passionate and you're so . . . I mean, these relationships feel like the beginning and end. You don't see that you've got fifty years of this stuff left, sixty years, whatever.

JMM: A father . . . it's just so hard to imagine.

Speaker 2: Like I said earlier, we are a big family of hunters, went deer hunting. Now as far as seeing a gun or something like that doesn't bother me. I own guns, but for . . . trying not to be too graphic, but if I were to go hunting and shoot an animal, I don't know how I would react if I saw that, if that makes sense.

JMM: That makes perfect sense.

Speaker 2: With the way he did it, I mean, once he pulled that trigger, it was over. There was nothing left. Well, it says on his death certificate that death was instantaneous, and it would have been. And had he not . . . of course, I never in a million years would have dreamed that would have happened.

I didn't think there was any ammunition there for the gun. I thought it was all locked up . . . I think it was there, it was available. If the gun hadn't been there, if I had had it and had it locked up and he hadn't had the gun, I don't know. Maybe he would have drank enough to just pass out and the next morning woke up with a bad headache or sick to his stomach and that would have been it. It was there. It was handy, it was lethal, and it was quick. Honestly, can't we do more to make people store their guns in a gun safe?

THE MAN CARD

Iᴺ 2010, Bᴜsʜᴍᴀsᴛᴇʀ Firearms unveiled an advertising campaign for its popular .223-caliber semiautomatic rifle, the civilian version of a fully automatic weapon used by US soldiers in Afghanistan and Iraq. The campaign invited men to have their "Man Cards Reissued" by answering a series of "manhood questions" and then, presumably, buying the gun. Ads appeared online and in leading gun and ammunition magazines and were first tied to a popular promotion in which sweepstakes winners received rifles along with cards certifying that their manhood had been "restored." As the gun website AmmoLand described it,

> Inspired by the overwhelming response to Bushmaster's "*Consider Your Man Card Reissued*" sweepstakes, today Bushmaster Firearms announces the latest part in the series; the Man Card online promotion. To become a card-carrying man, visitors of Bushmaster.com will have to prove they're a man by answering a series of manhood questions. Upon successful completion, they will be issued a temporary Man Card to proudly display to friends and family. The Man Card is valid for one year.[1]

Many of the questions on the Man Card quiz read as predictably stereotyped: "Do you think tofu is an acceptable meat substitute?" "Can you change a tire?" "Have you ever watched figure skating on purpose?" Other questions unsubtly invoked menace: "A car full of the rival team's fans cuts you off on the way to the championship game. What do you do?" After users completed the quiz, their Man Card arrived by download, e-mail, or post.[2]

The Bushmaster campaign flew under the radar of mainstream attention until December 14, 2012, when a young man named Adam Lanza fatally shot twenty children and six adult staff members at Sandy Hook Elementary School using a .223-caliber Bushmaster XM15-E2S rifle. Suddenly, the playful links between .223 rifles and masculinity became public liability.

In the days and weeks following Sandy Hook, the Man Card campaign emerged as a lightning rod for critiques about the relationships between male identity and high-capacity firearms. Three days after Sandy Hook, the *Huffington Post* highlighted the subtext of the campaign: "The fact that a company is selling deadly weapons based on the premise that it will up the purchaser's 'man cred' is disturbing in itself . . . the message that it sends about what it means to be a man in America is even more so." Buzz-Feed detailed "Bushmaster's Shockingly Awful 'Man Card' Campaign," while blogger and columnist Jessica Valenti tweeted an image of a Man Card and wrote, "This is an ad for the gun Adam Lanza used to murder 20 children & 6 adults. We need to talk about American masculinity." "Not man enough?" CNN asked several days later. "Buy a gun."[3]

Condemnations like these highlighted the correlations between masculinity and guns that so often play out after high-profile US mass shootings. And in this case at least, the critiques had an impact—in the weeks following Sandy Hook, Bushmaster quietly pulled most of the Man Card ads and took the promotional website offline.[4]

In the midst of the furor, many critics overlooked another, highly loaded component of the Man Card campaign: its explicit claims not just about masculinity but about privilege. On the flip side of the novelty Man Card, fine print explained that the bearer held "Rights and Privileges. . . . Today he is a man. Fully entitled to all of the rights and privileges duly afforded."

Privileges seems a particularly interesting word choice. The term generally implies special advantages or immunities available only to a particular person or group and not to others. Privileges thus connote benefits enjoyed by the few and beyond the reach of the many. As it turns out, usage of the term *privileges* fell considerably since its heyday in the early 1800s, a time when most English-speaking people had little trouble separating the rich and powerful from everyone else. For example, according to Google Scholar, published use of the term *privileges* appears as follows between 1800 and 2008:[5]

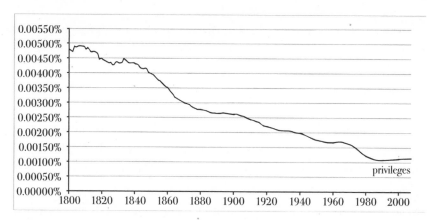

Source: Google Ngram Viewer, accessed May 06, 2018, https://books.google.com/ngrams
/graph?content=privileges&year_start=1800&year_end=2008&corpus=15&smoothing
=7&share=&direct_url=t1%3B%2Cprivileges%3B%2Cc0.

If the corpus of English-language written communication is any guide, the concept of a right reserved to elites has steadily declined for two-plus centuries. But there it was, twice, on the wallet-sized Man Card. "Rights and Privileges." *Privileges duly afforded.* A word and concept calling back to an unequal, inegalitarian past.

The advertisers surely must have known (or should have known) that "privileges," in the context of a promotion for semiautomatic weapons, could not help but invoke race in addition to masculinity. This is because for much of American history, laws and customs "duly afforded" the rights, advantages, and immunities of civilian firearm ownership for non-Hispanic US white persons in general, and non-Hispanic US white men in specific, and restricted them for everyone else. The privileges of white gun ownership meant that firearms emerged as particular weapons of white male authority in the Southern United States.

This notion of privileges provides entry into a third framework for understanding the relationships between guns, cultures, and everyday life in states like Missouri: the framework of *history*. The intersecting trajectories of guns, whiteness, and privilege help explain why firearms came to convey particular meanings to specific populations and address why people who feel their privilege was bestowed by guns might be so loath to give them up. History also becomes a tool manipulated by gun advertisers, corporate lobbyists, and politicians in order to further guns-at-any-cost agendas, even when faced with damning evidence of harm. Ultimately, in an era when people seem divided about gun violence prevention legislation to the point where we can't even reach consensus on bump stocks after mass shootings, history allows us to step back and consider the larger symbolic meanings of guns.

In early colonial America, firearms were the armaments of white upper-class power and a benefit that upper-class whites bestowed on lower-class whites to separate them from people of color. In England, gun ownership was a right restricted to the wealthy—the principle being that anyone below the rank of gentleman found with a gun was a poacher. But in the New World, white men "were armed and had to be armed," as historian Edmund Morgan describes it. Upper-class colonial white people allowed poor white people to carry firearms to quell rebellions by chattel slaves or to repel Native Americans and pirates. Aristocratic whites then found a new reason to carry firearms—to quell potential rebellions by lower-class whites. Laws in seventeenth-century Virginia allowed white people to carry firearms and forbade African slaves and Native Americans from doing so. Meanwhile, the first US authorities in New Orleans after the Louisiana Purchase moved to exclude free blacks from positions in which they were allowed to bear arms.[6]

Armed white citizen militias emerged in Southern states during the Revolutionary War to such an extent that their rights to bear arms were enshrined in the founding documents of the new country. Article VI of the Articles of Confederation, drafted in 1776 and ratified in 1781, required that "every state shall always keep up a well-regulated and disciplined militia, sufficiently armed." The Constitution, signed in Philadelphia in 1787, granted Congress the power "to provide for calling forth the Militia to execute the Laws of the Union, suppress Insurrections and repel Invasions." The Second Amendment, adopted in 1791 as part of the Bill of Rights, stipulated that "a well-regulated Militia, being necessary to the security of a free State, the right of the people to keep and bear Arms, shall not be infringed." Like much of the original Bill of Rights, the Second Amendment originally extended privileges to white people but not to slaves and free blacks.[7]

Scholars of gun culture in the United States often assume that the inclusion of armed white militias in the Second Amendment reflected eighteenth-century tensions between the need for national defense and fears of government tyranny. Historians and gun advocates point to debates between Federalists such as James Madison, who supported a centralized US military, and largely Southern anti-Federalists who feared a powerful federal government with a standing army. John Lott, in his controversial book *More Guns, Less Crime*, writes that "the founding fathers put the Second Amendment in the Constitution" because "they believed an armed citizenry is the ultimate bulwark against tyrannical government." In this telling, the Second Amendment emerged as a compromise that guaranteed the rights of white people to form militias in defense of sovereignty, state, or country, even if national defense largely fell to the United States Army.[8]

However, legal historians such as Carl T. Bogus, Robert Cottrol, and Raymond Diamond place white anxieties about control of black populations at the center of these debates as well. In an extensively researched "hidden history" of the Second Amendment, Bogus finds that "the militia remained the principal means of protecting the social order and preserving white control over an enormous black population." Bogus also details how anti-Federalists stoked fears of slave rebellions as a way of fomenting white Southern opposition to the Constitution, forcing Madison to placate slave-owning Virginians and other Southern white people through the assurances codified in the Second Amendment. Meanwhile, Cottrol and Diamond offer an "Afro-Americanist reconsideration" of the Second Amendment that explores the impact of guns on "subcultures of American society who have been less able to rely on state protection."[9]

Gun laws that secured the rights of white gun owners and restricted those of slaves and free persons of color spread dramatically in the antebellum period of the early nineteenth century, as white concerns about violent "negroes" reached fever pitch in many Southern states. After Nat Turner's Rebellion in 1831, armed militias and mobs conducted mass executions in Virginia, and the state legislature passed a series of laws that forbade free black persons "to keep or carry any firelock of any kind, any military weapon, or any powder or lead." In 1834, the Tennessee Supreme Court revised the firearms provision in its state constitution on racial grounds: "the freemen of this State have a right to keep and to bear arms for their common defence" became "the free *white men* of this State have a right to keep and to bear arms for their common defence."[10]

Supreme courts in nearby states followed suit in the years leading up to and during the US Civil War by proclaiming that gun rights extended only to white "citizens." In 1840, the North Carolina Supreme Court ruled in *The State v. Elijah Newsom* that "if any free negro, mulatto, or free person of colour shall wear or carry about his or her person, or keep in his or her house, any shotgun, musket, rifle, pistol, sword, dagger or bowie-knife . . . he or she shall be guilty of a misdemanour, and may be indicted therefore." So-called Slave Codes in states such as Georgia, Mississippi, and North Carolina banned gun ownership by slaves and free blacks because, as the Georgia Supreme Court put it in 1848 in an argument that presaged the infamous *Dred Scott v. Sandford* decision, "persons of color have never been recognized here as citizens; they are not entitled to bear arms." Around this same time, the newly admitted state of Florida passed a law that allowed white citizen patrols to search the homes of "blacks, both free and slave and confiscate arms held therein."[11]

Racial divides in civilian gun rights widened during Reconstruction, with lethal consequences. The Fourteenth Amendment promised equal protection of the laws to all citizens starting in 1868, and indeed, a number of black Union soldiers returned from the war with rifles in hand. But in the South and Midwest, local laws and everyday practices assured that firearms remained a white prerogative. Many Southern states enforced what were then called Black Codes that contained vagrancy statutes or defined black Americans as less than citizens in ways that made it virtually impossible for freedmen, or free black citizens, to obtain firearm licenses or carry guns. Meanwhile, racial disparities in firearm ownership gave white terror groups, such as the White League and the Ku Klux Klan, maximum leeway to intimidate and spread fear among newly liberated and unarmed former slaves. These armed groups emerged as central to restricting black gun ownership and discouraging black participation in political and economic life in postwar economies in the South. As Adam Winkler aptly describes it in his terrific book *Gun Fight*, "few people realize it, but the Ku Klux Klan began as a gun control organization" that aimed to confiscate any guns that free blacks may have obtained during and after the Civil War and thereby "achieve complete black disarmament."[12]

Abolitionists turned activists such as Frederick Douglass argued that newly freed slaves deserved the right to defend themselves against nightriders and white lynch mobs because local authorities failed to do so. Yet black disarmament campaigns continued for decades, leading to a state of affairs historian David Schenk describes succinctly: "Without political agency, or the means of an organized community militia to generate such power, the realization of freedom and the rights of citizenship for African Americans remained unobtainable for nearly 100 years."[13]

Tensions surrounding armed white terror and black disarmament coursed through the periods leading up to and during the US civil rights era. Armed Klan intimidation of black families and congregations continued virtually unimpeded in many parts of the South through the mid-twentieth century. Meanwhile, African Americans who attempted to take up arms in self-defense against white supremacist intimidation met with violent resistance. Robert F. Williams, president of the Monroe, North Carolina, chapter of the NAACP in the 1950s and early 1960s, became a vocal proponent of "the right of Negroes to meet the violence of the Ku Klux Klan by armed self-defense." With no protection from law enforcement, Williams advised African Americans to "arm themselves as a group to defend their homes, their wives, their children" because, as he contended, the Constitution bestowed the right to own a gun for the defense of a person's home or property on all Americans. "If the United States Constitution cannot be enforced in this social jungle called Dixie," he famously proclaimed, "then it is time that Negroes must defend themselves even if it is necessary to resort to violence." Violent white protests ensued after the Freedom Ride passed through Monroe, and Williams and his family fled to Cuba after being pursued by the FBI on fabricated kidnapping charges.[14]

Similar fates met other high-profile leaders who took up Williams's call for armed black self-defense. Mainstream condemnation followed Malcolm X's claim in 1964 that "Article number two of the Constitutional amendments provides you and me the right to own a rifle or a shotgun." Republican politicians, including California's Ronald Reagan, swiftly moved to enact expansive new gun-control measures when Huey Newton and the Black Panther Party for Self-Defense advocated carrying guns in public— as permitted by California law at the time. Reagan claimed that he saw "no reason why on the street today a citizen should be carrying loaded weapons." Fear of black people with guns also suffused a congressional report produced after a summer of urban unrest in 1967, which drew "the firm conclusion that effective firearms controls are an essential contribution to domestic peace and tranquility."[15]

It would stand to reason that racial imbalances in legal gun ownership would level out during the latter twentieth and early twenty-first centuries. After all, the late 1960s saw the beginnings of a series of ostensibly color-blind political and cultural shifts that aimed to democratize how Americans bought and sold firearms. On one side of the emerging gun divide, the modern gun control movement took shape after the high-profile assassinations of John F. Kennedy, Robert Kennedy, and Martin Luther King Jr. An unlikely coalition of politicians and activists drove what in retrospect would be the crowning achievement of the movement, the Gun Control Act of 1968. Although President Johnson saw the act as far from sufficient: "We must continue to work for the day when Americans can get the full protection that every American citizen is entitled to and deserves, the kind of protection that most civilized nations have long ago adopted," he said at the signing. But the law nonetheless brought new levels of federal oversight to the buying, selling, and tracking of guns, seemingly guaranteeing equity in the market.[16]

Meanwhile, starting in the 1970s and 1980s, the corporate gun lobby began its steady climb to dominance by proclaiming that gun ownership was an unalienable constitutional right bestowed to all Americans (in other words, the same argument made by Malcolm X). The NRA's well-documented transformation from a sporting and rifleman's organization into a powerful corporate lobby rested on a then radical reinterpretation of the Second Amendment. The "new" NRA took on long-standing assumptions that the amendment served as a guarantee of gun storage for well-regulated and disciplined militias for common defense, and it aggressively promoted the notion that the Constitution guaranteed the gun rights of individual citizens.

The gun lobby supported Ronald Reagan's successful run for the presidency in 1980 and funded the campaigns of senators such as Orrin Hatch, who in 1982 chaired the Subcommittee on the Constitution that produced a report titled *The Right to Keep and Bear Arms*. The report claimed to uncover "clear—and long-lost—proof that the Second Amendment to our Constitution was intended as an individual right of the American citizen to keep and carry arms in a peaceful manner, for protection of himself, his family, and his freedoms." This type of language also appeared in the so-called Firearm Owners' Protection Act of 1986, which invoked "the rights of citizens . . . to keep and bear arms under the Second Amendment." Over the next three decades, forty-four states would pass laws that allowed gun owners to carry concealed weapons in public.[17]

The political emergence of the NRA went hand in hand with the exponential growth of the US gun industry and the numbers of guns it manufactured and sold. By some estimates, America's privately owned gun stock increased by 70 million between 1994 and 2014. By 2015, American citizens owned 255 million guns, or more than one for every adult in the country—far and away the highest rate in the world. As *Vox*'s German Lopez explained it, Americans made up "about 4.43 percent of the world's population [in 2015] yet owned roughly 42 percent of the world's privately held firearms." In short, changes to the politics and economics of firearms meant that many more Americans could buy guns and that there were many more guns for people to buy.[18]

However, despite an insistence on universal rights and the promise of unencumbered gun purchases, legal gun ownership remained concentrated in white populations well into the twenty-first century. Dramatic expansions in gun sales and ownership effectively meant that white Americans in states such as Missouri remained disproportionately armed. According to polling data from the Pew Research Center's 2014 Political Polarization study, whites were more than twice as likely as African Americans to own and carry firearms. While the survey showed expanding demographics of gun ownership across the United States, it also supported the notion that non-Hispanic white, male, self-identified conservative Republicans over the age of thirty-five overwhelmingly owned and carried the most guns in the country. An extensive 2015 Harvard-Northeastern survey similarly found that white men comprised the majority of US gun owners, and particularly the majority of so-called gun super-owners whose firearm collections included between 8 and 140 handguns and long guns.[19]

Why did legal gun ownership remain highly concentrated by race and gender? Researchers tracking US gun trends suggested numerous practical explanations: Perhaps white men in places like Cape Girardeau hunted more often than did other people. Perhaps white men kept firearms because of connections to military service or felt more "comfortable" around guns because they had grown up in households with firearms. Perhaps black communities more likely supported gun control. Or perhaps the trends also symbolized three hundred years of history in which owning firearms and carrying them in public marked a privilege afforded primarily to white men.[20]

Racial tensions surrounding gun ownership lurched into full view in the 2010s, when Missouri and a number of other Southern, midwestern, and westerns states passed so-called guns everywhere bills. Such legislation legalized what were previously considered extreme gun-rights positions, such as the right to openly carry firearms in public spaces. A number of these bills also ended gun-free zones in places like parks, airports, and hospitals and allowed people to purchase even high-capacity firearms without a permit or training.

White men often emerged as the embodiment of these armed liberties. In 2014, for instance, white Missouri open-carry advocates asserted their self-claimed rights to carry anywhere and everywhere by parading through the African American areas of downtown St. Louis brandishing handguns, long guns, and assault rifles. When "guns everywhere" came to Cape Girardeau, a gun-toting local resident named Kevin Alexander told the *Southeast Missourian* newspaper that the legislation would "frighten people and it's going to do a lot of things, but for me, it's going to protect myself and my family."[21]

A white man in Cumming, Georgia, made national news in 2014 when he circled a parking lot overlooking a youth baseball game at a county park and menacingly displayed his holstered weapon—eerily presaging a shooting that would occur in Alexandria, Virginia, three years later at a practice for the 2017 Congressional Baseball Game. A number of parents asked the man to stop acting in a frightening manner, but instead, he allegedly pointed to his firearm and shouted, "See my gun? Look, I got a gun and there's nothing you can do about it!" Terrorized parents and players barricaded themselves in a dugout, and local 911 operators received twenty-two calls over the next twenty minutes. However, when police arrived at the scene, parents were startled to learn that the gun-toting man was wholly within his rights because of new legislation in the state that expanded so-called stand-your-ground rights and eliminated many gun-free zones, such as at county parks. "We support the constitutional right to bear arms," Forsyth sheriff Duane Piper told the media while explaining that the man did nothing illegal. "A park is one of those places where you can openly carry a weapon," added Deputy Doug Rainwater. "A lot of parents with their kids at Forsyth Park don't understand that in Georgia you do have that right."[22]

In 2015, police in Gulfport, Mississippi, cited open-carry laws in the state for their initial failure to detain a white man who frightened Walmart shoppers when he ambled through the store loading and racking shells into his shotgun. And in 2016, a *Washington Post* reporter followed a fifty-one-year-old white man named Jim Cooley as he strolled through the aisles of the Walmart in Winder, Georgia, buying groceries while wearing a "Trump Wants You" T-shirt and with an ATI Omni-Hybrid Maxx AR-15 semiautomatic rifle strapped to his back.[23]

These and other anecdotes played into the time-honed notion that gun laws validated the moral rights of white people, and often white men, to own firearms and carry them in public spaces. And they highlighted ways that the racial divide in guns, gun ownership, and societal reactions to armed civilians retained and derived meaning from historical connection to the tensions between white supremacy and black disarmament. "See my gun?" these white men and the laws that supported their public display said in varying ways. "I got a gun and there's nothing you can do about it!"[24]

Predictably, tales of black men who paraded their guns in public under the full protection of the law were few and far between. Instead, much like responses to Robert Williams and Malcolm X, armed black men often elicited public anger and fear. A sixty-two-year-old African American man named Clarence Daniels entered a Walmart in Tampa, Florida, with a legally owned pistol strapped to his waist, only to be tackled and put in a choke hold by a white vigilante who held Daniels to the ground while shouting, "He's got a gun!"[25]

Media frequently carried tragic stories of black men like Anthony Lamar Smith, Jermaine McBean, and Alton Sterling shot dead by police in the stand-your-ground, open-carry states of Missouri, Florida, and Louisiana, respectively, because of the threats they seemed to pose by carrying guns. "Florida Deputy Cleared in Killing of Black Man by 'Stand-Your-Ground' Law," read a headline in 2016 above an article that detailed how "a Florida judge dismissed manslaughter charges Wednesday against a sheriff's deputy who fatally shot a black man armed with an air rifle, citing the state's stand-your-ground law." The legislation protected the deputy who *felt threatened* by a black man with an air gun at the expense of the African American victim he shot.[26]

"Implicit bias" became the language commentators used to describe these differing responses to armed white and black citizens in public spaces—the assumption being that police officers and other people reacted differently to white and black gun carriers based on differing reflex assumptions about race. "When black faces and 'bad' words are paired together," a *Mother Jones* article that invoked neuroscience to explain implicit bias explained, "you feel yourself becoming faster in your categorizing . . . the trouble comes when the brain . . . forms negative views about groups of people."[27]

But the implicit bias framework often overlooked the different historical narratives embedded in American racial assumptions about guns. From before the birth of the nation, American laws, mores, and traditions coded armed white men as defenders and armed black men as threats. Not just the bodies were racialized; so were the guns as well.

Historical constructions also provide themes used and manipulated by staunchly pro-gun politicians, lobbying groups, manufacturers, and advertisers in their attempts to allow the selling of ever-more guns, primarily to white people. Take the mythology of the John Wayne–style gunslinger, frequently cast as central to twentieth- and twenty-first-century white mythologies about guns. The NRA long sponsored a Gunslinger of the Week award for football players and promoted images of white, Western, gun-toting cowboys at its annual convention. In 2017, journalist Francis Clines visited the NRA National Firearms Museum in Virginia and found that "a poster figure of John Wayne, the mega-hero of Hollywood westerns, offers a greeting here at the gun museum's gallery door as he holds his Winchester carbine at the ready." (Wayne himself once said in an interview that "I believe in white supremacy until the blacks are educated to a point of responsibility.")[28]

These and other associations are built on myths of white settlers and cowboys who tamed the Wild West, guns in hand, during the nineteenth-century westward expansion. In these tales, virtuous white settlers fought off Native American savages, or sheriffs and outlaws dueled on windswept streets in frontier towns, in ways that came to function as central components of modern-day narratives about frontier America. However, in his book *Gun Crusaders*, sociologist Scott Melzer exposes the role of white men with guns on the nineteenth-century frontier as a mythology not of the 1800s but of mid-twentieth-century popular culture. Guns were "unquestionably part of white westward expansion," Melzer writes, "but the role of firearms in expansion has been greatly exaggerated," and in reality, many settlers who traveled west found little use for firearms in their daily lives. Most settler communities valued cooperation and law and order and thus banned guns in public spaces unless a person was taking a gun for repair, hunting, or going to or from a military gathering.[29]

Even Dodge City, Kansas, despite its reputation as a town of shoot-outs and chaos, had a mere five killings in 1878 at its peak of violence "due to a lack of duels and six-shooter pistols." According to Melzer, white Protestant gunslinger heroes were largely invented by writers such as Zane Grey and Louis L'Amour and by 1950s-era movies such as *The Gunfighter* and *Gunfight at the O.K. Corral*. Gun makers, pulp magazines, dime novels, Western movies, and tourist towns "were important contributors to the romanticizing of the gunfighter myth," he writes, "and the producers of these goods benefitted from its widespread acceptance."[30]

The elevation of privileged white male protectors also coursed through gun advertisements in the decades leading up the Man Card advertisement. For much of the twentieth century, gun manufacturers promoted firearms as useful tools that aided responsible sportsmen or hunters. Companies like Bushmaster marketed their products in publications such as the *American Rifleman* as if they were sports equipment, akin to fishing gear or golf clubs.

But starting in the 1980s, the rhetoric shifted around the same time that the rereading of the Second Amendment found its way into legislation and the new NRA emerged; gun manufacturers began promoting the notion that their products help men recover their status, power, and respect. By the early twenty-first century, gun advertisements in publications such as the NRA magazine *American Rifleman* used language that seemed ripped right out the racial histories of guns in America. "The Armed Citizen, Protected by Smith & Wesson," read one campaign—recall that Southern states long-denied gun rights to African Americans because they were not allowed to be "citizens." Campaigns for the Tavor semiautomatic rifle claimed that the gun would "restore the balance of power" for men who owned it. Glock ads told men that owning their guns restored "the confidence to live your life." And of course, there was the Man Card.[31]

Communication studies professor Leonard Steinhorn maintains that this shift from firearms as utilities to firearms as totems of manhood and symbols of white male identity emerged because the gun lobby and gun manufacturers positioned guns as responses to yet another crisis of masculinity in post-1960s America. "It wasn't long ago when broad-shouldered white men dominated our culture, and their very status as breadwinners gave them power and pride," Steinhorn writes. According to Steinhorn, working-class white men long benefited from racial and gender discrimination that gave them a monopoly over manufacturing and construction jobs. Starting in the 1960s, the civil rights and women's movements brought increased competition into these marketplaces, while at the same time wages and the availability of manufacturing jobs declined precipitously. These changes in the economic and social order left working-class white men feeling bypassed, humiliated, and "victimized" by "usurpers" such as women and people of color. "So how do these white men restore the strength and prestige of their idealized past?" Steinhorn asks. "Through guns, which instill fear particularly among the urban and educated elites who hold the levers of power and status in society today."[32]

Surveys of American opinion suggest that these associations between armed protection and idealized whiteness were reflected more than in just advertisements or images—they also shaped the ways that Americans imagined *why* they needed guns in the first place, with marked shifts just in the past two decades. For instance, a whopping 67 percent of US gun owners cited "protection" as their primary reason for owning a gun in a 2017 national survey by the Pew Research Center, while just 38 percent claimed that they used guns for "hunting." These numbers represented inversions of 1999 survey results, when 49 percent of gun owners cited hunting as the reason for owning a gun while just 26 percent said they owned a gun for protection.[33]

This shift coincided with the emergence of the so-called new way of the NRA that promoted guns as primary means of self-defense in an increasingly unsafe world, even as crime rates fell considerably over this same period. "The surest way to stop a bad guy with a gun is a good guy with a gun," NRA executive vice president and CEO Wayne LaPierre famously proclaimed in 2014, while at the same time warning gun owners to remain on the lookout for "terrorists and home invaders and drug cartels, carjackers and knock-out gamers, rapers" and "haters." In a particularly unkind historical appropriation, the NRA based its controversial 2017

"Save America" campaign on a symbol lifted from the Black Power movement: the clenched fist.[34]

Similar themes emerged when sociologist Angela Stroud asked white, permit-holding gun owners in Texas to define what they meant by "good guys with guns." The men Stroud interviewed without fail portrayed people like themselves—other "responsible," white, permit-holding gun owners. Stroud describes an interview with John, the leader of an all-white concealed handgun license (CHL) class, who designated good guys as armed, white "Boy Scout pack leaders and . . . soccer and baseball [coaches] . . . PTA members . . . my students are the kind of people who are gonna pull over if there's an accident on the highway . . . active members of the community, contributing and doing what they can."

By contrast, Stroud found that persons of color appeared in the responses only to illustrate the logics whereby white people needed guns in the first place and never as good guys who might require guns for their own protection. John warned of a racialized "criminal class" that aimed only to steal and rob if not thwarted by armed "good guys." Other members of John's CHL class similarly justified their positions, describing anxieties about imagined dangerous neighborhoods and racial others. As a man named Adam explained to Stroud, "You hear about carjackings . . . let's just say you pull up to a convenience store and there's some certain people outside that make you feel a little nervous, then you've got your gun there . . . to make yourself feel more comfortable."

"Well, there was this car with like, four . . . um, youth guys," a woman named Ruth added. "They weren't white, Caucasian, they were . . . darker skinned, I guess. Dressed in really baggy [clothes] . . . I wish we had a gun with us."

For Stroud, examples of white people who carried guns to protect against racial others were particularly important because most of the racialized altercations never actually happened. Rather, white gun owners *imagined* these encounters based on anxieties about persons of color. In such stories, gun ownership became a defense of internalized notions of racial order as well as an external personal safety.[35]

Privileges ultimately lay the foundation for politics. Guns became the totems for particular versions of white identity politics that rose with the Tea Party and soon encompassed the entire GOP. In his successful 2016

Missouri gubernatorial campaign, controversial conservative Eric Greitens won an election in which he handed out "ISIS hunting cards" at campaign rallies and filled the airwaves with ads showing himself firing a "Gatling-style machine gun" into a lake. That same year, presidential candidate Donald Trump toted rifles onstage at campaign rallies in an attempt to woo the support of the NRA and told a newspaper that he carried a firearm with him "at all times."[36]

Looking back to the complex histories of guns and race in America is not meant to disparage anyone's right to feel safe and secure. Protecting self, family, and community represents a core human drive. "Hey, Mr. Robber, hold on a second . . . the police will be here in seven to nine minutes, and then we'll get back to this," a permit-holding man named Gil told Stroud when she asked him if he believed that the police or 911 might help him were he ever to be the victim of crime. "Or are you gonna be dead by the time the cops get there?" To Gil and many others, guns function as weapons, totems, and transitional objects that promise autonomy, protection, and self-reliance.[37]

And let's be honest: privileges, writ large, have benefits. Privilege is associated with safer neighborhoods, longer life spans, better schools, more cordial relationships with police, healthier diets, and any number of other positive characteristics and outcomes. In a gunfight, it's probably better to be the guy sanctioned to carry a firearm than the guy barred from doing so.[38]

At the same time, investing such deep authority into externalized objects is complicated. Psychiatrists like me sometimes think that men who outsource their sense of power onto external objects—and particularly onto objects shaped like guns—do so in ways that convey deeper, gendered insecurities about potency and perhaps even racial insecurities or projected guilt. Projecting such profound gender and racial meanings onto objects might then render men subject to the maneuvers of marketers, sellers, lobbyists, politicians, and other manipulators of common sense. Of course, guns are also incredibly dangerous, but the danger they pose to people who own and carry them and to their families becomes harder to acknowledge or recognize when these objects of potential self-destruction carry such weighted connotations.

If nothing else, the history of gun privilege thus opens another way for thinking about the complexity of undertaking gun research in places like

Missouri. "Think logically about your health," a researcher like myself might say. "But you're talking about our deepest privileges and biases and insecurities," might be the reply. "And you want to take that away?"

Put another way, the Man Card represented a footnote in a two hundred–year American history that coded firearms as larger than the sum of their actions, stocks, and barrels. Firearms connoted tools that claimed to help white men maintain privilege or restore it when it seemed under threat. This notion of armed supremacy was then codified into laws and everyday practices and passed down through generations. The nostalgia and the power helped armed white populations feel like they circumscribed and protected themselves, while at the same time enforcing and justifying all sorts of imbalances and segregations.

But the nostalgia imbued in the object often made it harder to see how, when taken to permitless, open-carry extremes, expectations of duly-owed power brought with them the potential to make even white lives more perilous and less safe. Gun logic required imagining danger around every corner; losing the Man Card needed to remain a constant threat. Over time, the dominant skill set and survival strategy for coping involved neither compromise nor negotiation. Rather, the response to change in many parts of the country always depended on building more castles and buying more guns.

INTERVIEW:

WE GOTTA TAKE UP ARMS

Interview excerpts, March 15, 2017, Ladue / St. Louis. Speaker 2: white male, 55, IT tech, son of gun dealer.

JMM: Your father sold guns, and you also grew up in a community that valued them?

Speaker 2: For sure. I grew up in the St. Louis area, but in a small town nearby. It's mostly rural community, and gun ownership was extraordinarily common. Mostly shotguns and mostly for hunting. But learning how to skin a deer was as much a rite of passage as learning how to use a baseball mitt. It was just something that we did as a culture, this culture, hunting and fishing and things like that was normal, a commonplace.

But it's funny, my family didn't have guns. We were in a neighborhood, like a subdivision, a typical suburban like subdivision. So we were raised a different way.

I think the irony was my dad was an ammunition executive—my dad worked for Winchester Ammunition—and his predominant target market was police departments and military. His job was to arm police departments, but he was never a guy who had strong opinions about gun control or gun ownership—or at least not ones that he shared with me. So we didn't grow up with firearms at all, despite my father earning his living in the munitions industry. I guess we had BB guns, but that was it.

JMM: What was his explanation, or your understanding for why he sold guns and there was a lot of guns in your culture but you guys didn't own guns?

Speaker 2: I wish I had an answer for that. I think he just never thought it was a big deal and probably didn't want guns in our home since he saw what they could do.

Truth be told, my dad didn't purchase a gun until two, three years ago. Then suddenly he became very pro-gun and very pro-gun rights about two, three years ago in the context of the Ferguson uprising.

Which, you know, dominated national headlines, as you know, but was particularly salient in the St. Louis area because it was happening there. There was this weird sort of mentality amongst the rural white folk that we gotta take up arms because the protesters could be coming for us. There were stories about I-40 and I-44 being blocked off at midnight because bands of revelers—*revelers* is the wrong word; rioters or whatever—looters were taking to the streets, and they were going to expand beyond the confines of the ghetto and come into West County and shit like that.

So around that time, my dad bought a gun, even though he still lives in rural Missouri—in a different part than the one we grew up in, but still lives in the St. Louis area—and my best friend from high school, who lives nearby, bought a pistol for my dad and began like intense instruction in the use of firearms.

It was so disturbing to me because I walked into Dad's house—I don't know how well you know that area, I know you're a Missouri person from long ago; he lives in a very safe suburb—and I walked into his house, and he and his wife were loading bullets into magazines on the living room floor while the music was playing, and I just thought, *What the fuck has happened in St. Louis?*

But there was this mentality, but it was in the context of Ferguson that again prompted my close high school friend to buy weapons for him and his wife and start teaching his kids about this.

JMM: When you say your dad became pro-gun also around that time, what kinds of things did he say about his rationale for suddenly owning a gun in the home?

Speaker 2: He was singing the song of protection. I need it to protect my house, my wife, my family. My dad and mom divorced probably fifteen years ago, and now he's remarried, and he's like, "I have to protect myself, I have to protect my wife because I think this is a real possibility that this is the world changing."

So constant referral to the "world" as if it's not what we used to think it was, the "world" and it's changing and radical Islam and Ferguson. I think it had a lot to do with the sort of zeitgeist of the sort of anti-police protests that began in Ferguson but extended through Baltimore and Wisconsin, other states where there were other shootings. North Carolina, where these things were happening and you were seeing these on the news, it was confirmatory evidence. "See, it's not just an isolated thing in Ferguson, Missouri; this is what we have to do as white Americans."

JMM: You're suggesting it was racially motivated?

Speaker 2: I would say that. Dad wouldn't, because I wasn't raised in a household where race was discussed much. But I wasn't raised in a household that was overtly racist to my recollection. It wasn't discussed much, but it was never disparagingly discussed. This certainly had a racial undertone feeling, and it did for my friend too, who again would say, "Racist? That's a joke. Are you kidding? I'm an educated professional; many of my good friends are black," and while that's true, they would be the friends in his consulting firm. You know what I'm saying?

The people would say . . . I guess the idea when there was a perception that your own safety and the safety of your family was really at play, then that would trump the niceties associated with race discussion. I think it is. Is that to say there's racism brewing under the surface in all of this? Probably. Probably. But it was something you instructed your kids against, raised your kids against, and espoused against. But then all of a sudden, it's like, "Okay, shit's getting real now," you know what I mean?

PREVENTATIVE MEDICINE

To SUMMARIZE WHERE we've come thus far: questions of risk emerged powerfully in the survivor stories people told in Cape Girardeau— where grieving relatives searched for warning signs they may have seen or preventive actions they might have taken. Yet these very same questions were rendered elusive by the social, political, and historical frameworks surrounding gun research and ownership. The promise of restored or defended authority represented by guns sat in uneasy repose with the knowledge vacuum about firearm risk prediction and prevention, invisibly shaping ways in which white citizens of Missouri lived and died.

Of course, in some other universe, coming up with better formulations of gun risk in places like Missouri would be entirely possible and even desired. Moreover, risk calculation is largely straightforward for pretty much any other topic except guns. Risk is an algorithm, a formula, a recipe. Risk is an exposed nail, unsecured scaffolding, a toxic vapor in the air. Risk is something people want to avoid.

Statisticians often calculate risk by multiplying probability times loss, or the likelihood of occurrence of an unwanted event by the consequence of that event. Such calculations help nervous investors, for instance, who can then compute the impact of adding particular stocks to their portfolios using economic frameworks of risk versus reward. Epidemiologists and practitioners of evidence-based medicine learn to calculate statistics of *relative risk*, a term used to describe the likelihood of developing a particular disease after exposure to a pathogen. Researchers who want to assess the impact of a new medication, vaccine, or surgery divide risk in an experimental group by risk in a control group to calculate what they call *risk ratio*. In these ways and others, risk becomes quantified, material, and known.[1]

But risk becomes exceedingly difficult to evaluate when the variables blink on and off, seemingly vital facts are painted into the primer, and usual ways of building consensus disappear from view. Without a firm set of findings on which to base best practices, risk becomes an abstraction onto which people project anxieties, biases, and fears. One person looks at the canvas and sees the *Mona Lisa*, another sees *The Scream*, yet another sees nothing but empty whiteness.

Politicians and lobbyists then manipulate the knowledge vacuum surrounding risk to balkanize everyday people on matters of life, death, and mundane daily routine—matters about which, if left to their own devices, people could probably forge consensus. All the while, scientific assurances that might help people feel mastery over events unforeseen or appliances untested function instead as variables left up for grabs. The forces that promote (and indeed, often gain financially from) polarization grow ever-more powerful, while hardworking people who live at various points along the oft-manufactured pro-gun–anti-gun continuum are left to fend for themselves.

Polarization then leads to an often-absurd state of affairs. Calculations of risk produce ever-safer cars, medications, bike lanes, and building codes. Yet the very idea of even studying risk becomes a risk itself when the conversation turns to guns, laying the groundwork for decisions that seem at odds with individual and national well-being. Gun-industry trade organizations fund leading gun suicide–prevention programs—and then force them to restrict mention of the potential risks posed by firearms. So, too, in December 2017, newspapers carried stories suggesting the profound failure of gun policies (or lack thereof) in Missouri. "Kansas City's Terrifying Year of Homicides—the Worst in 24 Years," read a headline in the *Kansas City Star*. That same month, the *New York Times* reported that homicide in New York plunged "to a level not seen since the 1950s." Yet instead of asking the seemingly obvious questions—Did the fact that New York restricted gun ownership relate to its success? How can we model these strategies elsewhere?—GOP politicians in the US Congress championed a so-called concealed-carry reciprocity bill that would allow guns from places like Missouri to flow more freely into cities like New York.[2]

The absurdity is furthered by another reality, one that will be our focus for much of the remainder of the Missouri section of this book: research that even attempts to use established statistical methods to assess the relative risk of firearms is roundly critiqued as unscientific by the same people who try to block funding for gun science.

Consider, for instance, the response to two studies by a leading group of public health scholars who studied the potential effects of different forms of gun legislation by comparing Missouri to Connecticut. The scholars—Cassandra Crifasi, John Meyers, Jon Vernick, and Daniel Webster of the Center for Gun Policy and Research at Johns Hopkins University's Bloomberg School of Public Health—chose these two somewhat comparable states because of their opposite trajectories on gun regulation over the latter half of the twentieth and early twenty-first centuries.

To recall, Missouri had a long tradition of gun ownership in rural and hunting communities. At the same time, the state closely regulated handgun sales in an attempt to assure that licensed dealers or private sellers sold firearms only to low-risk persons. From 1921 until 2007, Missouri enforced a permit-to-purchase (PTP) law that required anyone wanting to purchase a handgun to apply in person at a local sheriff's office. There, potential buyers would undergo an interview and a series of background checks to assess risk factors such as past convictions for violent crimes, being under a restraining order for domestic violence, or heightened risk of suicide.

Several lifelong Missouri residents with whom I spoke explained what it was like to buy and sell firearms under the PTP process. As they put it, the regulations were far from intrusive for gun buyers and represented rote components of everyday transactions surrounding guns. "It was no big deal at all," a retired lawyer from Joplin who grew up working in his parents' pawn and gun shop told me. "We never thought anything of it, just took a few minutes. Kind of made sense to have someone track the guns in town."

Missouri state lawmakers repealed the PTP law in 2007, and most remaining gun-purchase checks and regulations fell like legislative dominoes in the years thereafter. As noted earlier, 2014 legislation allowed anyone with a concealed weapons permit to carry guns openly in cities or towns that otherwise banned the open carrying of firearms. In 2016, the Missouri legislature passed "permitless carry" legislation, created new "stand-your-ground" laws, and expanded Castle Doctrine protections.[3]

By comparison, Connecticut had a largely uneven history of gun-control legislation until 1995, when its lawmakers passed PTP legislation mandating that all handgun buyers undergo background checks and complete safety courses. Legislative actions regulating the sale, possession, and use of guns and ammunition then expanded. In 1999, Connecticut pioneered a program of what is called "risk-based, temporary, preemptive gun removal," authorizing police to temporarily remove guns from individuals when there is "probable cause to believe . . . that a person poses a risk of imminent personal injury to himself or herself or to other individuals." After the Sandy Hook shootings in 2012, the state passed gun laws billed as among the "toughest in the country," including new bans on assault rifles and high-capacity ammunition magazines, and mandatory background checks for all gun sales alongside expanded background checks.[4]

The relevance of a comparison between the two states would thus seem clear. Missouri and Connecticut modeled two polar opposite approaches at the core of larger debates about guns in America: whether more or fewer guns and gun laws led to more or less crime. In other words, did easing restrictions governing purchase and transit of firearms decrease crime in Missouri, or did allowing more guns in public pose a threat? Did people in Connecticut suffer fewer gun suicides or accidents because of the stricter legislation, or did criminals run amok in ways that put law-abiding people at risk? Did gun legislation in one state or another change the ways people lived and died—and if so, how?

People usually ask these kinds of basic questions about most any type of legislation when they want to know if what their politicians did had the impact they wanted it to or if unforeseen or unintended consequences altered the calculus of reward versus risk. Legislation, after all, is rarely perfect in its first iterations and requires constant assessment to gauge whether it should be improved, amended, repealed, or replaced.

This was the approach taken by the Hopkins group, which published two high-profile comparative studies that compared the effects of the removal of PTP legislation in Missouri and on the potential effects of differing approaches to guns between Missouri and Connecticut. In the absence of other types of federally funded databases, the group relied primarily on death data—via WISQARS, police homicide statistics, and the National Association for Public Health Statistics and Information Systems (NAPHSIS).

In the first study, published in 2014, the group used police homicide statistics to focus mainly on Missouri, and, after extensive tracking, "estimated" that the repeal of Missouri's PTP law was associated with

> an increase in annual firearm homicides rates of 1.09 per 100,000 (+23%) but was unrelated to changes in non-firearm homicide rates . . . the law's repeal was associated with increased annual murders rates of 0.93 per 100,000 (+16%). These estimated effects translate to increases of between 55 and 63 homicides per year in Missouri.

These claims built on an earlier paper by Webster, which found that the repeal of Missouri's PTP law was likely associated with increased "diversion" of guns to criminals.[5]

Then in a 2015 study, the group used advanced statistical modeling to compare the potential effects of PTP laws on gun suicide rates in Missouri and Connecticut between 1981 and 2012. This second research paper involved a labor-intensive process of compiling data on all recorded suicides in Connecticut and Missouri over the roughly thirty-year time period, and then dividing these lists into firearm- and non-firearm suicides and pre- and post-PTP law changes for each state. The group then compiled similar data for a series of comparable states that did not implement PTP law changes over this same period, and statistically controlled for a number of state-level factors often associated with suicide rates, such as unemployment, poverty, demographics, and the presence or absence of strong mental health treatment systems. Among the key findings, as published in the journal *Preventive Medicine*:

> Connecticut experienced a drop in its firearm suicide rate coincident with the adoption of a PTP handgun law that was greater than nearly all of the 39 other states that did not have such a law at that time, and Missouri experienced an increase in its firearm suicide rate following the repeal of its PTP handgun law that was larger than all states that retained their PTP laws.[6]

The analysis ultimately estimated a 15.4 percent reduction in firearm suicide rates associated with the implementation of Connecticut's PTP law and a 16.1 percent increase in firearm suicide rates associated with Missouri's PTP repeal. The authors found no such trends in modes of suicide other than that by gun.

Both studies were relatively straightforward. Before and after. Compare, then compare again. Run some analyses, make some charts and tables. Estimate trends. This represented sound scientific practice. The framework, after all, had precedent:

> When one does research, it is most appropriate to take the simplest specifications first and then make things more complicated. The simplest way of doing this is to examine the mean crime rates before and after the change in law. Then one would examine the trends that existed before and after the law. This is the pattern that I've followed in my earlier work, and I've followed the same pattern here.

Thus spoke John Lott in *More Guns, Less Crime*.[7]

Given the disparities between the two states, the John's Hopkins researchers concluded in the 2015 paper that

> the findings of the study are relevant to physicians as it provides further evidence that reducing access to a firearm can prevent suicide. Physicians who treat patients at elevated risk for suicide can counsel patients and family members about the link between access to a firearm and suicide risk and the potential benefit of reducing firearm access. The study also highlights the value of a population-based approach to suicide prevention. . . . A PTP law that would restrict access to handguns for individuals with a history of severe mental illness, criminal behavior, domestic violence or substance abuse, or by simply delaying access to a firearm during a time of crisis through an application review period could prevent suicide.[8]

Note the passivity of these conditional sentences. Physicians *can* counsel patients and family members. A PTP law that *would* restrict access to handguns *could* prevent suicide. The phrasing is in no way declarative, or in any way suggests that the researchers advocated taking away anyone's guns. Instead, the argument conveys a measured position taken by scholars who knew they addressed just one possible intervention into a sensitive topic, and without the usual support of multiple other studies on the same topic in top journals as there are with every cause of unnatural death except guns.

A cautious tone also appeared in the literature that accompanied publication. "Crifasi cautions the findings do not indicate a clear causal relationship," read a press release put out by Johns Hopkins. Crifasi specifically highlighted that "factors other than handgun purchaser licensing may have [also] contributed to the decline in suicides."[9]

The restrained claims did little to blunt critiques from gun-rights advocates. Writing for Fox News, Lott accused Webster and the media of "cherry picking" data to elevate the risk of PTP repeal in Missouri. In the *National Review*, self-described Second Amendment and American exceptionalism scholar Charles Cook slammed the group's "iffy" methodology while claiming that "correlation doesn't equal causation" when it came to links between gun policy changes and gun deaths. Critic Robert VerBruggen lambasted an overreliance on death data to understand the impact of gun legislation, as well as the overall framework of "looking at states before and after they implemented gun-control measures." Brian Doherty, author of the book *Gun Control on Trial*, castigated the use of conditional tense, such as Webster's claims that gun laws "appear to reduce" gun fatalities.[10]

Gun-rights advocates basically raised the same concerns about the research as did the researchers themselves. Most of the points they made came straight out of the authors' discussions of the limitations of their own studies. Critics also failed to mention that the overreliance on death data, speculative methods, and tentative language resulted in large part from the broad-ranging effects of the ban on federally funded gun research. Or that the potential weakness of gun violence prevention research paled in comparison with the cavernous absence of even the most basic evidence demonstrating the health *benefits* of guns.[11]

In summary, people who reflexively shouted "Gun research doesn't add up!" were often the same people who supported a ban on effective gun research. It was as if they reprimanded plants for not flowering during a drought while at the same time blocking the trucks that delivered water. They did so without ever once suggesting they would support research that might better test not just the comparisons between Missouri and Connecticut but also the pro-gun positions that they themselves promoted.

For all their criticisms, gun advocates overlooked the most glaring problem with the suicide research: its lack of analysis of race. "The analyses controlled for a number of factors previously associated with suicide rates," Crifasi and her colleagues wrote in the article, "including unemployment; poverty; demographics (percentage of the population that was male, black, Hispanic . . .)." The authors further cited Missouri's but not Connecticut's "racial demographic composition" as a factor in need of statistical control.[12]

Such framing was curious because race functioned as a central component of the earlier 2014 homicide paper by the Hopkins group. "Homicide is the second leading cause of death for people aged 15–34 years in the USA and the leading cause of death for black males in this age group," read the very first sentence of Webster and Crifasi's 2014 analysis of the effects of PTP repeal on gun homicides in Missouri.[13]

The focus on race in the 2014 study but not in the 2015 study subtly conveyed the notion that homicide was a race problem but suicide was a policy one. Intended or not, race meant black homicide in Missouri but not white suicide in Missouri, Connecticut, and all other states where white men made up the majority of self-inflicted gun deaths. Blackness, as an analytical category, thereby remained front and center in discussions of violent crime. Whiteness remained controlled for and invisible.

Framing race as such likely allowed Crifasi and her colleagues to smooth out statistical differences between distinct geographic locales. But doing so also precluded the authors from addressing questions directly relevant to Cape Girardeau, stand-your-ground laws, the Castle Doctrine, and the Man Card: What if risk emerged, not just from the presence or absence of guns or policies? What if the guns and the policies rendered whiteness itself as a risk?

INTERVIEW:

THE BIGGEST HEART

Interview excerpts, December 20, 2016, Cape Girardeau. Speaker 2: white female, age 54, aunt.

Speaker 2: We just decided to push up Christmas this year and do things completely different than what we are accustomed to doing them because of what we've experienced in the last two years. Losing my nephew has been definitely taking a toll on my entire family.

JMM: What kind of things have you done differently?

Speaker 2: Well, we normally always celebrated Christmas on Christmas Eve. This year, we just decided to do it early and instead of having the big family gathering at the home, where all of the memories are.

JMM: That sounds really brave. Did it go okay?

Speaker 2: Yes, it did. We had my brother's daughter, who is the sibling of my nephew. My deceased nephew. I think it made her much more comfortable also because she didn't have to be there and see everything in the house that reminded her of her brother. Not that we're trying to forget him by any means, but it's hard to be happy and celebrate a joyous occasion when everything you look at reminds you of what you've lost.

JMM: I think those reminders are the definition of what it means to be a survivor, right?

Speaker 2: Right. My sister's daughter is only eleven. She's been extremely traumatized by the loss of her brother because she was there two years ago when it happened. Not there when he actually shot himself, but she was at school. They went and got her and brought her home immediately. She was there in the middle . . . she was there amongst all of the trauma and turmoil and the police, and it just wasn't a good thing. Not that it ever is a good thing, but she is in counseling.

I blame the Ritalin personally. Twelve-year-old kid, he just didn't seem happy. He wanted to sleep a lot. I don't think his problem was ADHD. I really think that he was misdiagnosed. I think that he was depressed, and I know when they were arguing about the Ritalin. . . . The doctor said this is for ADHD, but this is also for depression. I just don't think that he had ADHD. I think that he was depressed . . . he just felt like he didn't have any other way out, and that's my honest opinion.

Like I said, there's some speculation that maybe it was an accidental suicide. I don't see that. I say speculation because there were four bullets in the gun and he took three of them out. There were three bullets laying on the bed, on the opposite side of the bed from where he committed suicide.

JMM: Did you know how he got it or . . .

Speaker 2: Oh, yeah. His stepfather is a gun fanatic. There were four semi rifles under their bed that were not loaded, a Bushmaster and some others, but there was a 9mm Sig Sauer under the pillow that was fully loaded with a full clip and then an extra clip laying on the bedside nightstand. Then on his mother's side of the bed, there was a .38 Special fully loaded. The kids had access to all of it. We teach the kids about gun safety. They know not to touch them.

JMM: Was it one of those guns that he ended up using?

Speaker 2: Absolutely. It was the .38 Special.

JMM: It sounds like guns are a big part of their life.

Speaker 2: Yes . . . I even have pictures of them holding guns, posing at holidays.

He clearly had some things going through his head that he didn't share with us. That is a huge guilt for us, that we didn't catch that. That's where our guilt comes in because we might have been able to prevent some of this. After he committed suicide, we started checking out his Instagram pages; he clearly was a disturbed young man. We maybe could have prevented . . .

JMM: What's the process of trying to move on or trying to make sense of it?

Speaker 2: I don't know if you could ever make sense of it. I really don't. I have found peace with it, and my family is trying to find peace with the fact that we know that my nephew is in heaven. It was just all senseless in my opinion. I know for sure one thing that could have been done was those guns could have been locked up.

JMM: Yes, that was a question I was going to ask. Has this changed your views about guns or the role guns play in people's lives?

Speaker 2: It absolutely has not changed my view about guns. This does not make me anti-gun.

But part of me blames the parents. You don't leave two handguns, fully loaded, laying on a nightstand in a bedroom. If you choose to leave loaded weapons laying around your house and one of your own kills themselves with it, then why are you not criminally responsible? I don't understand that.

JMM: I'm struggling to answer your question because I can't think of why.

Speaker 2: I get that. It's not a crime to have a loaded weapon in your home, but as a parent, it is your responsibility to protect your child at all times. Leaving loaded weapons laying around your house is not protecting your child. I would certainly be a huge advocate of making it a law that if a child kills themselves with a loaded weapon in a parent's home, the parent is criminally responsible. . . . He had the biggest heart.

WHAT WAS THE RISK?

T WO QUESTIONS STUCK in my mind as I neared the end of the Missouri research. By that point, I had traveled through the state and conducted
multiple interviews, studied the history, and reviewed the scientific literature. I learned a great deal about what it meant to live surrounded by guns
in "gun country," began to understand why guns conveyed complex historical meanings, and assessed the strengths and limitations of scientific
research.

But the hovering questions that my findings seemed to point to were
the same ones glossed over by Crifasi and colleagues and by the critics
of their work. Did being a white citizen of Missouri put a person at higher
risk of firearm suicide? Did that risk change after Missouri loosened its
gun laws? In other words, was risk not merely individual and psychological but collective as well?

So I initiated my own brief data analysis. I realized I was wading into
the same data—particularly via the WISQARS database—that Crifasi
and her colleagues used and thus was inviting some of the same critiques.
Just to say it again, I believe we should press ahead with firearm research
whenever we can because I don't think that anyone on any side of this gun
control debate is well served by censorship or the absence of knowledge—
save the organizations and industries that benefit from polarizing Americans and making us think we hate each other or will never reach consensus
on difficult issues. I also believe we should be talking to each other more

openly about the deep meanings and fears that the guns have come to sym-
bolize. And at this writing at least, WISQARS is an open-access database,
so anyone is free to follow through the analysis I describe here or analyze
their own trends.

Data research is best done in teams, and I am very lucky to have an
outstanding group comprised of a statistician, a graduate research assistant, and several devoted undergraduates (all of whom I thank in the
acknowledgments section of this book). We began by setting research parameters using WISQARS. As a reminder, WISQARS is an interactive online database that compiles data on fatal and nonfatal injury across the
United States. Its information comes from a variety of sources but primarily from the National Vital Statistics System (NVSS) operated by the National Center for Health Statistics (NCHS). Here is the website: https://
www.cdc.gov/injury/wisqars.

Once open, we chose "Fatal Injury Data" from the pull-down menu—
and were immediately greeted with a litany of caveats, such as, "There was
a coding error in the 2014 file that increases the number of unintentional
firearm deaths," it explained. And later, "Year-to-year death data for a given
state can sometimes be affected by unexpectedly large numbers of death
certificates with the underlying cause coded as 'other ill-defined causes.'"[1]

Of course, this made sense. Categorizing an "intentional" cause of
death is difficult under any circumstance, and particularly so when the
pathogen kills in milliseconds. Did the deceased mean to pull the trigger
in a silent moment of despair, or was he acting out? What did intention-
ality even mean in a setting in which loaded guns remained in plain view
day and night? The difficulty of putting death into categories is ever-more
complex because of stigma against mental illness or concerns about life-
insurance reimbursements that might tempt coroners or doctors to list
cause of death as anything but suicides or accidental shootings.[2]

We chose "Fatal Injury Reports for National, Regional, and States,"
and "Suicide" and "Firearm" as the main parameters, or dependent variables. We then ran searches by switching around a number of other independent variables, such as, *Region/State, *Sex, *Age, *Years, *Race and
*Hispanic/NonHispanic. These final items reflect the somewhat confusing
nature of census categories. For reasons that hardly seem to make sense,
the most recent census lists White, Black, American Indian/Alaska Native,

Asian/Pacific Islander, and Other list as "Races" and then separately lists Hispanic/Latino as an "Ethnicity." There are various, oft-problematic reasons for these somewhat random racial and ethnic distinctions, but for this study, we took them at face value.[3]

We ran sequential searches that tracked gun suicides in the United States by race/ethnicity, gender, state, region, and year. We began our data analysis by making sure that we were on the same page as Crifasi and her colleagues. So we first looked at overall firearm suicide trends in Missouri and Connecticut, adjusted by what is called the *crude rate*. A crude rate is, roughly, the total number of deaths among residents of a specified geographic area, divided by the total population for the same geographic area for a specified period, and multiplied by 100,000. Crude rates allow for the most basic form of comparison across different populations and locales. For instance, Missouri has several million more people than Connecticut. Crude rates adjust for this difference.

Data tracking gun suicides in Missouri and Connecticut between 1985 and 2015 roughly followed the same trends as those reported by Crifasi and her colleagues in their analysis of the years 1981 to 2012. Crude suicide rates in Missouri generally declined until 2007, then began to rise. Importantly, the steepest increases occurred in the period after the Crifasi study ended in 2012, when Missouri gun laws became more permissive. In 2015, the state's gun suicides rose to an all-time high of 10 per 100,000 people.

Meanwhile, gun suicide rates in Connecticut followed a slow downward trajectory starting in the mid-1990s and generally hovered in crude rates between 2 and 3 per 100,000 people through the end-period of analysis.

We next undertook a quick multistate comparison, which revealed that these trends held when comparing Missouri and Connecticut to some of the other states commonly thought of as "loose" or "tight" states regarding gun violence prevention legislation. For instance, Texas and Florida also promoted open-carry, permitless-carry, stand-your-ground, the Castle Doctrine, and other legislation that loosened gun statutes. Meanwhile, New York, a state with consistently tight gun laws, reflected trends in Connecticut. A comparison of gun suicides in these states between 1999 and 2015 looks like this. Note how Missouri sets the curve:

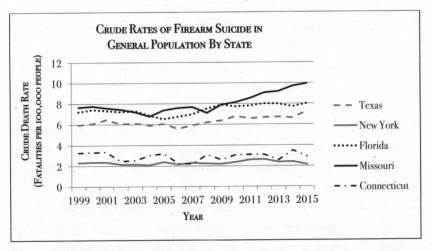

Source: WISQARS Fatal Injury Data via the National Vital Statistics System, organized by the Centers for Disease Control and Prevention, retrieved from https://www.cdc.gov/injury /wisqars/index.html.

Again, Crifasi and her colleagues controlled for race and gender, meaning that they combined citizens in Missouri and Connecticut into aggregate groups. Given the history of white men and guns detailed earlier in this chapter, we aimed to further break down the trends by race and gender. The charts we produced added depth to the Johns Hopkins analysis. For instance, white non-Hispanic men topped every other group for gun suicide in every year since 1985, surpassing the average of all other men combined, and trended even higher after the PTP legislation. On the opposite page is a chart that compares white men with the aggregate of all men, African American men, and white women. And below that is a similar breakdown for Connecticut.

The Missouri graph shows that white male firearm suicides remained atop suicides by everyone else, and particularly so starting in the mid- to late 2000s, around the time that Missouri began relaxing its gun regulations. White male suicides trended downward in the state from the mid-1990s until 2007 and then rose steadily until they hit their highest points on record in 2014 and 2015, at over 20 deaths per 100,000 white men. Meanwhile, firearm suicides by persons of every other demographic group showed what is called *random variability*, spiking occasionally but otherwise demonstrating relatively lower levels and no consistent increases or decreases over time.

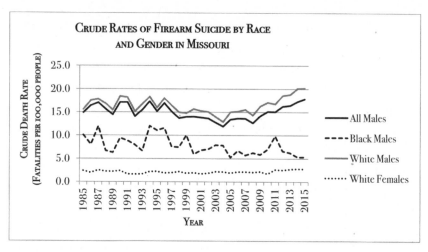

Source: WISQARS Fatal Injury Data.

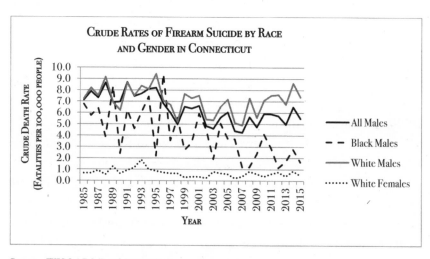

Source: WISQARS Fatal Injury Data.

By contrast, the Connecticut graph showed more varied trends. White male suicides peaked at 9 deaths per 100,000 people in 1994, again right before the state enacted tougher gun legislation, and then jumped up and down for the next twenty years but followed an overall trend of decreased death over time. Gun suicides by other groups of men fell considerably over the same period. For the most part, gun suicides by women, and particularly women of color, remained so low that they barely made it onto either graph.

Perhaps most important, the graphs powerfully suggest that white male suicide trends served as primary drivers of overall suicide rates in each state. Rates of white male suicide in Connecticut bounced around but generally declined after the PTP legislation and risk-based, temporary, preemptive gun removal interventions in the late 1990s, catalyzing an overall decline in gun suicides in the state. Meanwhile, in Missouri, rising rates of white male suicide paced overall steady increases in death by self-inflicted gunshot—a reality made clearer by the ways that the "all men" line so closely followed the white male line. White men, in other words, set the aggregate for everyone else.

In many ways, these trends are unsurprising. Once again, it's widely known that firearms are a primary means of suicide for men in general and white men in particular. However, the data opens up questions in addition to providing answers. Why were Missouri's suicide rates high to begin with, if the state boasted such strict gun regulation prior to 2007? (A good part of the answer: there were already many more guns in Missouri than Connecticut, and PTP did not affect all gun sales.) Did the disparity in suicide rates reflect different state economics, mental health systems, illegal gun markets, or other factors? What types of guns did men use for suicide? (WISQARS makes no distinction between handguns, hunting rifles, or AR-15s.) In this sense, how valid is the connection to PTP legislation, since PTP laws often regulate handguns but not other types of firearms?

Even with those important caveats, these race and gender trends are nonetheless remarkable, particularly regarding white male suicide in Missouri. One might assume, for example, that liberal gun laws in the state would make it possible for every person of every background and identity to buy a gun. As suicide researchers generally think of gun suicide as an act linked to access, it would stand to reason that gun suicide rates would rise for everyone accordingly. In reality, white men in Missouri outpaced everybody else, and at rates that far exceeded the percentages of actual white men in the state.

In 2015, white men comprised roughly 40 percent of the population of Missouri but were victims of nearly 80 percent of gun suicides. Put another way, non-Hispanic white men outpaced Asian men, Hispanic men, African American men, Alaskan men, and men of pretty much all other backgrounds at rates that appear as follows if you compare white men to all other men *combined*:

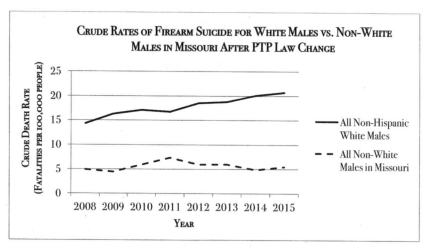

Source: WISQARS Fatal Injury Data.

The same Missouri patterns held, not surprisingly, when we compared white men to women. White men outpaced women of all backgrounds at rates that barely fit onto one graph, as shown on page 102.

Undoubtedly, regional differences factored into differing white male gun suicide rates in Missouri and Connecticut. The two states have historically dissimilar gun and hunting cultures, distinct mental health systems, and divergent state economies—and the studies cited above took many such factors into account. But it is hard to dismiss the suggestion that differing gun policies catalyzed different white male suicide rates between Connecticut and Missouri: PTP, mandated background checks, closed gun-show loopholes, required permits, limits on assault rifles, and other legislation in one state; the Castle Doctrine, open-carry, concealed carry, campus carry, and permitless carry in the other.[4]

Studies of gun violence prevention often try to assess the impact of particular initiatives like background checks or gun buyback programs, with varied degrees of success. The results of these studies are then used to support larger arguments for or against "gun control." But it's important to remain skeptical of any one study that tries to assess the effect of any one policy or act of legislation. The databases are far from perfect, and there are already so many firearms in circulation in the United States, practically one for every person, that no initiative will show immediate effect in parts of the country where there are already many guns. Perhaps most important, many studies seem to ask the wrong question. Instead of asking, "Did this one

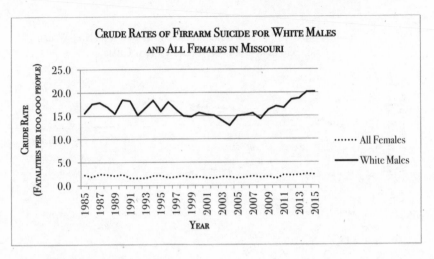

Source: WISQARS Fatal Injury Data.

initiative work?" why not instead pose the question, "What would life have looked like if pro-gun legislation had never taken effect?"[5]

So, as a final analysis, we imagined for a moment that, starting in 2007, Missouri followed the same path as Connecticut, where guns remained legal but Second Amendment rights coexisted with regulations governing the purchase and carry of firearms, and gun suicides responded accordingly. To do this final analysis, we switched to a more sensitive data analysis called an *age-adjusted death rate*, which controls for the effects

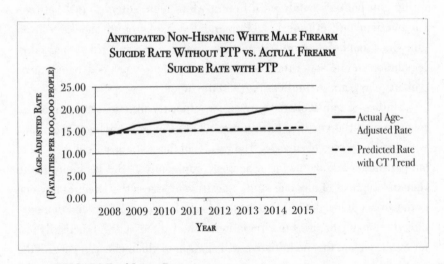

Source: WISQARS Fatal Injury Data.

Year	Actual white male gun suicides, MO	Hypothetical white male gun suicides, MO	Difference*
2008	343	374	(31)
2009	391	376	15
2010	412	377	35
2011	404	377	27
2012	447	377	70
2013	453	377	76
2014	486	378	108
2015	501	388	113
Total	3,437	3,023	413

* Differences in the totals are due to rounding.

Source: WISQARS Fatal Injury Data.

of differences in populations according to age distributions—accounting, for instance, for ways that one state or another might have more infants or elderly persons who might skew data on life expectancy. In that alternate reality, the post-2007 graph for white male suicide in Missouri might look something like the graph on the previous page.

In this calculation, the top line represents the post-2007 suicide rates for white men in Missouri while the bottom line represents the age-adjusted rate if trends in Missouri more closely followed those in Connecticut. The white space between the two lines represent lives that might have been saved by alternate political decisions and resultantly different everyday practices.

Calculated another way: The aggregate gun suicide rate rose by 15.48 percent in Missouri but only by 6.56 percent in Connecticut in the eight years after PTP removal (2008–2015). If rates of white male suicide in Missouri instead rose by the Connecticut rate of 6.56 percent per year, then Missouri's aggregate rate between 2008 and 2015 would have increased to 15.62 per 100,000 per year rather. Instead, that rate was up to 20.17 per 100,00 by 2015, as indicated by the graph above. In terms of actual lives, the differences between this hypothetical world and reality appear as follows:

In other words, the space between the actual line and the alternate-reality line conservatively suggests that the loosening of Missouri's gun laws equated to 413 additional white male suicide deaths over the years 2008–2015. Over these eight years, this averages to an additional 52 white male deaths per year on top of Missouri's already high gun suicide rates.

To put these additional white male deaths in perspective, 52 deaths in a year would exceed the reported gun deaths by defensive use, home invasion, or accidental shooting in Missouri in every year since 2012. The 413 deaths over eight years equals the total number of reported gun deaths from mass shootings in the entire United States in 2015. The number of additional deaths in Missouri between 2008 and 2015 dwarfs the number of Americans killed by terrorist attacks over this same period. According to a terrorism tracker produced by the nonpartisan New America Foundation, "in the fifteen years after 9/11, jihadists have killed 94 people inside the United States." According to US State Department reporting, 145 Americans died by "overseas terrorism" between 2007 and 2015, for an average yearly mortality rate of 18, while 70 Americans died via "domestic terrorism" over this eight-year period, for an average yearly death rate of 8.75. (According to WISQARS, the total number of persons killed by terrorism in Missouri between 2008 and 2015 was zero.)[6]

Suicide can happen to anyone, anywhere, at any time. "The thought that I might kill myself formed in my mind coolly as a tree or a flower," Sylvia Plath wrote in *The Bell Jar*. Even trained psychiatrists and psychologists have great difficulty predicting which of their patients will take their own lives. At the same time, it seems highly plausible that at least some of this tragic loss of life could have been averted by different barriers to means, different economies, and more sensible legislation. In other words, the white space between the lines represents lives that might have been saved by different politics.[7]

Ultimately, what do all these lost lives mean?

One way to think about the accrued loss of life is via a statistic that public health researchers call *PYLL(75)*. PYLL stands for "potential years of life lost," and *75* represents the average life span in the United States. PYLL calculates the average number of years that a person would have lived had he or she not died prematurely by unnatural causes. Researchers calculate the PYLL for individuals by subtracting the person's age at death from the reference age. For example:

- Reference age = 75; age at death = 6 months;
  PYLL(75) = 75 - 0.5 = 74.5
- Reference age = 75; age at death = 80;
  PYLL(75) = 0 (age at death greater than reference age)

When added up, these individual numbers become building blocks for larger calculations of premature mortality by specific causes within specific populations. A researcher can estimate the total number of life years lost by Hispanic teenagers who die in automobile accidents in Wyoming, or by middle-aged Asian Americans who overdose in Indiana. Or, for our purposes, by white men who die by firearm suicide in Connecticut and Missouri.[8]

Without a database like WISQARS, subtracting the ages of all gun suicide victims in Connecticut and Missouri from 75 would take a very long time, but the site logs the ages of death and does this calculation for you. With a few clicks, we learned that the PYLL(75) for white, non-Hispanic white men in Connecticut who died by suicide by firearm was

1999–2006: 16,133
2008–2015: 16,577

In other words, the PYLL(75) grew only by 444 total years lost over the sixteen-year time period, or at a growth rate of 2.75 percent. By contrast, PYLL(75) for white non-Hispanic men in Missouri who died by suicide by firearm was

1999–2006: 72,307
2008–2015: 84,884

In the eight years after the loosening of PTP and other gun regulations, Missouri suffered 12,557 more lost years of white male productive life than over the prior eight years. That represents a 17.39 percent increase in white male time—time spent working, playing, raising families, *living*— that was instead lost to gun suicide.

Once again, comparing the differences between the states' respective rates revealed the steep cost of gun suicide. Had the PYLL(75) in Missouri risen by the 2.75 percent seen in Connecticut, then the years lost in Missouri from 2008–2015 would have totaled 74,295 instead of 84,884. The difference between actual and hypothetical lost years due to white male gun suicide in Missouri was *10,588*. In essence, *loosening gun policies in Missouri went hand in hand with the loss of over 10,500 years of productive white male life in the state over the subsequent seven years.*

Cost itself is another way of understanding the difference between Missouri's white male gun suicide rate and Connecticut's. According to WISQARS, the average cost of a firearm suicide involving a white male in Missouri in 2010 was $1,004,007. This number averages expenses such as medical and emergency services along with loss of work and income. Using 2010 prices, admittedly a conservative estimate, we could then multiply that figure by the fifty-two average annual deaths to estimate that white male gun suicide cost Missouri $52,208,364 per year. When we multiply $1,004,007 by the 413 hypothetical deaths in Missouri, we learn that the white space between the lines cost the state roughly *$414,654,891* between 2008 and 2015.[9]

Ultimately, all of this math comes back to risk.

I thought once again about the refrigerator magnets. Threatening or talking about wanting to hurt or kill oneself was a risk factor listed on the magnet that group leaders handed out to participants at the Cape Girardeau meeting. Withdrawal from friends, family, and society gained mention, as did feelings of hopelessness, increased alcohol or drug use, aggressive behavior, and dramatic mood swings. And for good reason—mental health researchers identify these and other fluctuations from the norm as warning signs that suggest potential suicidality.

But as I did the math, I began to appreciate that risk factors listed on refrigerator magnets are based almost entirely on individual psychological factors and stressors that assess how a particular person acts or how they feel. However, risk factors for gun suicide (unlike homicide) rarely ask people to assess risk based on who a person *is*, what they *are*, or where they *live*.

The math revealed, however, that being (white, male) and living (in a place like Missouri) emerged as profound risk factors between 2008 and 2015. For instance, when you add it all up, the relative risk of dying by self-inflicted gunshot for a white man in Missouri versus a white man in Connecticut looks like this:

	DEATHS	POPULATION	AGE-ADJUSTED RATE
All white non-H men in MO, 2008–2015	3,437	19,289,162	16.93
All white non-H men in CT, 2008–2015	716	9,921,415	6.50
Increased risk			2.60

And the relative risk of dying by self-inflicted gunshot for a white man in Missouri versus a nonwhite man in Missouri looks like this:

	DEATHS	POPULATION	AGE-ADJUSTED RATE
All white non-H men in MO, 2008–2015	3,437	19,289,162	16.93
All black non-H men in MO, 2008–2015	182	2,772,280	7.11
Increased risk			2.38

In other words, the math shows that white non-Hispanic men in Missouri were 2.60 times more likely to die by firearm suicide than white non-Hispanic men in Connecticut, and 2.38 times more likely to die by firearm suicide than nonwhite men in Missouri.

These kinds of odds place death by self-inflicted gunshot as a category whose relative risk functions within the same orbit as risk factors for more well-known causes of death. For instance, a quick WISQARS relative risk analysis reveals that rates of non-Hispanic white male death by gun suicide roughly equaled mortality rates for car accidents, diabetes, Alzheimer's, influenza, and pneumonia. Much has been made about opioid addiction in rural America and its impact on white men. But the aggregate death rate for white males by unintentional drug poisoning in Missouri between 2008 and 2015 was 17.51 per 100,000 people, while the rate for self-inflicted gunshot was 17.82.

Meanwhile, over those same seven years, a white man in Missouri was eleven times more likely to die by gun suicide than in an accidental house fire and fifteen times more likely to die by gun suicide than by "natural/environmental" causes, such as from flood, earthquake, tornado, or by falling from a ladder, electrocution, smoke inhalation, or dog bite. Perhaps most important, the aggregate death rate for white men dying from firearm homicide was 2.56, meaning that white men in Missouri were seven times more likely to turn guns on themselves than to be fatally shot by intruders in their castles or assailants against whom white men needed to stand their ground.[10]

Recall the idealized stereotype of armed white maleness promoted by the Man Card and validated by much of American history. Armed white maleness connotes rights, privileges, and a place that, if not atop the hierarchy, was not at the bottom either. The promise of armed white male privilege also bolsters the appeal of NRA-backed politicians and their increasingly popular pro-gun agendas in places like Missouri.

The allure of this notion of armed white male power makes sense in many ways. Who wouldn't be tempted by a platform that claimed to increase one's own privilege, power, safety, and authority? However, again, the math and the graphs suggest the dangerous, mortal underside of linking privilege so closely to instruments of warfare and of then supporting politicians and policies that allow these instruments to be ever-more easily allowed into people's everyday lives and intimate spaces. The data overwhelmingly suggests that more guns mean more deaths, and particularly so for the very people whose privileges and potencies Man Cards and pro-gun policies claim to restore.

This brief data study ultimately highlights the extreme difficulty of balancing Second Amendment rights and time-honored gun traditions on the one hand and public health on the other, particularly in places like Missouri. There and elsewhere, prevention programs often focus on people's access to guns during fleeting moments of despair and on the relationships between access to guns and the risk factors listed on magnets and similar everyday resources.[11]

For instance, a new suicide-prevention program in Missouri asks gun sellers to watch for "potentially suicidal" gun buyers. "Trust your instincts," a flyer from the program tells retailers. "You are under no obligation to sell a gun to anyone . . . when you delay a sale due to concerns about suicide, notify the police and nearby dealers." This type of intervention rests on the common-sense assumption that the risk of gun suicide lies in individual minds, moments, impulses, and access. In outliers. Sweaty, jumpy people shopping nervously for guns in a crowd of calm good guys. Eyes-aglazed people who appear suspect or suspicious.[12]

But the data raises the prospect that the risk of white male gun suicide may also reside in larger structural levels as well. Like Greek soldiers inside the Trojan horse, this risk is embedded in the stereotypes and fantasies of armed white male supremacy on which gun markets and marketers thrive in the first place. This risk grows in relation to policies that make it even easier for white citizens to purchase, carry, and display guns, or narratives that warn "good guys" that their guns are always in danger of being taken away.

In these ways and others, risk functions as a product, not of the outlier but of the invisible mainstream. And the quest for best ways to limit guns to people in moments of despair suddenly opens into a series of much larger questions. How in the world might we go about changing white masculinity? Or can we open a space to talk about why white men feel they need guns in the first place? What threats do they imagine, and what safety or reassurance do guns represent?

Put another way, the data hints at the possibility that white male gun suicide may be a side effect of both loose gun policies and conceptions of white masculinity, in addition to the effects of troubled individual minds. And that in this sense, white men writ large make a Faustian bargain in order to accept the larger benefits of gun ownership more broadly.

Again, increasingly loose gun laws mean that pretty much everyone in Missouri enjoys equal and expanded opportunity to own and carry a gun. Yet within this brave new world, the same demographic that often pushes for and supports expanded access has come to occupy an increasingly hazardous category of potential demise. White men die by their own guns two and a half times more often than do their nearest demographic, and exponentially more often than they do at the hands of dogs, bears, ladders, carjackers, intruders, terrorists, or other predators combined.

As this process plays out, the peril to white men comes not just from the instrument, the impulse, or even the legislation. Rather, privilege itself becomes a liability. White men themselves become the biggest threats to . . . themselves. Danger emerges from who they are and from what they wish to be. Over time, the data suggests, "being a white man who lives in Missouri" then emerges as its own, high-risk category.

INTERVIEW:

THE WHYS AND WHAT-IFS

Interview excerpts, December 16, 2016, Cape Girardeau. Speaker 2: white female, 44, daughter.

JMM: As I mentioned before, I'm doing research on gun suicide. I know you and I talked about this a bit before, but maybe you could just tell me a little bit about your own history with this issue.

Speaker 2: Well, for my family in particular, growing up in the Midwest, we had always had firearms in our home. I still do. . . .

I don't blame the firearm for the loss of my father, first of all. Strong military family, NRA from the beginning. We own lots of guns, go to the range. That's not gonna change. Got my gun from my dad, in fact. Take my kids to shoot all the time.

But of course I feel it was a very shocking trauma of course with my dad using that particular means to end his life. It's pretty lethal. That was a shocking means, I believe. Because it was a self-inflicted gunshot wound to the head. It was pretty traumatic in that itself. That to me was really just as shocking. I think it left just a second trauma, just thinking about. . . . Reading the police report and just. . . . It was just so much more traumatic as far as the lethal means of it. I think it was really traumatic to me especially, being a woman.

JMM: What is your understanding of what led up to it?

Speaker 2: I wonder that all the time, all the time. I had talked to him four hours before he died, and he was in great spirits and planning a barbecue for the next day for us to come over and have fun. It sounded fantastic. It just sounded wonderful. Like I said, hindsight now, I know that he had basically set the stage of what he was going to do that night. Kept asking me, "When are you coming over? When are you coming over?" I said, "I'll be there. I'm on my way." I lived about an hour away. I was on my way to the house. When he took his life, he called my mom. Got her on the phone and asked her if there was any way to fix the marriage. She said no, and that's when he shot himself.

I think maybe if he would have been more of lucid mind, even though I've done enough research at this point that I know that at that point . . . I don't know this for a fact, but I would hope that he would have been a little bit more lucid to the thought of, *Maybe if I think about this a couple more seconds, I'll change my mind.* That's wishful thinking from a suicide loss survivor. . . . We always want to believe that something would have changed their mind, but we don't know. The whys and what-ifs. You know.

I was on my way there. Had I got there ten minutes earlier, had I not stopped and got my son a Happy Meal, maybe I would have been able to save him. There's those maybes. It's tough. It is a lot of guilt.

JMM: I can totally understand; it's like trying to make sense of something that just makes no sense, and especially when it's a parent.

Speaker 2: Oh, absolutely. In the beginning, I felt abandonment. It totally destroyed my family. It took me a long time. For many years, I felt very alone and ashamed. I was very ashamed of it. I wouldn't tell people the truth when I met them and they'd ask, "Oh, you're so young. Your dad is deceased?" "Yeah, he had heart problems." It was a long time before I could come to terms with . . . it was a lot of education, really.

JMM: We all seem to be so polarized about this, but over time, have your views about guns changed in any ways as a result of your experiences?

Speaker 2: Yes, it is really all over the place, to be quite honest. I've seen it gone in both directions. Some people have all the guns destroyed. Some people just are adamant, it wasn't the gun's fault. That's kind of where I fall. I just have never—I guess just because they were always in our home, I don't know. It's no different than a kitchen knife in my opinion. It's a weapon for defense, self-defense. Self-defense is the way I've always looked at a firearm. That's just the means that my dad chose to use. It's unfortunate. We've just always had them. My brother's an avid hunter. His children, he has boys. They're avid hunters. My son's an avid hunter. It's just part of our life.

JMM: That makes total sense.

Speaker 2: I do not know honestly that much about it if there's some kind of a background check or anything, my daughter's telling me. She's fifteen. She's like, "There is a background check, Mom. There's a background check." She must know more about it than I do. I'm not aware of that, honestly.

But I think there should be. I think there should be definitely some sort of background check involved in buying firearms. I do believe there should be. I don't think you should be able to walk into any kind of shop and just buy a firearm and walk out. Not just with suicide reasons but just with the things that we're seeing in the work today as far as schools being shot up and different things. I personally feel like there should be some kind of background check done. I don't know what extent or who even would set that whole thing up.

TRIGGER
WARNINGS

Back in Cape Girardeau, I walk slowly toward the parking lot outside the library after the support group meeting. Dawn and Billie will drive me back to my motel, but the two linger in the lobby, chatting. In the moment of quiet, I reflect a bit more about the group, the pain, the bravery I had seen.

I can't help but think that so much of the tension that survivors describe, in the group and in my interviews, arises from the difference between individual and structural explanations of gun suicide. Survivors are stuck between warning signs they might have seen or should have known on the one hand and predetermined factors built right into the laws, traditions, and culture of their communities.

Only in retrospect do individual-level warning signs shout out "This was a risk factor!" as if flashing red lights. Did you not see your father sliding into depression? Why did the doctor prescribe Ritalin? How did we allow him to date that awful girl? In the minds of survivors trying to make sense of the unimaginable, these and other searing questions serve as grounding frameworks that suggest A led to B, a direct line from the doctor, the illness, the bad date to the loss.

Of course, life rarely stands still to allow us to spot subtle warning signs amid a constant flow of daily events. However, in retrospect, those flashing individual factors seem impossibly clear. Individual factors thus serve as the basis for a guilt known only to survivors, a gnawing sense that "our loved ones might still be alive if only we had been more attuned."

Guilt then functions as more than self-beratement—it also promotes the altogether human fantasy that the act of suicide, like the guilt itself, is under our control.

Perhaps some of the pain results from the flip side of this type of daily observation. A nagging question asks whether there were aspects of our loved ones that we did not know. Secret lives, or thoughts, or parts that they kept hidden from us? Perhaps their worlds spun independently from our own?

Then there are the structural factors. Understandably, survivor narratives often express anger about structural factors when consumer products are involved in injury and death. *What do you mean you knew about the faulty airbags? How on earth did you build power lines so close to our homes? Did you not test for these awful medication side effects beforehand?* Such reasoning channels indignation upward at corporations and careless wizards hidden behind curtains. Structural factors can also lead to cold comfort in the form of lawsuits, settlements, or admissions of culpability.

More than anything else, the group and the interviews suggest how complicated, confusing, and ever-more painful survival narratives become when death comes from the barrels of guns—for reasons even in excess of the fact that laws generally protect gun manufacturers from liability claims. Yes, perhaps we should have done more to secure it, lock it, keep it away. And yes, perhaps the product should have come with tamper-proof packaging, a safety cap, or some other form of trigger warning meant to circumvent disaster. At the same time, people have been told for most of their lives that these products are us, circumscribe us, privilege, defend, and define us. That questioning these products and their role in our lives is a form of heresy. That blaming the gun or the politician or the policy is what liberals do. That giving even an inch on guns means that the squatters and the migrants will overrun the plantations and the farms.

There is an undeniable power in this form of us-versus-them logic in places like Missouri. Here, guns function as totems, symbols of belonging and of self- and community protection, revered sources of power. Perhaps in part for these reasons, survivor narratives often sound as if spoken in a strange code, in which causality sometimes loops on itself, twists and turns, and comes out sideways. *He died by gun: I am not allowed to blame the gun: I blame myself.* Or perhaps, *I have a gun for protection: I could not protect him: you cannot protect him.*

I have no illusion about the potential impact of policy on the problem of gun suicide. I probably came to Cape Girardeau thinking that gun traditions might merge with fancy upstream policy solutions like background checks, smart guns, gun violence restraining orders (GVROs), or PTP laws. And perhaps in some other world, like the world I'll inhabit when I leave, that makes sense. But right now, in a cold parking lot in the middle of night in the middle of somewhere, these interventions feel like small drops in a massive bucket that keeps getting bigger. Potential solutions feel so far away, and particularly so because of politicians and a political system that block even the slightest attempts at compromise and enable ever-more bullets and ever-more guns.

My experience in Cape opened windows into complex relationships between the people, the place, their histories, and their guns. Guns mark forms of family and privilege that the white Missourians with whom I've spoken cling to as an inheritance. Guns also represent trauma multipliers that turn passing moments of desperation into agonizing and permanent loss for individuals and for communities. Joined together, guns come to embody, truly, double-edged swords, inasmuch as the same people and communities who benefit from imagined privileges represented by their guns also live closest to suicide enablers in moments of desperation.

More guns may or may not lead to less crime—the jury seems very much still out on this oversimplified assertion. But on a December night in Cape Girardeau, at least, more guns seemed to connect to disproportionally more despair.

Dawn reaches me first, and I'm glad to see she has the car keys. She presses a button on the key ring, and the automatic locks jump to attention. We get into the car, and she revs the engine in order to get the heater going. We sit waiting for the car to warm and waiting for Billie. The group is Billie's baby in so many ways. She is always the last one to leave the meetings.

Dawn turns to say something to me but turns back to face the windshield before speaking.

"You know, I do think there needs to be some kind of middle ground, to be honest," she says. "People here love their guns, but we can't just have guns everywhere all the time. It's just creating chaos and, you know, not making us any more safe.

"I would never say that in the group, though."

PART 2

TENNESSEE

UNAFFORDABLE

DONALD TRUMP CAMPAIGNED for president on a promise to "terminate" the Affordable Care Act (ACA) and replace it with "something terrific." As the first six months of his administration unfolded, he often repeated that vow—and Republican lawmakers set about the work of coming up with a health care bill that was terrific. Debates, proposals, and uncertainty swirled through the halls of Congress as "repeal and replace" lurched into motion, fell from the weight of real-world implausibility, and then arose again and again like acid indigestion.[1]

A constant theme emerged from the almost unimaginably dysfunctional process of trying to sink people's health care with no real alternative in place: every single GOP proposal, initiative, or inaction carried negative consequences for Southern white working-class populations who formed the core of Trump's support base.

"Trumpcare Is Already Hurting Trump Country" warned the lead editorial in the *New York Times* on May 19, 2017. The opinion piece detailed how the mere threat to dismantle the ACA prompted major insurance companies to stop selling policies or raise premiums significantly. A subsequent House bill further endangered health coverage for at least 24 million people by cutting spending on Medicaid and eliminating subsidies that helped the poorest Americans buy insurance. The editorial argued that

> what's bizarre about the Republican strategy is that it is likely to cause
> the most damage where many of Mr. Trump's supporters live. Rural and
> suburban areas are more likely to lose insurers and see big premium in-
> creases if Obamacare goes down, because companies have less incentive

to stay in markets where there are fewer potential customers and where it is harder to put together networks of hospitals and doctors.

The *Times* piece pointed to trends in several Southern and midwestern states. "In places like Iowa, Nebraska, and Tennessee, companies such as Aetna and Wellmark are so spooked by the uncertainty that they are considering abandoning the market."[2]

This argument reflected not just a potential result of repealing the health care law but an existing fact: many Southern and midwestern states failed to embrace the ACA from the outset, refusing to expand Medicaid or promote robust insurance marketplaces, and thus relied on single insurers to provide coverage. Washington's threats to cut subsidies threw health care for entire states and regions suddenly up for grabs. The result, to understate, was uncertainty. "No one feels optimistic about the market," Tennessee insurance commissioner Julie Mix McPeak later claimed.[3]

Uncertainty grew with every Republican attempt to bury the ACA and then with the administration's overt efforts to undermine it. By the summer of 2017, publications like *Mother Jones* published charts that predicted how many more people might be uninsured under each Republican health care bill, as if the numbers were betting lines for college football games. By the fall of that year, the *Wall Street Journal* and other publications detailed how a series of pending presidential executive orders could gut health insurance markets while making it easier for insurers to offer plans that were "skimpier" than what the ACA allowed, circumventing rules laid out by Congress when it passed the law in 2010. Then, among Trump's first comments after passage of a sweeping tax reform bill in 2017 that also ended the ACA's so-called individual mandate: "We have essentially repealed Obamacare," he said, "and we will come up with something much better."[4]

From early on in the repeal process, commentators and journalists frequently assumed that people would not allow it and that political loyalty would change when their well-being was at stake. Citing 2017 Kaiser Family Foundation and Gallup polls, the *Times* concluded that "61 percent of Americans already know where the fault should lie: with the Republicans" and that "Senate Republicans ought to keep these polls in mind as they come up with their version of Trumpcare."[5]

Yet as I watched the Trumpcare roller coaster play out, I could not help but think of research that my colleagues and I conducted in Tennessee over the preceding years—research suggesting that political identity and loyalty were more complex than the media assumed, and especially so in the Southern and midwestern states that solidly supported Trump at the polls.

Yes, survival and well-being represent core human drives, and protecting the health of yourself and your family remains sacrosanct. Most people, for the most part, want access to affordable health care in order to do so. However, I had seen firsthand how many voters in Trump country felt the burden of centuries of history that charged the idea of government intervention in general, and into health care specifically, with race and class politics—often accompanied by overt xenophobia and racism. Even with the ACA, where the programs simply provided government oversight in support of private companies and commercially made pharmaceuticals, public welfare spending was taboo for many white lower- and middle-income voters. When the ACA came along, the GOP deftly played on this history to instill loyalty for positions that often rendered white working-class bodies expendable. Challenging such loyalty would take much more than editorials, opinion polls—or even better health care plans.

I came to this conclusion between 2012 and 2016, when Trumpcare was not yet a figment of even the wildest GOP pipe dream. Over this span, my colleagues and I conducted health-related focus groups with self-identified white and African American men in Tennessee. We asked the men about their opinions regarding health and illness, the ACA, and health insurance more broadly.

Tennessee was an important site for several reasons: chief among them that, while the state was home to leading US health insurance companies, such as HCA Holdings, its politicians also continually blocked the ACA and Medicaid expansion for state citizens. Health insurance coverage rates thus remained low for many lower- and middle-income Tennesseans when compared to expansion states; health care coverage in many ways became an export product as a result. As of February 2017, seventy-three of ninety-five counties in the state had only one insurer offering health care plans, putting these counties at peril if the insurers decided to pull out. For the early part of that same year, the city of Knoxville had no insurer. "As a state we already did not have a lot of options," an article in the *Tennessean* explained. And "now, 16 counties are facing having no [insurer] options in 2018."[6]

Our focus groups explored people's attitudes about the ACA. As this section of the book details, we found jarringly different attitudes among racial groups. African American men largely supported the ACA because the legislation potentially helped "everybody" and because they felt that anything would be an improvement over Tennessee's crumbling health care delivery system. But many white men, like Trevor mentioned in the introduction to this book, voiced a willingness to die, literally, rather than embrace a law that gave minority or immigrant persons more access to care, even if it helped them as well. Many white men also complained about the fiscal cost of the ACA, while neglecting the cost their opposition exacted on their health.

In many ways, the frameworks surrounding rejection of the ACA in Tennessee differed considerably from those underlying gun expansion in Missouri. The gun debate centered on protection, privilege, and *individual* responsibility. It set people in castles and instructed them to stand their grounds. Health care, meanwhile, promoted networks, safety nets, and other metaphors that highlighted real or imagined *connections* among bodies and communities. The central tension of political debates against the ACA rested in the ways that GOP politicians tried to set people apart and mistrust each other, even as diseases and pathogens showed little respect for social categories of race, class, or political orientation. Where guns invoked anxieties regarding risk, health care produced highly charged fears about cost.

And yet, guns and health care were aligned for reasons beyond the fact that they emerged as core components of rightist GOP platforms—and often in ways that precluded compromise or negotiation. Our focus groups highlighted another important similarity in the conversations surrounding pro-gun and anti-ACA politics in Southern and midwestern US states: both asked working-class white Americans to put their own bodies on the line in order to "defend" conservative ideologies.

In a variety of complex ways, white populations frequently justified their support for anti-ACA positions not through the benefits that expanded health care might have for themselves or their families but through concerns about threats to their status and privilege represented by government programs that promised to equally distribute resources or imagined health advantages. We often found that no ivory-tower health-policy explanation of the ACA's potential benefits came close to challenging concerns about ways that health insurance came from the administration of an African American president or placed white Americans into "networks" with immigrant and minority populations.[7]

At the same time, as this section of the book details, the success of anti-ACA politics in places like Tennessee came at high mortal costs for the on-the-ground white Americans who supported, embodied, and paid a heavy toll for their rejection of Obamacare.

COST

O N AN UNUSUALLY warm night in February 2015, I'm sitting with twelve white men around a rec room table in a transitional low-income housing project in Franklin, Tennessee.

The room smells of desperation, heightened all the more by decades of cigarette smoke entombed in the furniture, walls, and floor. Fluorescent lights buzz quietly overhead; individual tubes occasionally flicker on and off. A vending machine that sells twenty-five-cent cans of soda hums in the corner. Above it hangs a small television bolted to the ceiling. Even the table has seen better days, its brown surface frayed to khaki-colored cork at the corners.

This space feels like a respite stop at the end of the road, which in many ways it is. Low-income housing represents the last frayed netting that tries to catch men as they fall from whatever safety their lives once represented toward homelessness and the streets. Tennessee is a state without much safeguard in that regard. Residents pay no state income tax, and many social services suffer as a result. Which is to say that the social lattice is weak, has many holes, and often fails to catch men, such as the ones with whom I'm speaking, on their way down.

Men end up here for a variety of reasons. Some lose their way because of addiction; others because of lawlessness. Most of the men I meet on this night end up in the no-exit room with the twenty-five-cent soda because of illness—a chronic cough that one day produces blood, or the gradual emergence of blurred vision and numbness in the toes, or chest pain, stomach pain, or shortness of breath. For many people, these symptoms mean a trip to a doctor who might diagnose a dreaded but potentially treatable condition, such as infection or diabetes or colitis. But for these men, the diagnoses become primary tumors for larger, metastatic social and economic problems.

A few of the men recognized early warning signs and went for checkups. Their doctors found chronic illness, yet the diagnoses provided just enough opening for insurance companies to claim preexisting conditions and deny care. Other men didn't even bother, since the bureaucracy for getting to a clinic and then waiting in line for medications seemed worse than the illness itself. Symptoms fulminated as a result. Most of the men then fell into what policy experts dispassionately call the *doughnut hole* of coverage—meaning these men were just well enough to maintain menial employment, working hourly on assembly lines or at odd jobs. The income from these jobs put them just above the level of poverty—at the time, $15,856 a year per person. Most of them thus no longer met state requirements for Medicaid. Insurmountable mountains of medical bills then followed.[1]

Franklin is a largely white and predominantly conservative town twenty-one miles south of Nashville. According to the US Census, 85 percent of Franklin residents identify as Caucasian, and many identify as Republican. The stretch of I-65 near Franklin is lined by gun-show billboards and a monument to Nathan Bedford Forrest, the first grand wizard of the Ku Klux Klan, complete with a row of Confederate flags.[2]

Not coincidentally, help seems up the road on this particular night. In Nashville, politicians in the Tennessee statehouse debate the implications of the ACA and a subsequent plan called Insure Tennessee, sweeping legislation meant to help Tennesseans much like the ones with whom I speak. Among its many interventions, the ACA aimed to close the doughnut hole by expanding Medicaid to people above the poverty line and protecting against insurance discrimination for chronic illness.

If the ACA wasn't a panacea for the dire financial and biological situations faced by the men in the group, it was close. But the men, much like the politicians up the road, will have none of it. The reason, the men tell me in so many ways, is *cost*. "The dang thing cost too much," says a man in his late forties who uses a walker to ambulate due to diabetic neuropathy. "We got enough debt in this country as it is." "It's a waste of our hard-earned tax dollars," adds a man in his fifties who wears a nasal oxygen cannula because of chronic lung disease.

Cost came up repeatedly in focus groups with white men that I conducted between 2012 and 2016, when deliberations about expanded federal and state health insurance effervesced nationally and raged with particular vitriol in Southern states. To be sure, cost was an entirely valid concern in the conversation about health care reform. The ACA was a large, ambitious, and expensive program, the specifics of which were subject to much debate. However, in rooms like the one in Franklin, cost meant neither the cost of illness nor the cost of debt. Instead, all too frequently, cost provided the logic for inaction, for keeping Tennessee's paltry and failing health care system as it was. Cost meant doing nothing.

Each group began with a straightforward set of questions: How would you describe your health? What types of things do you do to stay healthy? And so on.

When I ask these questions in Franklin, a fifty-three-year-old white man named Tom who worked an hourly job at a fast-food drive-through suddenly spoke up.

"I'm fifty-three, and I already had two heart attacks; I have a chronic cough," Tom tells the group. Tom listed a series of behaviors that he felt contributed to his ill health. "I'm fat, I smoke, my diet sucks. I work twelve hours a day flipping burgers, then I come back to my room, eat junk food, and watch TV and fall asleep. I'm a ticking time bomb, health-wise—I've got high blood pressure bad, just like my dad did, and he died young." Tom wears a backward baseball cap, loose-fitting shorts, and an oversized *Dawn of the Dead* T-shirt.

In a medical setting, any number of Tom's life choices and characteristics might be described as risk factors for his various ailments. Sedentary lifestyle, smoking, obesity, family history, and a diet high in fried, fatty foods are all linked to medical conditions such as diabetes, cancer, COPD, and heart disease. "High blood pressure can lead to heart disease and stroke—leading causes of death in the United States," the US Centers for Disease Control thus advises doctors to warn their patients. "But you can work to reduce your risk by eating a healthy diet, maintaining a healthy weight, not smoking, and being physically active."[3]

But to consider Tom's story only from a medical perspective misses a key element that would emerge repeatedly in our groups: the health effects of ideology. "I ain't supporting Obamacare—no way, no how," he said. "And I ain't signing up for it neither. The dang thing costs too much."

In the best of all worlds, cost would seem a fair trade-off for health. Of course, cost implies paying real money. But taking that money out of your pocket and exchanging it for well-being would seem to represent a good reason why you might want money in your pocket in the first place. Money pays for health at the individual level, in the form of doctor's visits or medications. Money buys health at the community level as well, in the form of well-maintained roads, highways, and other, safer social structures. Here and elsewhere, cost taps into the larger tensions represented by currency; something that we spend our lives trying to accumulate at personal levels, but that means little if not also invested into communal transactions that raise the value of society as a whole.[4]

And yet in a room in a housing project in the real world of the American South, cost also functioned as a proxy for the tensions of race, as questions of *Who is paying for whom?* and *Whose labor supports whom?* led to deliberations about ways to hoard health for some persons, while denying it to others.

IN THE NAME OF AFFORDABLE CARE

PRESIDENT OBAMA SIGNED the Patient Protection and Affordable Care Act—better known by the second half of its name—into law in March 2010, mandating a set of ostensibly consumer-friendly benefits meant to reduce financial burden to individuals and families. The legislation included free preventative care. As the official website announced at the time, "all new plans must cover certain preventive services such as mammograms and colonoscopies without charging a deductible, co-pay or coinsurance," and "a new $15 billion Prevention and Public Health Fund will invest in proven prevention and public health programs that can help keep Americans healthy—from smoking cessation to combating obesity."

The ACA also introduced new consumer protections. Again according to the website at the time, "insurance companies will be prohibited from imposing lifetime dollar limits on essential benefits, like hospital stays," while creating "a $5 billion program to provide needed financial help for employment-based plans to continue to provide valuable coverage to people who retire between the ages of 55 and 65, as well as their spouses and dependents." Vitally, the ACA also introduced support for previously uninsured persons and bolstered states' abilities to provide care for even the most vulnerable inhabitants: "states will be able to receive federal matching funds for covering some additional low-income individuals and families under Medicaid for whom federal funds were not previously available."[1]

In other words, the ACA sought to widen health care networks and control costs by regulating and expanding private insurance and promoting prevention, while at the same time broadening Medicaid eligibility and coverage. Even the most ardent supporters of the ACA agreed that the law was far from perfect and represented a series of first-step and often painful compromises between private interests and the public good. But most supporters also believed that the law would at least strengthen communal safety nets in ways that benefited the health of society writ large and particularly the health of lower-income persons—and that the first iterations could be improved and updated over time. Speaking to reporters several months after the ACA's passage, President Obama optimistically explained that "this law will cut costs and make coverage more affordable for families and small businesses. . . . It's reform that finally extends the opportunity to purchase coverage to the millions who currently don't have it."[2]

In June 2012, the US Supreme Court seemingly ended the political battle over the ACA's legitimacy when it upheld core tenets of the legislation. Writing for the majority, Chief Justice John Roberts endorsed the government's right to enforce ACA's "individual mandate" that required persons above certain income levels to purchase health care or face tax penalties. The Court thus sanctioned what might be considered fiscal principles of herd immunity—namely, that networks of health care and social support work best when most people participate in them.[3]

But the 2012 decision also provided enteric coating for a poison pill. While the Supreme Court decision assured enough money to keep the system afloat, it also undercut a core component of strategies to provide health care for lower-income persons. This was because the ruling also substantially limited the law's forced expansion of Medicaid. In its initial formulation, the ACA linked a host of federal payments to each state's participation in health care reform. Thanks in part to an amicus brief filed by a conservative Vanderbilt University law professor named James Blumstein, the court ruled that the ACA exceeded its constitutional authority by "coercing" states into participating in Medicaid expansion. The court held that Medicaid expansion was "optional" for states and that each state could make its own choices about coverage for the less fortunate.[4]

In some other universe, one might expect that Tennesseans like Tom would embrace the ACA in general and coverage expansion in particular. The reform's interventions directly addressed many of the medical conditions from which Tom suffered, as well as the social and economic stressors that rendered his access to treatment ever-more difficult and costly. Moreover, the notion of funding broad-ranging health care for people at the bottom of the economic spectrum carried particular resonance in Tennessee. Much as Missouri once supported effective gun violence prevention strategies, Tennessee once functioned as a Southern beacon for progressive approaches to health care for low-income populations.

In the early 1990s, for instance, the state launched an innovative health care reform program called TennCare, meant to expand access to health care and control rising costs. TennCare represented the first state Medicaid program to enroll recipients in managed care programs administered by private-sector organizations rather than in traditional fee-for-service plans, while at the same time offering health insurance to residents who did not have it. The program represented a novel public-private partnership designed to combine the strengths of government and business in order to expand care.

At the time of TennCare's rollout, Governor Ned McWherter proudly proclaimed that the program helped the state "slay the bear" of uncontrolled medical costs. A front-page headline in the *Knoxville News Sentinel* told how "TennCare Boosts Health Coverage to 94 Percent in State" above an article that detailed how the program raised funds to pay doctors, hospitals, and others who provide care for seriously ill patients, "such as those with AIDS or hemophilia—and the severely mentally ill." The program soon drew interest from other Southern states, in large part because, per the *Nashville Business Journal*, it seemed to "shift the cost of providing health care to the poor away from the state onto the federal government and health care providers"—specifically, passing 91 percent of the cost to the federal government, with the state paying the remaining 9 percent.[5]

TennCare proved highly popular at first, and enrollment quickly exceeded all estimates. Registration hit 1.2 million after just a year, forcing the state to limit eligibility. Over the following years, TennCare spawned a series of programs for mental health and substance abuse and a subsequent program, TennCare II, aimed more directly at cost control.

But with success came trouble. The need was too great; the people too sick. Tennessee offered little else in the way of supportive social services. Expenses soon soared past projections. A 1995 article in the Memphis *Commercial Appeal* urged a wait-and-see approach: "Getting TennCare to work the way it was supposed to will take time, patience and further reform." Physicians complained about low reimbursement rates, and some doctors refused to see TennCare patients. In 2000, the conservative Heritage Foundation called TennCare an example of "failed healthcare reform." A series of state-commissioned reports concluded in 2003 that TennCare was "not financially viable" without significant change. The program's annual budget rose from $2.64 billion in 1994 to more than $8.5 billion in 2005, an unacceptable bloat for a state that was at the same time in the process of eliminating state income tax.[6]

Insurers pulled out as revenues fell. So the state began to cut the program, and cut, and cut some more. It reduced benefits and services and limited coverage for prescriptions. It set far stricter limits on enrollment eligibility. Then it cut people—lots of people, jettisoned into the realms of the unsupported and the uninsured.

By 2012, the program was in dire straits. TennCare administrators resorted to health care lotteries to distribute the program's limited resources to the many low-income Tennessee residents whose annual incomes put them above the cutoff for coverage, but whose medical bills rendered them unable to afford to purchase private insurance on their own. As the *New York Times* described it in a 2013 article titled "Tennessee Race for Medicaid: Dial Fast and Try, Try Again":

> State residents who have high medical bills but would not normally qualify for Medicaid, the government health care program for the poor, can call a state phone line and request an application. But the window is tight—the line shuts down after 2,500 calls, typically within an hour—and the demand is so high that it is difficult to get through.[7]

Meanwhile, Tennessee fell to the bottom of US states in health care outcomes. "There really is a health care crisis in this state," Rick Johnson, CEO of the Tennessee Governor's Foundation for Health and Wellness, later claimed. "Almost 70 percent of the people in Tennessee are classified as overweight or obese, we have near epidemic rates of hypertension and stroke, very high rates of cardiovascular disease."[8]

In other words, rarely in the history of recorded time was there a state more in need of, or more ideally fitted for, the ACA and Medicaid expansion than Tennessee. Medicaid expansion would provide coverage for the increasing numbers of people who fell through the cracks due to the failures of TennCare. Expanding the state's health care infrastructure would also extend its capacity to serve doughnut hole populations. The ACA promised to offset the very costs that TennCare owed, inasmuch as the pooled funds of the federal government would effectively address TennCare's debt. Evidence also suggested that the framers of the ACA attempted to learn from the lessons of the failure of TennCare specifically by promoting cooperation rather than promoting competition. Indeed, the caveats of TennCare might have positioned Tennessee politicians as sage national leaders as a result of their experiences. As public health scholar Christina Bennett puts it, the nation had the potential to learn from Tenn-Care in order to "prevent similar problems in the national health care plan or in other state's plans."[9]

Perhaps most important, national health care reform was poised to help Tennessee deliver on its goal of quality care for all citizens. On paper, the ACA was like manna from heaven, if the manna was low-carb, loaded with antioxidants, and came in multiple pizza and ice cream flavors.

In the real world, of course, the ACA and Medicaid expansion met ferocious resistance in Southern states like Tennessee. This resistance was often articulated through anxieties about government interference in personal health decisions, and concerns about cost. Tennessee's Republican senator Lamar Alexander pushed to "repeal Obamacare" by defunding it, on the grounds that it was simply too expensive. Conservative Republicans in Tennessee similarly latched onto the idea of cost to resist any expansion of health care coverage in the state. Leading the charge was Lieutenant Governor Ron Ramsey, a onetime real estate auctioneer turned anti-government and anti-Washington crusader. Ramsey damned the 2012 Supreme Court decision as evidence of "a government unrestrained and out of control" and warned that Obamacare "will cost Tennesseans $1.1 billion in the next few years."[10]

Tennessee was not alone. Cost concerns took center stage in challenges to the ACA mounted by business organizations, state and local governments, and conservative advocacy groups throughout the South. Cost was at the fore of Missouri's Proposition C, which sought to deny the federal government the financial resources it required to enforce the ACA because "a person shall not be required by law or rule to pay penalties or fines for paying directly for lawful health care services" without need for insurance. Cost also emerged as a rallying cry for conservative media outlets. *Breitbart* mockingly imagined "sticker shock" linked to Obamacare with taxpaying Americans forced into welfare by hidden costs. Conservative politicians, such as Florida's Marco Rubio, repeatedly assailed Obamacare as a financial "risk" that the United States could not "afford."[11]

Make no mistake: concerns about cost reflected financial realities for many middle- and lower-income people like Tom, as well as for many small-business owners. A number of health economists raised alarms from the outset about rising premiums, decreased competition among health insurance companies, fees for refusing coverage, and decreased provider choice. "As the Affordable Care Act moves closer to full implementation," economist Jeffrey Dorfman wrote in 2013, "a lot of people who expected to receive a free lunch are discovering that they are instead getting stuck with the bill." By 2015, headlines in the *New York Times* announced that "The Experts Were Wrong About the Best Places for Better and Cheaper Health Care." "Obamacare Premiums Are Going Up," news reports announced in 2016, while citing a Kaiser Family Foundation report predicting "premium increases" in coming years. Researchers would even later argue that, because preventative care helped people live longer, it added additional costs to the system brought on by these added life years. These and other developments revealed an inconvenient truth: at the end of the day, population-level medical care is often more expensive than it is affordable, and particularly so in the United States. And, as physician and health economist Aaron Carroll succinctly puts it about health care, "sometimes good things cost money."[12]

At the same time, even before the ACA's rise and Trump-fueled fall from grace, many leading metrics suggested that, in terms of cost, men like Tom and states like Tennessee had little to fear from the ACA. Federal subsidies protected lower-income persons from the steepest premium increases. Numerous credible reports detailed ways that the ACA was working well, particularly for the poor. An expansive study by the Robert Wood

Johnson Foundation found that "widespread slowdown in health spending" saved the United States *trillions* of dollars and that the uninsured rate dropped to the lowest level on record. ACA-enabled coverage also extended health care to many immigrant and minority persons who were previously uninsured and ended up in emergency rooms under only the direst circumstances.[13]

In other words, cost was a real concern for lower- and middle-income persons and families, for the state, and for budget hawks who worried about rising debt (until, of course, they were asked to vote on the 2017 federal tax bill). Most supporters agreed that the initial iterations of the ACA represented first steps but that the program would need adjustment to control for fiscal realities that emerged as the massive program came to life.

However, the more I spoke to people like Tom, the more I came to realize the extent to which cost also seemed to tap into a host of deeper concerns that had less to do with dollars and cents and more to do with the unaffordable and often highly unhealthy American politics of race.

FOCUS

THE START OF a focus group feels like the first day of school after summer vacation. One by one, participants grudgingly filter into a room that tries its best to feel welcoming but that cannot hide its true intentions. Neat stacks of boxed meals sit on a table by the entrance. Another table contains an array of bottled sodas, water, or sweet tea. *Take me*, the meals and the drinks say. Only after accepting the seduction do the takers notice a less appetizing third table piled with stapled copies of confidentiality waivers, lengthy questionnaires, and bundles of Costco-grade cheap pens.

Men enter the room. They take their time choosing boxed meals even though the selections are limited to two, meat or vegetarian. They spend even more time choosing between one of the three drink options. Then they unflinchingly grab waivers, questionnaires, and pens and take seats around a table.

The group starts with a nervous quiet as the men eat, fill out the questionnaires, and stake out their positions in a roomful of strangers. The leader opens the conversation. "I would like to thank you all for coming this evening. We're here to talk about health."

Focus groups came into vogue during the World War II era. In fields like business, politics, the social sciences, and motivational psychology, experts used the groups to assess what was called the *reason behind the reason*. Psychologist and marketing pioneer Ernest Dichter reportedly coined the term *focus group* when he convened groups of strangers and asked them camouflaged questions about their product preferences to understand the meanings conveyed by brand names and consumer objects. Early focus groups assembled people at a New York YMCA and asked

139

them about after-workout cleanliness, leading to a new slogan for Ivory soap. Groups of young middle-class girls shaped the promotion of the first Barbie dolls.[1]

In their present iteration, focus groups often function as methods of interactive social-science research. Volunteers (often paid) discuss their attitudes, beliefs, or opinions about products, political candidates, ideas, innovations, or pieces of legislation. Our groups assessed Tennessee men's attitudes about health and health care reform. We particularly wanted to gauge the language and implicit associations through which people such as Tom rejected the notion of the ACA even as they themselves suffered from some of the very medical conditions and profound economic stressors that the reforms ostensibly aimed to address.

We advertised for participants by posting flyers at community centers, churches, clinics, and gyms throughout middle Tennessee. "Volunteers Wanted for Research Study," the notice read. "We plan to conduct focus groups with men ages 20–60 in Nashville and surrounding areas about how they define health and make decisions about health. . . . Participation is voluntary and confidential. . . . In recognition of their time and contribution to the project, participants will receive a meal and a $30 Visa gift card." This framing yielded hundreds of potential participants, some of whom cared deeply about health and others who cared deeply about Visa gift cards and free meals.

We organized participants into groups of twelve to fifteen, deliberately sorting men by a host of factors in ways that subtly built uniformity into the proceedings. We wanted participants to feel automatically part of a group and thus comfortable enough to share their opinions and biases. For example, the groups in our study were comprised only of men. Men are notoriously bad at talking about their health, identifying their own health problems, or visiting physicians. We surmised that our subjects might feel more comfortable sharing around other men—especially when discussing the ACA's potential applications to men's health issues like prostate cancer.[2]

We also roughly matched participants by income level. A great deal of research links men's health behaviors and attitudes with their socioeconomic status. As the authors of an epidemiological study of socioeconomic differences somewhat dryly put it,

Determinants of socioeconomic differences in health behaviors are poorly understood but are likely to include characteristics of the physical environment (for example, places to walk, availability of healthy foods), social norms (for example, smoking levels in the community, eating habits), and the costs of health protective behaviours. Individual knowledge, attitudinal, and motivational factors stemming from educational access, life experiences, and the general level of health consciousness expressed within the local social environment, are also relevant.[3]

We further divided participants into separate groups of white and African American men. This final division was perhaps the most important because differing historical trajectories shaped white and black experiences with health care and health insurance in the US South. A once slave-owning state, Tennessee long mandated separate and unequal health care. White hospitals and clinics refused to treat African slaves and free blacks through the Civil War. In 1881, Tennessee passed the first segregation legislation in the postbellum South, a law that required railroad cars separated by race, setting a template for the Jim Crow era. Reconstruction-era discrimination against African Americans by medical schools and teaching hospitals in Tennessee was so extreme that in 1876, black physicians opened one of the nation's first African American medical schools, Meharry Medical College in Nashville, to serve the black community.[4]

Tennessee is home to large parts of the American health insurance industry. Yet health insurance itself also carried racial valence in Southern states like Tennessee. Through much of the nineteenth century, insurers covered African Americans as property rather than as people. In 1856, for example, the Charter Oak Life Insurance Company offered "slave insurance" for white slave owners. For just two dollars, whites in Tennessee could purchase a twelve-month policy on "a 10-year-old domestic servant that would yield $100 if the slave died. Policies for older slaves, like a 45-year-old, were more expensive, costing the slave owner $5.50 a year." Historian Michael Ralph describes Civil War–era slave insurance as central to the formation of US health and life insurance industries and a way that owners of capital sought to shield themselves against the risks associated with the loss of an individual's capacity for labor:

The same period which witnessed the demise of formal enslavement saw the debut of structures that protected the privilege of people whose wealth and power suddenly threatened to come undone: this would include sharecropping and convict leasing.[5]

Thus, topics of health care and health insurance in Tennessee were already imbued with historical tensions long before the ACA, as questions such as *Whose life is worth saving and insuring?* or *Whose bodies are seen as risky?* coursed through larger debates.

History was also important because much of the South had responded to prior federally mandated social or health plans along racial lines. Again, in the mid-1960s, Senator Strom Thurmond of South Carolina—as he defected from the Democratic Party to the GOP—menacingly warned that the Civil Rights Bill of 1964 would lead to "upheaval of social patterns and customs," leading to violent revolt by white Southerners. Similar patterns of Southern opposition emerged when the Truman administration introduced the concept of mandatory national health insurance in 1945 and when the Johnson administration introduced Medicare and Medicaid in 1965, eliciting widespread white concerns that Southern hospitals would have to integrate in order to receive funding.[6]

Conversely, providing equitable, community-based health care historically signaled a form of empowerment in black communities. For instance, sociologist Alondra Nelson details how the Black Panther Party supported free medical clinics for black Americans as part of its broader strategies for advancing social justice. Panther leader Bobby Seale saw the clinics as more than window dressing: "When donors visited the Black Panther Party, they came and saw our real programs, a real clinic, with real doctors and medics, giving service to people."[7]

America's racial history was often inflected in the debate over the ACA. Surveys of national data suggested vastly differing opinions among racial groups regarding the law, in large part because of differing attitudes about the federal government in general and President Obama in particular. As one example, political scientist Michael Tesler described a "spillover" effect in which racial attitudes about President Obama shaped American opinions about health care reform. According to Tesler, the ACA expanded an already deep divide between black and white Americans' support for government programs, whereby African Americans became "overwhelmingly" supportive of the ACA while white Americans increasingly believed that "health care should be voluntarily left up to individuals" rather than the federal government.[8]

Meanwhile, certain right-wing critics openly likened ACA resistance to the stand taken by the Confederacy during the Civil War. As the conservative website *Freedom Outpost* described it under a headline warning that "Federal Agents Will Enforce Obamacare," "in a move that is reminiscent of the tyrannical actions of Abraham Lincoln that led to the War of Northern Aggression, Barack Obama says that he will not wait on states to enforce Obamacare."[9]

Our research in focus groups aimed to chart how this gulf in attitudes about health might impact health behaviors and attitudes in addition to beliefs about the ACA. Did racial differences influence men's everyday health decisions about diet and exercise? Would white men in the South prove more willing to embrace health care reform when faced with mounting evidence that their health in particular was worsening?[10]

Given the emphasis on masculinity and race, we decided that a same-race man would lead each group. My colleague Derek Griffith, a public health researcher who identifies as an African American man, led groups of men who similarly self-identified, while I watched via video. And I, a self-identified white man, headed groups of men who considered themselves to be white, while Derek watched remotely. Each group also included a graduate student assistant who sat in the corner and oversaw the taping and logistics.

Every group followed the same script. The men ate and filled out questionnaires with basic information about medical histories. Then the leader posed a series of open-ended questions. Themes included health and health decisions (e.g., *What do you do to maintain your health? Who is not healthy?*), manhood, and autonomy (*As a man, to what extent is your health within your control?*), and, most important for our purposes, health politics and opinions (*What role should the government play in promoting your health? Who or what is to blame for America's health problems?*).

We met in church basements, men's dormitories, libraries, break rooms, low-income housing projects, and community centers in once Civil War–contested towns like Nashville, Franklin, and Murfreesboro. The men we spoke with included a lawn-care service owner, a retired dentist, and a FedEx deliveryman—as well as any number of men who had not held gainful employment in some time because of illness, addiction, or life circumstance. One man came to a group wearing a leather biker vest that broadcast his identity as a Tea Party Patriot.

Talking to groups of men in the South is a particular experience if you're a Northerner. Overt religiosity and conservatism emerge in deep twang. Men often tell you what church they go to when they introduce themselves ("Born and raised here in Murfreesboro, and I go to First Baptist Church, me and the wife too"). A bravado of what sociologist Michael Kimmel calls Southern "muscular Christianity"—crucifix necklaces and forearm tattoos, elaborate facial hair—abuts formal mannerisms and a "yes, sir" or "'preciate that" in every reply. A somewhat contradictory relationship to authority also manifests: men decry government or elitist interference or colonization in one breath and express deep brand or corporate loyalty ("I love my McDonald's") in the next. On the whole, many Southern men embody what historian C. Vann Woodward once called the "divided mind" of the South, in which Southerners, and Southern white men in particular, seek the material gains of modern America while still holding fast to mores, prejudices, or historical traumas of their regional pasts.[11]

For all the divisions and the bravado, early sections of the focus groups showed the commonality through which men of various backgrounds, shapes, and sizes defined, and struggled to maintain, health. Derek or I would ask the same broad questions at the start of each group: What is health? What does being healthy mean to you? What do you do to maintain your health? In every group, we spent the next fifteen minutes discussing the food that men did or did not put into their mouths or the exercises that the men did or did not do.

"I don't eat fried unless it's wings; I'll never give up wings. That's what I think of when I think of health," a forty-one-year-old white man who worked as a welder told a group that I led in a community center meeting room. "I love potato chips and [points to a boxed meal] it's probably the last serving I'll get for another month," a small-business owner told another group that I ran in the meeting room of a library in a well-to-do suburb. He added that health is "really about discipline for me. It's actively controlling what I'm putting in my mouth. I try to walk at least three to four times a week."

We met a number of men like Tom, who swore by fast food. We also encountered men who sought to adopt healthy eating habits even when faced with limited options. "[Health is] a balanced diet pretty much, a lot of vegetables, you gotta eat your fruit, and try to pretty much stay away from a lot of bread," a skinny, heavily tattooed man and self-described "twenty-nine-year-old unemployed recovering addict" told me. "It's such a fast pace people just grab so much fast food and everything," added a forty-one-year-old man who worked in a refrigerator manufacturing factory. "I remember back when my grandparents . . . they ate a lot of fried foods and grease and stuff, but they'd go out in the morning at sunrise and work till sunset so they worked it off and they lived to be in the nineties, you know."

Men in Derek's groups defined health similarly. "I eat a lot of grape-fruit; I eat a lot of salads," a thirty-two-year-old tech store manager explained. "I feel like I'm in good shape. The only thing I gotta do is stop smoking these cigarettes." "Health, yeah, it's also how much you eat," added a forty-four-year-old security guard. "I mean, you eat certain types of foods during the day, fast food. I eat late in the evening, but my main thing at night is sugar and those carbs that store that sugar and you don't burn them off, so I try to avoid those." A thirty-one-year-old factory worker detailed how "I'm not gonna eat a Big Mac, Filet-O-Fish, or any kind of fried thing like that; I'll eat protein shakes in the evenings." A forty-two-year-old man who lived in low-income housing described his health as a "balanced diet pretty much, a lot of vegetables . . . In the morning, I let them go ahead and get them carbs and eat real good because in the evening time your body tends to slow down, you know . . . for me it's just all about, you know, how you're eating, breaking your meals up throughout the day."

Many of the men we spoke with saw their health as largely dictated by their own actions or inactions. *To what extent is your health within your control?* we asked. Men of both races generally linked their health to their own agency, as manifest through what they ate or what they did. One man told me that "I eat vegetables and fruit, and you know I might even work out. I'm forty-one, and I haven't been to the doctors in at least ten years." "If you have a heart attack or something like that, it's obviously something that you're not doing maybe properly," added another man in the same group. "Basically, it depends on how you live your life," a man told Derek. "If you live a healthier life and do the right things—eating right, getting the proper amount of sleep, getting regular physicals annually, and living right—it depends on you."

The associations between diet, health, exercise, and autonomy made sense on several levels. Many men interpreted cultural and public health messages through powerful frameworks of individualism and personal choice. *I am what I eat and what I do*, the men conveyed, *and my health reflects choices that I, and I alone, make*. As a fifty-six-year-old small-business owner put it in a group that I ran, "What goes in and what comes out of my body, I have 100 percent control of . . . and nothing prevents me from being healthy."

Another common theme emerged across groups: despite good intentions, life circumstances rendered healthy lifestyles exceedingly difficult for many men. *What is the status of your own health?* we asked, and *What prevents you from being as healthy as you want to be?*

The narratives of lower-income men in particular reflected how larger structures, such as institutions or economies, shaped health outcomes far more than dietary practices or individual choices. "I have HIV," a white man in his midforties told me. "I've been living in the street. If I went to a shelter or to a church, they might say, 'Don't come back until you have a doctor's note saying you're cured of this disease.'" "I work fourteen-hour shifts in a factory seven days a week, got no time to work out," added another. "We ain't got no Krogers or fresh food or vegetables in our neighborhood," a man told Derek. "Also, you may wake up one morning, and you say, 'Well, I can't find a job.' Next thing you know, you do something, go to jail; and then hell, your mind wasn't strong enough, see, you made a mistake. You sit behind bars. Next thing you know, you're depressed."

Had we just talked about food, diet, and exercise, the hour-long groups would have passed with ease. White men and black men might have sounded largely the same when it came to the desires and frustrations of staying healthy within a social milieu that constantly pressured people into eating more, worrying more, and exercising less.

But the tone changed, in racially distinct ways, when the conversations veered into the politics of health.

SOCIALISM

S IMILARITIES AMONG BLACK and white groups usually ended around min-
ute twenty. To that point, men of various backgrounds sounded similar
refrains about the vicissitudes of trying to stay healthy in a world filled
with drive-through windows and cheap hamburgers, and the atmosphere
in the rooms remained causal and jocular as a result. "I'll tell you how to
live a healthy life," an older gentleman explained to me. "Judge Judy says,
'Keep it in your pants,' and dear old Dad said, 'If you can't afford them,
don't make them.'" The room erupted in laughter. *This thing is a piece of
cake*, I imagined men in my groups thinking. *Easiest thirty bucks I've made
all week, plus free lunch.*

Then questions got more pointed. *So*, the group leader might ask, *it
seems like we all want to make healthy life choices for ourselves. But who
else is responsible for protecting our health? For instance, what should the
role of the government be in promoting your health?*

For many white men in the South, the word *government* elicits an au-
tonomic peptic response. Like asking about "gun control" in Missouri,
phrasing a question about "government" in states like Tennessee hangs
heavy with historical inflections. For instance, *government* invokes the
Reconstruction period, when federal forces and Republican governments
"occupied" Southern states and pressured them into granting political
rights to newly freed slaves. At the time, *redeemers* became the term for
white Southerners who violently aimed to uphold white supremacy, in
opposition to the so-called carpetbaggers and scallywags who promoted
Reconstruction governments, black citizenship, and black political activity. Government also implies the bitter legacy of the civil rights era, when

many—though certainly not all—white Southerners viewed federal efforts
to desegregate schools, lunch counters, voting booths, and hospitals as
threats to the so-called Southern way of life.[1]

The word *government* gains particular charge when it collides with
words and ideas connoting individual autonomy or personal choice, such
as guns, money, or health. This was certainly the case for many participants in the white male groups. The words *government* and *health* hung in
the air like pathogens. Previously garrulous rooms grew quiet. And suddenly, race mattered.

In the basement of a low-income housing project on the outskirts of
Nashville, a rail-thin man in his midforties named Brian spoke his mind.
"I don't think really they [government] should have anything to do with
it [health], personally." His comments broke the uncomfortable silence
spawned by my asking about government's ideal role in health care. "I just
don't think they should be in the business of health care or trying to influence health care or doctors in any way whatsoever."

The men in Brian's group appeared down on their luck. Many had
fallen off life's rails due to illness, addiction, or unforeseen circumstance.
The housing project provided a home base as they fought their ways back
to stability. One man used a wheelchair because doctors recently ampu-
tated one of his feet due to uncontrolled diabetes. Two men pulled green
oxygen canisters on wheels, like strange docile pets.

Earlier, Brian described an ongoing struggle with shortness of breath
that resulted from emphysema. "I've been smoking since I was eleven, so
it's a long time." Like many men in the group, he relied on various forms of
assistance to deal with the physical and financial implications of chronic
illness. "I used to work as a welder," he told the group. "Now I have to use
the air conditioner on 24-7 no matter what, and I've got like nine different
kinds of breathing medicines."

"How do you manage?" I asked.

"Well, I'm broke," he replied, "and I would be dead without Medicaid or the VA . . . I mean, people are without any kind of health care and
they're going to die. And . . . I don't think certain drugs they should charge
as much as they charge and probably even be free."

Brian clearly understood how he benefited from Medicaid and VA programs, but when the word *government*—without specifying state, federal,

or other—entered the conversation, he decried intervention or assistance. "No government, no way."

"Wait, I'm confused," I interjected. "Ten minutes ago, you said that government health care saved your life. What happened?"

A good deal of Brian's response cataloged real-world frustrations with bureaucracy. Long lines, long waits, lost hours. In his experience, this bureaucracy thwarted his authority and autonomy. "Go to the doctor and spend my day wrapped in red tape."

But the crux of Brian's resistance resided in dogma. "And in my opinion," he continued, "and like with Obama, it's just a form of like socialism or, you know, communism or something like that."

Of course, accusations of socialism and communism functioned as central components of conservative critiques of health care reform. "Obamacare is pure socialism," the bombastic TV host Bill O'Reilly decried, several years before Bernie Sanders made democratic socialism fashionable again. Yet in the heat of the room, with a jury of twelve white men seated around a table, it became increasingly clear just how deeply anxieties about race suffused these ideological resistances. Again and again, mentions of government, ACA, health care expansion, or system reform elicited white male anxieties about the usurpation of health and economic resources by irresponsible, lazy, and often racialized others.[2]

"And a lot of people use this Obamacare that use the state up when there's a lot of people been sick, but there's a lot of people that's not sick. They go to two or three doctors, you know, and just use the shit out of it, and then when somebody really needs it, they ain't there for you to get," the elderly man in the wheelchair said moments after Brian's claims about socialism. Not ten minutes earlier, this same man had told the group that "I've done had five heart attacks . . . I've got seven stents in . . . My antibiotics would cost me $700 without help."

"Yeah," one of the men pulling an oxygen tank added, "there's a lot of people that use welfare, the welfare department and stuff that needs to get jobs, quit having children, and really get buckled down now. I mean, I'm not saying everybody; I'm just saying there's people that have ten and twelve kids. There ought to be a cutoff point somewhere there."

"Well," the man in the wheelchair replied, "it's generation after generation."

"Well, I'm just saying," the man with oxygen responded, "they're using it up. It's about time something . . . it's not going to be there anymore."

Several moments later came an unprompted exchange about government, health, immigration, and politics among the group. The interaction went as follows—participants are labeled *R* for "Respondents," and I am listed as *I* for "Interviewer":

I: Does anyone have anything to add about government and health?

R1: It's all about the Democrats want to see a social system where people can go and get affordable free care.

R10: Democratic Party is socialist now; they're communists.

R6: No, I wouldn't call them communists.

R1: I wouldn't even call them socialists at this point; they may become that way. But the Republicans are like, they want people to pay their fair share—

R6: Exactly.

R1: —the people of America as far as the health care system. At least they're trying; the Republicans don't handcuff them like they do everything else.

R9: But it, everything, but the worst thing is, is that what really pisses Americans off is that we are pocketing all the Mexicans, all the, all the illegal, mother, mothertruckers, their houses, their cars, their food stamps, everything they want, we're paying for it.

R2: It's true.

I: I'm confused—how do you think that relates to health care?

R9: Yeah, listen, there's a lot of jobs Americans are not going to do; they just ain't going to do it. You're not catch nobody in there picking no peppers. These Mexicans come over here, pick peppers and stuff, that's if they got to work . . . that's fine, but they're coming over here and living and don't have a piece of nothin'.

R7: Yep.

R2: The Spanish will do it because they're used to living in seven, seven people in a room and making beans, you know, beans and rice for supper. And they come over and eat pork chops instead.

R9: We're paying for everything for them.

R2: Because they come over here and have babies.

R10: Yeah, if they're illegal, they'll go to the Medicaid system.

R2: Yeah, they get to.

R10: They have a baby, they go to the emergency room.

R9: They'll, they'll try to even con you out of your own freaking social security number.

R2: And I'll tell what's really bad because Americans can't even, some of us can't even get, you know, like try to get help SSDI and stuff, we can't get but they can.

R5: We're starting to sound like Donald Trump rallying.

R2: If you was born here, you was born here.

This conversation took place in early 2016, a moment when the American political spectrum seemed rife with possibility. Multiple candidates contended for each party's presidential nomination. Donald Trump's upstart bid was still seen as a sideshow or a distraction, just the latest iteration of Ralph Nader or Ross Perot.

Yet something felt truly startling about the ferocity in the room as the group narrative shifted from jokes about McDonald's and keeping it in your pants to racially and ethnically charged invective. Answers to seemingly straightforward questions about health behaviors and attitudes revealed a group psychology that identified health risks on welfare mothers, Mexicans, gangs, and other abject others who undermined the system. *We are the guardians of our own health*, the group mentality implied. *But socialism and communism undermine us, cost us, and ultimately link us . . . to them.* The narrative then constructed barriers of inside and outside. *If you was born here*, the message conveyed, with *here* implying not just the United States but also the white, anti-communist South, then *you was born here*.

I recall looking reflexively to my research assistant, a twenty-three-year-old medical student named Brian Smith who silently operated the AV equipment. Our eyes met. In that moment, we later confirmed, we were asking ourselves the same question: *Holy shit, could Trump actually win?*

To be sure, the men in this particular group, what we later called the *Trump rallying group*, likely felt themselves to be competing against other socioeconomically disadvantaged persons for precious resources. Behind concerns about people on welfare using it up and mothertrucking Mexican immigrants draining Medicaid (even though undocumented immigrants did not qualify for the program in the first place) lay anxieties about limited funds, support services, and other essential commodities for which they might have to contest, should equal distribution become the law of the land. Perhaps this was a lesson they learned from TennCare. In a state that forced health officials to hold lotteries to distribute benefits, there were not enough benefits to go around.

Perhaps capitalism had once dealt fairly with men such as these. *Work hard and the superstructure will take care of you*, it said. *We'll cover your salary and your family and your health care and your pension in exchange for your body and your life.* But now there was no such bargain, and particularly in so-called right-to-work states like Tennessee, where the health of individuals was increasingly subordinate to the health of corporations. Even the best blue-collar wages were often not enough to get by, let alone allow anyone to join the evaporating middle class. Whiteness, to again reference historian David Roediger, became the currency through which the men laid claim to their dwindling benefits. Conversely, candidates like Donald Trump preyed on these men's fear of losing even more of their dwindling privilege and security.

Socialism and communism carried racial implications as well, inasmuch as they connoted the breakdown of racial boundaries and hierarchies. Southern hospitals desegregated with extraordinary speed after the passage of Medicare in 1965, despite Ronald Reagan's predicable critique that the program functioned as medical "socialism." Civil rights–era white protesters argued that "race mixing" was a symptom of "communism" in ways that played out in racist Southern discourse well into the twenty-first century. "You mean to tell me," Tennessee pastor Donny Reagan asked in 2014, "that Communism has infiltrated our message, not through Stalin, not through Mussolini, but through mixed marriage?"[3]

Thus, lower-income men in the South espousing racist and anti-immigrant views was not hugely surprising. But the ways they did so, in the context of conversations about health, exposed tragic ironies. Here were men who depended on assistance for stents, antibiotics, operations, or oxygen tanks decrying the very networks that potentially provided lifesaving help. Their expressions of whiteness and white anxiety seemed in so many ways to work against their own self-interests; to live free *and* die sooner.

Importantly, though, these lower-income men were not the only groups I led that linked a rejection of the price of health care expansion with ideological concerns about losing racial privilege or having to pay for racial or national others. To a degree, similar concerns arose in every single group of white men.

Resistance to government involvement in health care was not universal. One of the participants in a middle-income group I led near Murfreesboro spoke in support of government assistance. "I think they're going in the right direction," said the man, in his fifties and wearing a "US Army Vet" baseball cap. "I mean, nothing's perfect, you know, but I think Obamacare, I think it's a good thing. I mean, looking at countries like Canada and Great Britain, it's worked for them . . . I like it when the government gets involved in important issues like that."

But even in the middle-income sessions, the overarching consensus of the group shifted away from governmental assistance and toward the "right kind of insurance," and Donald Trump:

> R5: I can really care less about the government, you know, to be honest with you. Obama, he ain't going to get nothing accomplished.
>
> R4: Set us trillion dollars in debt.
>
> I: Who's that?
>
> R4: Obama. About a trillion dollars.
>
> R5: I don't know anything about Obamacare, don't want to, I don't want to know about Obama. I'm about sick of hearing about that; I'm about sick of hearing about him, to be honest with you.
>
> I: He's in his second term, right?
>
> R5: Well, thank God.
>
> I: And you feel he's not looking out for your interests?
>
> R5: He's not, he's not. I don't think he's looking out for this country.
>
> R3: It's better not doing anything at all, that's just my personal opinion.

R7: I think we've got to get out of everybody else's business, start taking care of our damn own—stay at home, letting you mow your own grass.

R5: And that way there would be more money out there for the right kind of insurance, you know. There would be more money for the right kind of insurance for, for people like us to be taken care of. Why are we over in Korea and China and everywhere we don't have no business being? It ain't none of our damn business.

I: Are there politicians or parties that might do a better job looking out for your interests?

R4: I like Donald Trump. He's the mos' arrogant SOB I ever seen in my damn life. That's the kind of president we need, tell the world where to stick it.

R2: I've never voted in my whole life. I'm registered, and I'm going to vote for Trump.

Meanwhile, white men in higher-income groups couched their anxieties in somewhat more nuanced terms. I met with a group of small-business owners in a library in a well-off Brentwood neighborhood. They answered the government question with similar disdain. No sooner had the words *government* and *health* left my lips than a man in his fifties who owned an electronics store proclaimed, "My personal beef with the government is that it's just the old adage that the government, every time they get involved in something and it's something that works, they're gonna screw it up or it's just too many cooks in the kitchen, so to speak."

"We're responsible for our health," added another man who later revealed that he was a pastor. "So I think inside this room you probably— we'd like the government to stay out of it. I think that's what we would really prefer and take responsibility for our own lives."

Once again, concerns about autonomy closely aligned with concerns about the costs marginalized others might inflict upon the men in the room. "We have hundreds of people killed every day when two gangs get together," a physician's assistant—who to that point had been silent— chimed in, seemingly to a question he posed in his own mind. "People kill there, two gangs shooting it out. You're talking about what would happen in a totalitarian government that said you can't have McDonald's or anything like that. We've already seen how that works."

"Going back to the people that are poor," the electronics man interjected, "they go buy the potato chips and eat the junk food with their food stamps and then . . . "

"Yeah," added a man who owned a lawn-care service. "A lot of the people that I know that are in poverty are not healthy . . . the vast majority of them are very overweight, and the children are overweight."

"And how do you know they're not healthy?" I asked.

"Well," the man continued, "just by their physical appearance, generally speaking, although you can look at their facial expressions, their faces and look at the coloring of their skin, that type of thing."

EVERYBODY

ONE MIGHT REASONABLY expect African American men in Tennessee to harbor even more skepticism about government intervention than their white counterparts. White men often phrased their anxieties about government through ideological language that described events they feared *might* happen ("The government could be watching us right now")—in somewhat the same ways that white gun owners who spoke to sociologist Angela Stroud imagined fictional black aggression toward white people to justify open carry of firearms.

But many African American men did not need to imagine speculative fears—they could recount firsthand experience with governmental intrusion or neglect. The African American men in our groups described being pulled over, hassled, or unfairly surveilled by police. Many lower-income black men also recounted ways that local governments denied basic services to their neighborhoods or failed to provide, support, or improve key infrastructures. Black men of all income levels described the profound generational impact of mass incarceration. "A lot of black fathers been on the street or been in the hood or got incarcerated."

For these and other reasons, black men frequently folded their skepticism about government into a broader recognition of social injustice. In one group at a community center in a middle-income suburb of Nashville, a thirty-two-year-old man proclaimed that "me personally, I don't feel no politics, politicians, and none of their peers." Soon thereafter came a heartbreaking exchange about what it meant to live and survive in a system that often felt hostile to who they were rather than what they did:

R2: The first issue for being a black man in the United States is we
    have a lot of restrictions against you. . . . First of all, you're
    not gonna get the same opportunities as everybody else. I
    have been in situations where my color has made a part of me
    getting a promotion or me being chosen to take over or lead
    something or being a part of something. Black people still has
    racism against them in the United States; it's doing it behind
    your back.

R9: The odds are already against us being black men, and we al-
    ready are targets. We already are set up for failure; the world
    is designed for us to fail. We don't get the same chances. I'll
    probably still be in my same position five more years before
    they even consider giving me a raise. They don't wanna see us
    getting ahead, and then when we do get ahead, they target us
    because they feel like all of us are drug dealers. If I'm driv-
    ing a nice car, "Why he got that? Well, I'm about to pull over
    and harass him." Racial profiling. Malice intent. They do all
    that to knock us off our character. We're taught this from the
    beginning.

These men, in other words, lived as "outcast[s] and stranger[s] in mine
own house," as W. E. B. Du Bois once described the doubly conscious
experience of black America in which internalized identity coexisted with
the thousand cuts of everyday restrictions and subliminal racisms.[1]

When the conversations turned to government interventions in health
and health care, many black men described precisely the same medical
and economic stressors as did white men and detailed the same struggles
to stay healthy. Some even voiced concerns similar to those raised in white
groups that people gamed the system in ways that drained resources. "I
kind of agree with some of the stuff that Republicans have said," one man
in his midforties, who himself identified as a Republican, said. "It's like a
lot of the times the people who are considered lower class or poor, a lot of
them, is in my family. You know, a lot of them are the ones to be the ones
that sit back and say, 'Hey, I'm gonna live off government.'"

But black men consistently differed from white men in how they conceived of government intervention and group identity. Whereas white men
jumped unthinkingly to assumptions about "them," black men frequently

answered questions about health and health systems through the language of "us."

For instance, when Derek asked, *Who is responsible for your health?*, practically every group looked around the table and then looked within. A group of men in a low-income housing complex on the outskirts of Nashville—in the very same complex where we convened a group of lower-income white men on a different night—responded as follows:

> R7: Well, we as African Americans, we are not as healthy as we need to be because we don't put our health first. So as a people as a whole, we need to start thinking healthy.
>
> R2: It's the fact that our educational level isn't so high and some of the environments that our boys grow up in.
>
> R1: It all depends on how your circumstances be and how you work your way out of those circumstances.
>
> R6: Our parents, our family told us that black men, African American men don't like going to the doctor and we never did go, but as time went on we started changing that, so we're getting wiser.
>
> R7: Something that we as African Americans we don't do enough of, and do it in a constructive way.

For these men and others with whom we spoke, questions about responsibility and health elicited responses using *us, we, our*, and other autobiographical monikers that connoted communal responsibility. *We* implied populations forged by race and ethnicity—we as African Americans—as well as by assumed common attitudes and experiences—"our family, our parents." We, as *Chicago Defender* editor Robert S. Abbott once put it, implied "the Race."[2]

Through this framework, black men in Tennessee generally provided profoundly different replies about government intervention into health and health care than did white men. When Derek asked the dreaded question—*What should the role of the government be in promoting your health?*—responses were far less skeptical:

> R1: I don't think that the government needs to control everything, but I do think that they need to control certain things. The

people always say let the free market dictate what societies think. Well, we let the market dictate for society, and then look at what happened. We had the crash, so the government had to step in and set rules and regulations on what the market can do. If you don't, it would have happened again.

R6: I'm for Obamacare because in a country as big as ours, I don't see why we can't have affordable health insurance for everybody. I'm for it.

A number of men voiced support for the ACA or understood its critics through reference to President Obama himself. A fifty-two-year-old postal worker claimed that "I'll say once he get elected the first time, that put all black men on notice that we can strive to get to that level."

"Yep, we got a black president," a sixty-nine-year-old retiree added. "Whoever thought that was going to happen? But that's what we fought, and that's what we died for, that's what we went prison for. So if you can get a black president, then don't tell me you can't, you can go Harvard, you can go to get, you know, tech, open you a business."

Similarly, a thirty-three-year-old mechanic explained how "with the Obamacare, you have a lot of people with health care now; they don't want to give him credit for that, simply because he's black and that's the same that Reagan or someone had implemented way back several years ago."

Other respondents reasoned their support for health care reform for far more practical reasons: they saw it as beneficial, largely because they assumed that government services were ultimately more useful than they were tyrannical.

R10: Obamacare makes it easier for us to get insurance and also get a doctor . . . and poor people benefit. Now they take their kids to the doctor.

R6: I think Obamacare is giving you a right to protect yourself too. You know what I'm saying—you go in the hospital, they ain't going to work on you. It's tough if you ain't got no insurance.

R1: Like for instance, my sister-in-law, she moved from Maryland. She got sick and lost her job . . . my wife is trying to get her insurance so she can go into the hospital and she done have a stroke.

> R7: Everybody should have health care. . . . People are now getting educated more by going to their doctors, going to get active in their facilities, going to get active at church and after they're home, then you know. It's all about, one it's like a domino effect, one pushes the other.

Themes of protection extended outward as well, inasmuch as many men saw government as an arbiter against excesses or injustices of corporations:

> R5: It's the responsibility of the government to protect the citizens from entrepreneurs . . . the vegetables and the fruits and that we eat are covered with pesticides, and so someone has to protect the citizenship.
>
> R1: As a society, so that's the government's role to make sure that people who are trying to get that extra buck don't kill us in the process.

In other words, where white men reacted astringently to the thought of "intervention" into health care, black men saw health care "expansion" as a net benefit and government as a fail-safe, albeit a far from perfect one, against predatory illnesses, persons, or corporations.

Issac Bailey, author of the memoir *Proud. Black. Southern.*, argues that many African Americans adopted political compromise as a practical necessity. As Bailey writes, African American communities time and again saw

> incremental change improve their lives. That's why they embrace Martin Luther King Jr. without question while revering Malcolm X from a distance. That's why they are much more enthusiastic about the Affordable Care Act—which has helped minority Americans the most—than white progressives who have either been lukewarm or, in some cases, even hostile to health reform because they don't believe it was radical enough.[3]

Did the black men's responses represent this lineage of pragmatism? Or did the differing attitudes about the ACA voiced by black and white men reflect different historical relationships to government, health, and health care?

At the same time, if divergent histories of white and African American communities in the South were the sole factors that determined views on utility of government, it would follow that racially distinct narratives of perceived benefit or self-interest emerged. This certainly appeared to be the case for white men, whose anti-government ideologies created crystal-clear categories of *us* versus *them*. *We define us by what we have*, these groups implied, *and we define them by the fact that they want what is ours*.

Black men's responses were far from monolithic. Yet on the whole, the anxiety central to the white groups—a constant pressure to bear and embody the cost of staying on top—remained absent when black men spoke. Instead, unburdened by ideologies of supremacy or the invective of fallen greatness, black men narrated health care as a benefit—rather than as what the historian Roediger called a wage.

Thus, when Derek asked a group of men in a middle-class suburb *So who benefits from Obamacare?*, the responses sounded like this:

> R3: Everybody.
>
> R9: Everybody.
>
> R3: Everybody, if you ain't got no insurance, number one. But everybody under sixty-five. You know what I'm saying.
>
> R6: The kids and all of us.
>
> R5: Especially the low income. They, they mostly really gain from it, seriously.

Similarly, the responses in a group of lower-income men sounded like this:

> R1: Everybody. That's the two things that is not racist—speeding and health care. They don't care who you are—speeding or sick, they don't care—they, you're going out or you're going in. They don't discriminate for your health or speed. So that's the two things.
>
> I: Whose, okay, any other thoughts about who benefits from Obamacare?

R5: I think society does; I think society does in that it keeps it, with people having insurance, it keeps the cost down for everyone.

R6: Yeah, because people are healthy because of the checkups and things like that, so I think everyone, I think, as a society, I think we all do by having people insured.

R7: Someone has to protect the citizenship, not just black people but protect us as a country, you know.

Everybody. Society. The citizenship. For these men, health care was a utility shared by all, for the benefit of all. Where white men often defined government involvement as a risk or debt, many black men saw a communal safety net as an investment. Expanded health care enabled well-being for highly practical, seemingly nonideological reasons: health care allowed more people to go to doctors and to do so before they became gravely ill, thus saving money and improving quality of life. This line of reasoning is often attributed to ivory-tower health economists who study the benefits of particular health policies through frameworks of economics or public health. In the African American groups, we found that many people on the ground felt the same.[4]

Moreover, for many black men, support also enabled knowledge ("People are now getting educated more by going to their doctors, going to get active . . . like a domino effect") and boosted community and communal safety. Perhaps most importantly, this framework allowed black men to view health care reform as having value for society as a whole, rather than for any particular racial group. As one participant put it, "I think everyone, I think, as a society, I think we all [benefit] by having people insured."

DE-
PROGRESSIVE

THE ACA WAS supposed to work much like the African American interviewees imagined. Though far from perfect, the law would expand coverage in places where many low-income residents lacked access to affordable health care, while at the same time expanding consumer protections. President Obama detailed as much in a press conference three months after passage. "Would you want to go back to discriminating against children with preexisting conditions?" he asked while announcing the ACA-linked Patient's Bill of Rights. "Would you want to go back to dropping coverage for people when they get sick? Would you want to reinstate lifetime limits on benefits so that mothers . . . have to worry? We're not going back. I refuse to go back."[1]

However, the citizens of Tennessee did not see the benefit of this logic, and the health of men and women in the state almost certainly suffered as a result. If, as our groups suggested, two distinct racialized scripts surrounded health care expansion in Tennessee, then narratives of suspicion, disdain, and rejection prevailed over narratives of inclusion and common gain.

Initially, several powerful voices in Tennessee supported full implementation of the ACA. Expansion garnered backing from business communities, and particularly from large health insurance companies based in Tennessee, such as HCA Holdings and Vanguard Health Systems. Eight of Tennessee's chambers of commerce, including the Tennessee Chamber of

Commerce and Industry, signed letters and briefs arguing that Tennessee should expand Medicaid. Practically all of the state's major newspapers came out in support of the ACA as well. The *Jackson Sun* defined opposition to health care reform as "irrational and self-defeating."[2]

But the narrative of disdain would win out. In March 2013, GOP Tennessee governor Bill Haslam ominously responded to President Obama's "we're not going back" vow when he told a joint session of the state legislature that "I cannot recommend that we move forward." In a speech cheered by Tea Party lawmakers, Haslam justified his decision to opt out of Medicaid expansion by detailing concerns about "cost." The governor bowed to the concerns of Republicans like avowedly anti-government Lieutenant Governor Ramsey, who reiterated his arguments that "a federal government which can coerce its people to buy a product is a government unrestrained and out of control."[3]

That was far from the end of the process, however. Instead of expanding Medicaid, Haslam proposed yet another "Tennessee plan" for health care reform that involved using federal Medicaid money to buy private insurance for low-income residents of the state. Indeed, the governor spent much of the next two years working on a proposal that he called Insure Tennessee. In December 2014, Haslam introduced his initiative with great fanfare and claimed that it would "not create new taxes for Tennesseans and [would] not add additional costs to the state budget." In other words, Insure Tennessee was Obamacare minus Obama. As *USA Today* described it, this formulation catered to GOP lawmakers in Tennessee by taking power away from the federal government and instituting "real conservative reform." Insure Tennessee soon garnered support from academics, policy makers, leading philanthropists, and over two-thirds of citizens polled across the state.[4]

Haslam called for a special session of the legislature to debate the merits of his new plan. But despite the seemingly broad support, Insure Tennessee was effectively dead on arrival in early 2016, and once again, a health care plan sank under alarmist rhetoric about cost. "Insure Tennessee Doesn't Have a Chance," read a headline in the *Kingsport Times-News*. "Ramsey Tells Insure TN Supporters to Shove It," shouted the *Nashville Scene* above an article detailing how the state senate's conservative supermajority claimed that Insure Tennessee "would demolish state finances." "Did you pull that [bill] out of the trash can yet?" Ramsey later asked at a press conference. True to form, eight of the twenty members of Tennessee's House Insurance and Banking Committee cosponsored a competing piece of legislation that prohibited any form of Medicaid expansion in the state. Insure Tennessee never even made it to the floor for a full vote. All the while, state GOP politicians decried the ACA's price tag. "The Affordable Care Act is too expensive to afford," Tennessee Seventh District Republican congressman Marsha Blackburn repeatedly claimed at town hall meetings and in Fox News appearances in 2017, while arguing for an overall repeal.[5]

These claims were patently false. As lawmakers well knew, the federal government would have paid a whopping 93 percent of the costs of Medicaid expansion until 2022 and no less than 90 percent of the cost of covering people made newly eligible for Medicaid on a permanent basis. Nonpartisan groups such as the Congressional Budget Office (CBO) estimated that expansion would ultimately lead to a 2.8 percent increase in Medicaid spending for states like Tennessee from 2014 to 2022. Yet this increase paled in comparison to the net savings that state and local governments would realize in health care spending for the uninsured—up to $101 billion in uncompensated care according to leading health care consulting firms. In addition, the state would have received what was rightly called "a windfall of federal money" equaling an estimated $7 billion over five years. Even the AARP agreed. The American Association of Retired Persons released its own Tennessee study showing that Medicaid expansion would bring in goods and services valued at $17.6 billion and wages, salaries, and benefits worth $7.9 billion.[6]

The political rejection of expanded health care networks in Tennessee formed an unfortunate epilogue to our focus groups. Tennessee's conservative senate majority assured that our conversations with low-income men about the possible benefits of the ACA remained speculative. Like a martyr at the stake, health care remained unreformed.

What was the ultimate cost of rejecting the ACA and Medicaid expansion for the men in our groups in Tennessee? And what was the gain? These questions ran through my mind repeatedly in the months and years following our focus groups as Donald Trump rose to power and debates about health care remained at the center of American politics. Tennessee became a notional model, not for a Southern attempt to take care of all citizens but for an effective way to resist doing so.

It seemed plausible to consider that the white men in our groups gained something, inasmuch as the anti-reform position they advocated ultimately prevailed. These men were far from naive or ignorant about health care. In many ways, their anti-government rhetoric derived from genuine concerns about autonomy and did so in ways that made sense contextually. On myriad levels, white men gained group cohesion by "fighting back" against health care reform or retaining their own notions of status and privilege, even as they themselves suffered from conditions that required medical assistance. Putting their bodies on the line created categories of us versus them, defenders versus invaders. And perhaps the gain then accrued, not so much from a biomedical perspective but from what historians and theorists such as Du Bois have described as the psychological benefits of being white—or what historian George Lipsitz once termed a "possessive investment in whiteness."[7]

Resistance to health care reform also reflected venerable Southern traditions of opposition to change and particularly to perceived Northern intervention into racial norms and social orders. Historian Drew Faust describes "a kind of guerrilla warfare of the domestic, of the local" that Southern white populations waged in the Reconstruction period, in which whites "just refus[ed] to let society change in the ways that the architects of [Negro] freedom in the North might hope for." Resistance to government intervention provided a common cause, along with a strength in numbers that, as journalist Daniel Hayes writes about white men in Kentucky, "comes less from unity than desperation." For Hayes, desperation emerged from nostalgia for vanished, possibly mythical ways of life, in concert with the very real implications of NAFTA, Walmart, and "sustained economic violence at the hands of tyrannical governments of both parties." In an age of outsourcing and globalization, this resistance became one of white men's remaining marketable skills, deployed to guard the old ways through modes of resistance and self-sacrifice that made them perfect consumers and foot soldiers for the Tea Party, the National Rifle Association, and the Trump campaign.[8]

Perhaps a bit of perverse empowerment accompanied the pain. Not ironically, suffering in the name of subversion is a dynamic associated with slavery. Historians and literary theorists have explored how enslaved blacks in the South used their bodies as sites of opposition. English professor Saidiya Hartman details how "small scale and everyday forms of resistance" manifested through illness and pain shaped black identity, while gender studies scholar Barbara Baumgartner writes that the slave's broken body "serves as a key locus of opposition; it enables her to refuse to capitulate to further demands of servitude."[9]

Such correlations are not meant to downplay very real hardship and loss. Rather, they suggest that Southern white medicalized suffering occurred within historical and ideological frameworks that allowed white men to interpret ACA resistance in way that gave larger purpose to the act of refusing medical intervention. Pain affirmed group identity and a position in a hierarchy that, while hardly at the top, was not at the bottom either. No amount of Yankee logic, information, or public health would change that. Safety nets, provider networks, and other grids linked lower-income white men to onetime subordinates turned perceived competitors. Untreated pain, in this one sense, could be read as *gain*—or at least a victory for stasis.

Assessing the *cost* of ACA rejection, however, required no theory or philosophy, no historical context. Rather, the price of Tennessee's refusal to embrace health care reform was quantifiable.

THE NUMBERS
TELL THE STORY

To RECALL FROM the Missouri section, assessing the health impacts of gun policies required a fair amount of statistical guesswork because of federal bans on large-scale funded research. But research on health care faces no such constraints. On the contrary, an ocean of data and studies is available for researchers who track the effects of health care reform, or lack thereof, on populations.

Our statistical team dove into this data in the months following the focus groups. We compiled data from published studies, foundation reports, and federal databases to assess the implications of ACA- and Medicaid-expansion rejection for white and African American citizens of Tennessee. We quickly realized that, in order to evaluate the effects of Tennessee's decisions about health care reform, we needed to compare health and illness in Tennessee with trends in states that made different political choices. The decision on whether to implement Medicaid expansion seemed the best starting point for our analysis because it affected coverage for the most vulnerable populations in the state, including the lower-income men in our focus groups. We uncovered a host of useful studies and databases that tracked how state efforts to expand Medicaid affected *all-cause mortality*—essentially, the rates at which people die.

Of course, rates of death change due to any number of social or environmental factors. Plagues, wars, failed economies, and brush fires raise mortality rates, for instance, while new plumbing sewage systems, vaccines, or smoke alarms lower them. In an ideal world, effective health insurance plans also reduce mortality rates because they promote preventative care for lower- and middle-income persons, transforming illnesses such as cardiovascular disease, depression, respiratory disease, or neoplasms from death sentences into manageable conditions.

The math, then, becomes morbid subtraction: deaths by certain illnesses or pathogens at a time before an intervention, minus deaths after. Or deaths in an area that adopted Medicaid expansion, minus deaths in a comparable area that did not.

Such math lay at the heart of important studies conducted by Harvard health policy scholar Benjamin Sommers and colleagues. In 2012, Sommers published a paper that tracked changes to mortality rates in the five years before and after Medicaid expansion in Arizona, Maine, and New York, comparing each to a neighboring state that did not expand. The analysts studied a time before the ACA but provided a commonly used template that would be used to assess its effects on low-income persons, since the Medicaid expansion efforts were largely the ones adopted by the ACA. After extensive analyses, the research group found that expansion led to "significant decrease in mortality during a 5-year follow-up period, as compared with neighboring states without Medicaid expansions," particularly in adults between the ages of thirty-five and sixty-four, minorities, and low-income persons—an age range roughly comparable to the men in our groups. The authors ultimately found that all-cause mortality declined by a whopping 6.1 percent, or 19.6 per 100,000 people, after expansion, including a 4.53 percent decline for white residents and an 11.36 percent decline for nonwhite residents. Sommers concluded that "2840 deaths [were] prevented per year in states with Medicaid expansions" compared to similar states that rejected expansion.[1]

In a follow-up analysis from 2014, Sommers and his colleagues also found that mortality decreased by 2.9 percent in Massachusetts and by 2.4 percent in the state's white populations after the implementation of the comprehensive health reform known as Romneycare, a state-run health insurance program that provided the intellectual framework for the ACA. Sommers wrapped up his findings by arguing that more health insurance roughly correlated with less death because insurance "leads to increased coverage, and such coverage leads to better access and more utilization of clinical services, including office visits, with resulting gains in self-reported health status."[2]

The two Sommers analyses provided a useful starting framework for a first experiment: What would the mortality rates for white and African American populations in Tennessee look like if Tennessee had also adopted Medicaid expansion?

We pulled Tennessee's all-cause mortality rates by accessing a database called the Wide-ranging Online Data for Epidemiologic Research— or WONDER, for short. WONDER, like WISQARS (Web-based Injury Statistics Query and Reporting System), is an open-access information bank compiled and maintained by the CDC. We used WONDER data to plot all-cause mortality in Tennessee between 2011 (the first year of the ACA) and 2015 (the most recent year of federal data at this writing). Then we did a series of calculations to project what the data might have looked like had Tennessee expanded Medicaid and seen improvements like those

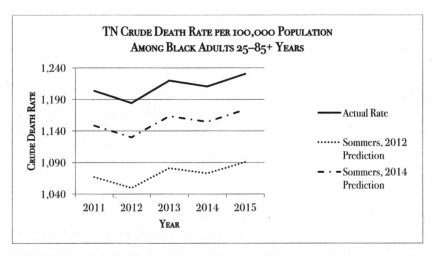

1. CDC WONDER Underlying Cause of Death Database, https://wonder.cdc.gov/ucd-icd10 .html.

2. B. D. Sommers, K. Baicker, and A. M. Epstein, "Mortality and Access to Care Among Adults After State Medicaid Expansions," *New England Journal of Medicine* 367, no. 11 (2012): 1025–1034, https://doi.org/10.1056/NEJMsa1202099.

3. B. D. Sommers, S. K. Long, and K. Baicker, "Changes in Mortality After Massachusetts Health Care Reform: A Quasi-Experimental Study," *Annals of Internal Medicine* 160, no. 9 (2014): 585, https://doi.org/10.7326/M13-2275.

Comment: CDC WONDER database was queried by year and gender; Tennessee; all categories of urbanization included; age groups 25 through 85+; all genders; non-Hispanic black; years 2011 through 2015; all weekdays, autopsy values, and places of death; all causes of death.

in Arizona, New York, and Maine (Sommers 2012) and Massachusetts
(Sommers 2014).[3]

We crunched the numbers and generated two simple but reveal-
ing graphs. The graph on the previous page shows mortality rates for
black, non-Hispanic adults ages twenty-five to eighty-five in Tennessee.
The top line in this graph represents the actual mortality rates for African American citizens of Tennessee from the WONDER database. The
other two lines theorize what the mortality rates might have looked like
had the rates for African Americans in Tennessee followed trends in the
Medicaid-expanding states tracked by Sommers. The middle line depicts
what might have happened to African American mortality following trends
in Massachusetts (2014), where expansion reduced nonwhite mortality by
4.6 percent. The bottom line represents mortality rates modeled on those
seen after expansion in Arizona, New York, and Maine (2012), where more
Medicaid coverage reduced nonwhite mortality by 11.36 percent.[4]

It is crucial to acknowledge that such comparisons must be made with
caution. Profound differences in health care systems, access to physicians,
education, infrastructure, and environment exist among these states. Even
with that in mind, this straightforward comparison uncovered some jarring
results. Most importantly, when we subtracted the number of lives represented by the two projections inspired by Sommers from the actual figures,
we learned that if Tennessee had expanded Medicaid, *between 1,863 and
4,599 black lives might have been saved from 2011 to 2015*. That staggering number is actually conservative: the figures did not account for the
many more African American citizens who grew sicker but did not actually
die during the time frame.[5]

The chart on the opposite page showing white mortality trends revealed equally jolting results. As before, the top line represents the actual mortality rates for white, non-Hispanic citizens in Tennessee between
2011 and 2015—a time when studies showed life expectancy for Southern
white populations decreasing overall. The other two lines depict what the
mortality rates might have looked like had death rates for white citizens
of Tennessee followed trends in Massachusetts (2014, middle line), where
expansion reduced white mortality by 2.4 percent, and in Arizona, New
York, and Maine (2012, bottom line), where expansion reduced white mortality by 4.53 percent.[6]

Subtracting the values of the Sommers-based projections from the actual figures suggested that between 2011 and 2015, *between 6,365 and*

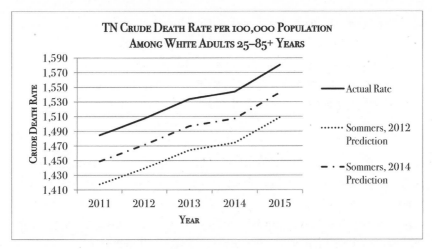

Sources: CDC WONDER Underlying Cause of Death Database; Sommers et al., "Mortality and Access"; and Sommers et al., "Changes in Mortality."

Comment: CDC WONDER Database was queried by year and gender; Tennessee; all categories of urbanization included; age groups 25 through 85+; all genders; non-Hispanic white; years 2011 through 2015; all weekdays, autopsy values, and places of death; all causes of death.

12,013 white lives might have been saved had Tennessee expanded Medicaid. Again, this projection does not capture the fact that health benefits from social programs usually grow over time as more people sign up and access preventative care.[7]

The experiment validated some of the more problematic claims made by white men in the focus groups. Medicaid expansion probably helped low-income minority populations *more*, and these populations felt greater life costs of not expanding. But rejecting expansion in order to deny benefits to minorities came at significant cost to white populations as well. To assess that cost, we finished our comparisons by adding up all the white and African American years that expansion might have saved. We calculated this by subtracting all the years that Tennesseans *would* have lived if the state expanded Medicaid from the actual average ages of death in the state—which happened to be 66.1 years for African Americans and 71.7 for whites. This final math produced another set of astonishing statistics about the potential cost of rejecting Medicaid expansion—even without yet accounting for Latino or immigrant populations:

- A minimum of 21,565 and a maximum of 28,933 black life years would have been saved if Tennessee had expanded

Medicaid between 2011 and 2015. This translated to
as much as *37.1 days of life per black Tennessean.*
- A minimum of 73,181 and a maximum of 138,115 white life
years would have been saved if Tennessee had expanded
Medicaid between 2011 and 2015. This translated to
as much as *14.1 days of life per white Tennessean.*[8]

On an aggregate level, Tennessee's failure to expand Medicaid potentially cost every single adult black and white resident of the state somewhere between two and five weeks of life. If this estimation in any way represents reality, then it places "failure to expand Medicaid" on a continuum among leading man-made causes of death in Tennessee.[9]

Next we asked questions about the competitive insurance marketplaces, or lack thereof, in Tennessee. Here we found it useful to compare trends in Tennessee with those reported in Kentucky, the Volunteer State's northern neighbor. Kentucky and Tennessee share a number of demographic, geographic, political, and historical similarities, particularly along the south-central Appalachian regions. But Kentucky broke with Tennessee and most other Southern states when it embraced the ACA and expanded Medicaid. In May 2013, then governor Steve Beshear, a Democrat, announced to much fanfare and predictable resistance that the state would expand Medicaid to cover most adults with incomes under 138 percent of the federal poverty level and support insurance marketplaces as well. Beshear called the expansion "the single most important decision in our lifetime" for improving the health of Kentuckians—who traditionally ranked near the bottom of the US population in nearly every health indicator.

Only three years after that announcement, Kentucky voters elected a new Republican governor, Matt Bevin, who ran on a promise to dismantle the ACA and Medicaid expansion. In June 2016, Bevin laid out plans to close the state-run Obamacare insurance marketplace and roll back Medicaid. Yet even in the data from late 2013 to early 2016, the effects of expansion in Kentucky posed a stark contrast to trends seen in Tennessee: 425,000 Kentuckians, representing fully 10 percent of the population, gained coverage in the first year alone—even though the Medicaid expansion did not go into effect until a year later. According to an in-depth study published in *Health Affairs*, the percentages of the state's low-income adults without insurance dropped from 40.2 percent to 12.4 percent as a result of expansion—one of the largest reductions in the country. Increasing numbers of Kentuckians visited doctors. The state also saw reductions in the numbers of people who skipped taking their medications because of cost or claimed to have difficulties paying their medical bills.[10]

Kentucky's adoption and Medicaid expansion produced yawning gaps in coverage between the two states. A wide-ranging 2015 report compiled by the US Department of Health and Human Services (HHS) tracked uninsured populations of each state in the years leading up to the ACA. We pulled Tennessee and Kentucky out of the extensive tables in that report and learned that the two states carried roughly similar percentages of uninsured persons for the five years leading up to ACA adoption. Roughly 16–17 percent of the population of each state under age sixty-five remained uninsured between 2009 and 2013, with Kentucky slightly outpacing Tennessee. In the first year of the ACA, even before Medicaid expansion, uninsured rates in Tennessee saw modest improvements. But uninsured rates in Kentucky plummeted.[11]

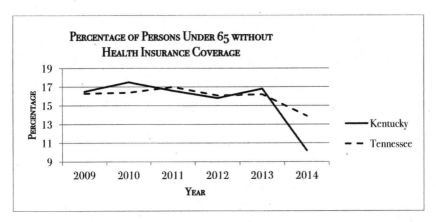

Source: National Center for Health Statistics, *Health, United States, 2015: With Special Feature on Racial and Ethnic Health Disparities* (Washington, DC: US Government Printing Office, 2015).

After the 2014 Medicaid expansion kicked in, these trends were particularly pronounced in lower-income populations as shown in the graph on the next page.[12] Here as well, these sharp divides carried further implications when broken down by race. For instance, in 2016, the Commonwealth Fund compiled data from the US Census Bureau and the Behavioral Risk

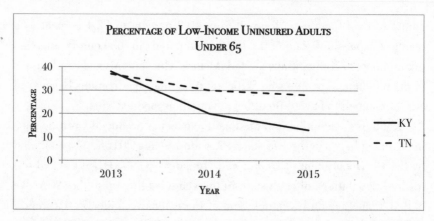

Source: S. L. Hayes, S. R. Collins, D. Radley, D. McCarthy, and S. Beutel, "A Long Way in a Short Time: States' Progress on Health Care Coverage and Access, 2013–2015," Commonwealth Fund, December 21, 2016, retrieved from https://www.commonwealthfund.org/publications/issue-briefs/2016/dec/state-progress-coverage-and-access.

Factor Surveillance System into a report that tracked health care coverage trends by state and by race from 2013 to 2015. We pulled Tennessee and Kentucky from that database and again saw stark differences between the two states. Predictably, Kentucky posted much sharper declines in the number of uninsured African American and Hispanic adults ages nineteen to sixty-four than Tennessee. These gaps accelerated after Medicaid expansion began in earnest in 2014. For instance, percentages of "Hispanic" persons with insurance in Tennessee fell dramatically behind those in Kentucky because uninsured populations fell dramatically in Kentucky but flatlined in Tennessee:[13]

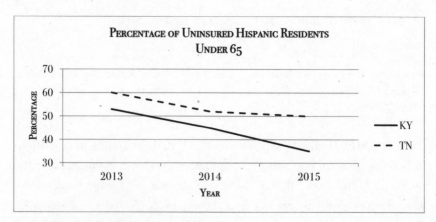

Source: Hayes et al., "A Long Way in a Short Time."

A similar dynamic appeared in African American populations:

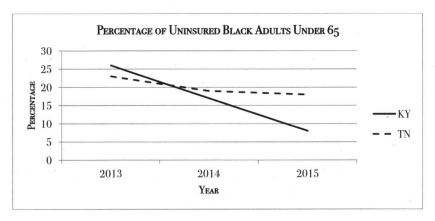

Source: Hayes et al., "A Long Way in a Short Time."

And here as well, blocking health care for "Mexicans" and "welfare queens" came at considerable cost to white populations in Tennessee. Percentages of uninsured white persons were largely the same between the two states in 2013, but a growing gap emerged after the ACA began to take effect:

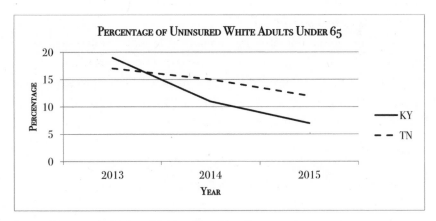

Source: Hayes et al., "A Long Way in a Short Time."

Moreover, with many white persons in both states living near or below the federal poverty level, Medicaid expansion widened the gap between coverage rates in Kentucky and Tennessee for low-income white populations in particular. Low-income white populations in Kentucky saw significant gains, while similar populations in Tennessee fell behind even 2013 levels:[14]

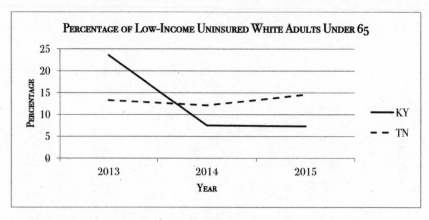

Source: Hayes et al., "A Long Way in a Short Time."

What did all of this mean? Did falling rates of health care coverage in Tennessee actually matter in the real world? Studies show a roughly 25 percent higher risk of death among uninsured persons when compared with privately insured adults. Insurance does not by itself prevent or cure diseases. However, we found a related phenomenon in our study of the available data: *not only did people in Kentucky have more access to physicians and medical care compared to Tennesseans, but Tennesseans paid more for what care they did receive.*[15]

The data showed that growing numbers of Tennessee citizens skipped routine office visits. At the same time, increasing numbers of Kentuckians saw clinicians for checkups and routine screenings. For instance, percentages of adults who went over a year without a routine doctor's visit rose in Tennessee but fell sharply in Kentucky:[16]

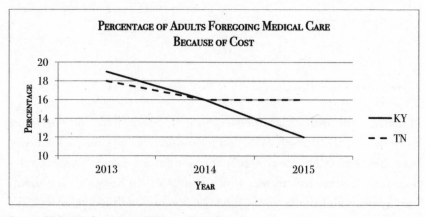

Source: Hayes et al., "A Long Way in a Short Time."

Adults in Tennessee were also dramatically more likely than adults in Kentucky to forgo health care because of cost:

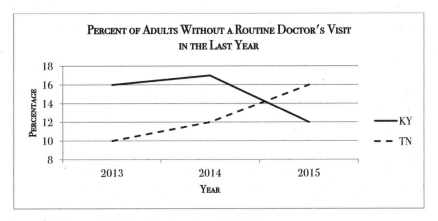

Source: Hayes et al., "A Long Way in a Short Time."

On the persistent question of cost, we found that health care expenditures in 2015 constituted 12 percent of the median income in Tennessee but only 10.4 percent of the median income in Kentucky—once again undermining the argument among ACA opponents that it was simply too expensive. Families in Tennessee contributed nearly $400 more per year to employer-sponsored health care plans than did families in Kentucky. Meanwhile, the average Tennessee employee in a 2015 employer-sponsored insurance plan paid $6,477 in premium and deductible costs; average costs were only $5,693 for comparable plans in Kentucky.[17]

Make no mistake, the picture was not entirely rosy. For instance, research would also suggest that higher rates of coverage correlated with greater emergency room use, thus increasing the cost of overall coverage. Yet when I compared gun suicides in Connecticut and Missouri, the spaces between real-life mortality figures and projections came to represent lives that might not have been lost under an alternate reality, in which politicians and policy makers made different decisions when they came to particular forks in the road. Here, as I considered the space between Kentucky and Tennessee, I saw yet another set of spaces open up between lines that had profound real-world implications. The more favorable lines represented Kentucky's brief embrace of a functional, if early and imperfect, health care reform. The less favorable lines represented Tennessee's perpetual rejection. The space between the good lines and the bad lines once again became the space of politics, brought to bear on the matter of people's bodies and lives.

These spaces once again represent ellipses between what was possible and what became real. The space that would have been filled upward, had Tennessee adopted the ACA or supported Governor Haslam's Insure Tennessee substitute, thereby leading to lower costs and better health outcomes. Or, conversely, the gap that began to close slowly downward in time, after Kentucky rejected the ACA in favor of Bevincare, a gap that would have closed even faster had any of the ill-fated Trump or GOP plans gone into effect in states like Kentucky that had seen improving outcomes under the ACA. This was because the "plans" put forth by Bevin, Trump, and the GOP may or may not have led to better health outcomes—but they indisputably would have done so by dramatically reducing the numbers of Americans with health insurance. As but one example, the CBO predicted that the coverage gap between the ACA and the first GOP health plan looked something like this:

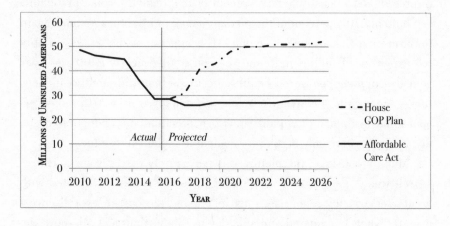

U.S. Census Bureau (actual); C.B.O. (projected)

Source: Congressional Budget Office, "H.R. 1628, American Health Care Act of 2017," May 24, 2017, retrieved from https://www.cbo.gov/publication/52752.

These spaces lay at the heart of the comparative arguments surrounding the Trump administration's troubled attempts at repealing and replacing the ACA. Critics of the ACA suggested that turning bad lines to good ones was not worth the cost. In the lead-up to the GOP's first attempt at repeal and replace, White House press secretary Sean Spicer repeatedly claimed that Trump's "marketplace solution" to health care would increase coverage and reduce cost "through negotiating with pharmaceutical companies and allowing competition over state lines." Trump himself, alongside joined by any number of straight-faced politicians, made the same argument, while suggesting that his health care solutions would tame the ACA's runaway costs. "With these actions we are moving toward lower costs and more options in the health care market," Trump announced in October 2017, while signing an executive order that scrapped ACA subsidies paid to health insurance companies to help cover out-of-pocket medical costs for low-income people, "and taking crucial steps toward saving the American people from the nightmare of Obamacare."[18]

These arguments, too, were patently false. Trump, Spicer, and others conveniently overlooked that Medicare, through its prescription drug benefit, already negotiated lower prices through private insurance companies that provided medicines to enrollees; in addition, the ACA already permitted insurance companies to compete across state lines. More broadly, the claims flew directly in the face of our data. Gutting Medicaid would surely decrease taxes for corporations and wealthy people. But those savings would come at potentially devastating costs to less affluent individuals and families living in expansion states such as Kentucky.[19]

The ACA was no panacea. High premiums, underinsurance, and high deductibles remained major issues in markets across the country. A joint poll by the *New York Times* and the Kaiser Family Foundation found that 20 percent of Americans under age sixty-five with health insurance still reported having problems paying their medical bills over roughly the same time frame as our data. Yet by comparison, 53 percent of people without insurance said the same.[20]

More importantly, research studies consistently showed Medicaid to be a cost-effective program for lower-income persons because it provided financial protections, increased rates of preventive screenings, and improved health. One 2015 study, plainly titled "Considering Whether Medicaid Is Worth the Cost," found that the benefit of providing Medicaid was "$62,000 per quality-adjusted life-year (QALY) gained" and that states that invested in Medicaid and its expansions saw an average net return of $68,000 per enrollee.[21]

The ACA also protected Americans from medical bankruptcies. Researchers estimate that over 60 percent of people who file for bankruptcy in the United States do so because they are unable to pay for medical costs due to a lack of health insurance or so-called underinsurance (insurance not sufficient to cover the costs of a major health incident). A 2009 study by a group of scholars in Boston, including a rising Harvard law professor named Elizabeth Warren, found that 62.1 percent of all US bankruptcies in 2007 were medical. Ninety-two percent of these medical debtors had medical bills over $5,000, or 10 percent of pretax family income, and the remainder met criteria for medical bankruptcy because they lost significant income due to illness or mortgaged a home to pay medical bills. Similarly, a 2013 insurance study found that over 35 million US adults had unpaid medical bills in collections, 17 million suffered lowered credit ratings due to high medical bills, and 15 million used up all of their savings to pay medical bills. Notably, research consistently showed that medical debt disproportionally affected persons with less than a college education and households that earn less than $50,000 per year—a warning sign for citizens of Kansas, whom we will meet in the following section of this book.[22]

Reduced personal earnings represented another potential cost of illness ameliorated by health insurance. The logic is straightforward: less insurance correlates with poorer health; poorer health correlates with fewer productive work years and more time off work due to illness or injuries.[23]

Ultimately, when it is all added up, the concerns about the ACA's cost yet again did not make sense when analyzed through the logic of life years, dollars, and cents. Politicians warned that expanded health care would take actual money out of the pockets of hardworking Americans in places like Tennessee or force them to pay for the ill-fated health decisions of others, when this was clearly not the case.

Moreover, this idea of cost also frequently assumed that health was fair and equitable—*I* pay what *I* owe, and *I* pay for the consequences of my own actions—and conveniently overlooked the deep unfairness of medical expenses. According to the World Health Organization, for instance, determinants of health largely result from community and communal factors in addition to individual ones:

> To a large extent, factors such as where we live, the state of our environment, genetics, our income and education level, and our relationships with friends and family all have considerable impacts on health . . . the

context of people's lives determine their health, and so blaming individuals for having poor health or crediting them for good health is inappropriate. Individuals are unlikely to be able to directly control many of the determinants of health.[24]

People often get sick despite their attempts to stay healthy. They get sick not because of their poor choices but because they happen to live near plastic factories or drink water tainted with lead, or because of radiation, global warming, or secondhand smoke. Yet this notion of health as a communal responsibility, a network, or an economy remained elusive in the dialogue of the white men in our groups and in the language of Donald Trump. Here, notions of cost sounded as if phrased through the Castle Doctrine, brought to bear on the castles of white bodies. *I smoke, I drink, I ride a motorbike without a helmet*, the logic implied, and *I alone reap the benefits and suffer the consequences. I am the master of my own autonomous house.*

Logics of cost made no sense in terms of dollars and cents. However, cost *did* seem to make sense as a metaphor, a symbol, or a proxy for talking about a much larger societal debt. Fear about money stood in for anxieties of connectedness in the contexts of health and illness. This coded language was spoken by politicians who were allowed to get away with false claims about health, as well as by white men with whom we spoke in Tennessee. In one example from our focus groups, white men believed that their costs rose due to the irresponsible actions of gangbangers, Mexicans, and minorities. But this logic completely overlooked that individual actions and health behaviors of white men might raise premiums for minority populations as well. Recognizing cost as such would have meant seeing the economy of health as a larger grid, or an inescapable net in which one person pulled and another person, many webbings away, moved.

Cost, in other words, functioned as a metaphor for concerns about a system that gravely threatened the sense of individualism underpinning particular white notions of health. This point is often overlooked by progressives who reflexively argue for government health care for all without taking account of the racial and historical intonations of federal health care networks in places like Tennessee. Here, seemingly self-evident arguments about communal well-being and shared risk engender specific forms of white anxiety. This was because, in our focus groups at least, cost connected everyone. Cost was an economy in which the well-being of white men always depended on the responsible actions of everyone else, including Mexicans and welfare queens. Debt in the context of health care suggested that, even though some owed more and some less, the health of white Americans was always and already beholden to others.

Again, this is not to suggest that health care is free, even in the best systems, or that we should build health care programs based on any type of racial resistance to joining social networks (as Trumpcare makes increasingly clear). Health care is expensive, and sometimes prohibitively so. Insuring more people adds to the expenditures of participating states, insurers, and the federal government. More wellness visits, mammograms, well-baby visits, chemotherapy, acute care, and other services mandated by the ACA inevitably cost money. And though the ACA and Medicaid expansion would have cost real money from *somewhere*, the dirty little secret of federally funded health care programs in states like Tennessee is that much of the actual expense would be borne by the taxes of . . . Northerners.

Were it truly a post-racial America, cost concerns might have raised certain existential questions about citizenship and responsibility: *What is life worth? What is our responsibility to each other? How can we balance individual behaviors and public wealth?* But in the real world, cost generated into a feedback loop that we recorded in some of our focus groups, where white Tennesseans used "cost" as a thinly veiled way to talk about race. Or as the politician, Christian minister, and political commentator Mike Huckabee put it: "We have a health care system that, if you're on Medicaid, you have unlimited access to health care, at unlimited levels, at no cost. No wonder it's running away."[25]

Yet the graphs suggest that expanded marketplace options yield competition rather than price-gouging and that investing in the health of everyone ultimately lowers a variety of costs for . . . everyone. People go to doctors sooner rather than in times of crisis. Healthy people buy into the system. Premiums for everyone begin to decline.

As a result, the shared financial burden that fell on individuals and families became relatively less in an expansion state than in a bordering non-expansion one. If, as Senator Orrin Hatch would poetically put it, Obamacare supporters represented the "stupidest, dumbass people," then these supporters in Kentucky were at least stupid enough to live longer lives with a bit more money in their bank accounts than their smarter, anti-Obamacare neighbors in Tennessee.[26]

Data thus suggested ways that rising tides of coverage buoyed everybody and in ways that promoted societies in which people felt more connected to each other rather than less so. As sociologists Tara McKay and Stefan Timmermans describe it in a landmark study, the ACA produced a series of intangibles that promoted "social cohesion" in communities that adopted the legislation, as well as positive health effects.[27]

Community investment thereby worked against the forces of structural racism that rendered the suffering of persons at the lower ends of the economic spectrum as uncovered and, all too often, invisible. Ralph Ellison described such suffering in the prologue to *Invisible Man* thus: "I am a man of substance, of flesh and bone, fiber and liquids—and I might even be said to possess a mind. I am invisible, understand, simply because people refuse to see me." The second-order social benefits of the ACA helped to "see" the unseen.[28]

But many white people continued to refuse to see. Tennessee refused to see the possibility and promise of change. Kentuckians, meanwhile, elected a governor whose primary message amounted to "If you are poor, I will take away your health care." Americans elected Donald Trump on a platform that openly aimed to wipe out gains seen in states like Kentucky and bring everyone down onto the graphs of Tennessee. "Repeal it, replace it," Trump shouted, "and get something great!"[29]

From economic or medical perspectives, these claims were made of little more than hot air. But from the perspective of race in America, they seemed all too familiar. Mirroring and amplifying the tensions of our groups, Trump essentially asked lower-income white people to choose less coverage and more suffering over a system that linked them to Mexicans, welfare queens, and . . . to healthier, longer lives. And we, as a nation, chose the bottom lines in the charts.

In so choosing, voters and politicians who claimed to bolster white privilege again turned whiteness into a statistically perilous category. Donald Trump and other leaders may have successfully appealed to long-held beliefs about white nationalism and supremacy. But the data suggests that the policies these politicians supported, and that their supporters voted for, effectively assured that white people, too, would pay more and suffer more and, ultimately, die more in the service of these larger ideals.

In other words, from a public health perspective at least, it seems more than possible that the policies and sentiments that aim to bolster the identity of whiteness also effectively turn whiteness itself into a heightened, perilous, and *ever-more-costly* category of risk.

PART 3

KANSAS

BENEATH THE SURFACE

I<small>T'S</small> A<small>UGUST</small> 2017, almost time for the school year to begin. The principal of a large Kansas public high school spares time for a quick interview in the fifteen minutes he has between meetings. He appears calm, and he walks into his office to meet me, in sharp contrast to the swarm of activity taking place throughout the building. Teachers busily organize their class-rooms. Students tack posters in the hallways, announcing upcoming rallies and events. Office staff scurry about. The energy is nervous, anticipatory, and seemingly all consuming. But the principal is unconsumed.

I make note of this as we begin our brief conversation. "You seem re-laxed," I say, "given all the commotion."

"Well, you know," he replies cheerfully, "I've been at this for a while."

The first part of our conversation details his plans for the coming se-mester and his thoughts about the future of the school.

But the mood shifts when the topic turns to politics.

"You know, this is always my favorite time of year," he says. "After the lull of summer, we're finally back in business. Everything starts again. I feel it, for sure.

"But these past years," he continues, "they've taken a toll on me, on lots of people. I went into this because I love Kansas schools. I just love what we do here. So many people feel ownership and pride."

He pauses. "But given the greatness of our schools . . . it's hard to understand, why have we stopped supporting them? If people only knew

191

the ways we've stopped supporting our schools. A principal's job used to be to provide vision. But now so much of what I do is shift money around. I take from here and put it there. Then I take from there and try to fill a gap somewhere else. Someday . . . this is going to catch up with us. . . . Probably already has."

I nod, not so much because I know the particular pressures he faces, but because I've heard these types of concerns before.

THERE'S NO PLACE LIKE HOME

KANSAS IS A state awash in nostalgia. Locals often talk about the *old* Kansas, the Kansas *we grew up with*, the land of yesteryear in which forward-looking citizens got along and got things done.

Perhaps it's the Oz effect. L. Frank Baum's 1900 classic novel *The Wonderful Wizard of Oz* and the iconic 1939 film adaptation imagined Dorothy's homesickness for black-and-white Kansas as the driving force behind her interactions with the strange Technicolor world of Oz. When the Scarecrow tells Dorothy that he "cannot understand why you should wish to leave this beautiful country and go back to the dry, gray place you call Kansas," she replies, "That is because you have no brains."[1]

Perhaps this nostalgia arises because many Kansas narratives are penned by Odysseus-style expatriates who, much like Dorothy, gain an appreciation for home through adventures in faraway lands. In his memoir, *One Soldier's Story*, Senator Bob Dole reflects that "I've often said that anyone who really wants to understand me has to go back to my hometown of Russell, Kansas—if not literally, then at least emotionally and culturally." For Dole, Russell represents the core of a hardworking, no-complaints ethos that served him well as a soldier and then as a politician. Similarly, Thomas Frank narrates his modern classic *What's the Matter with Kansas?*

from the perspective of a native son who moved to New York to pursue a career in publishing, only to return home as an adult.[2]

Or perhaps it's because Kansans perfected the art of what psychologists call *reaction-formation*, turning ennui-inducing endless plains and quiet cornfields into imaginary places of vibrant progress and rejuvenation. Postcards from the 1930s of a small mill town called Milford, Kansas, population 271 at the time, depicted a festive, cosmopolitan fountain of youth, while the slightly larger rail town of McPherson, with a 1940s-era population nearing 7,000, imagined covered wagons riding the plains into a booming industrial future.[3]

I, too, can't seem to shake my Kansas nostalgia.

After my father's military service, my family moved back to the Midwest. Our first home there was a ranch-style house in Shawnee Mission, a Kansas City suburb. My father was just starting out as a young doctor, and my mother went to school to become a psychologist, but we still had a backyard large enough for a full swing set and a makeshift baseball diamond. Blackberry bushes grew on the side of the house. For my brother's birthday party, my parents rented a horse named Buster to give neighborhood children rides around the yard.

In time, the house grew smaller and our family grew larger. Somewhere along the way, we moved into a more expansive turn-of-the-century house in Kansas City, Missouri. Our Missouri home was a mere two blocks from State Line Road, an innocuous-looking thoroughfare dividing the Kansas part of the city from the Missouri one. To the casual observer, State Line looks like any other road in any other town. But kids who grew up nearby knew the difference. The Missouri side of the road felt always unkempt. The Kansas side was cleaner. If you got a new bike, you wanted to ride it on the Kansas side, since the roads were smoother and better maintained. If you planned a summer party, you wanted to hold it in a park on the Kansas side as well, where you could count on well-mowed grass and clean facilities and bathrooms.

Then there were the schools. If you lived on the Missouri side, you grew tired of watching your friends move to Kansas around the time that they reached junior high. Everyone knew the reputation of Kansas public schools: excellent teachers, small class sizes, advanced curricula, and strong track records placing students into colleges. For these reasons, many parents felt a move to Kansas was worth the extra property and income taxes, which they viewed as an investment in their children.

The Missouri side suffered by comparison. Missouri public schools reeled under successive attempts to rectify deep racial inequities—the state had a larger African American population than did Kansas, and courts repeatedly found black districts underresourced and overcrowded. Through the 1970s and 1980s, plans for forced busing between black and white schools gave way to "optional" busing, which led to so-called inner-city magnet schools. These and other strategies proved effective means of integrating classrooms. But, as is often the case, integration came at a steep cost: the Kansas City school district experienced massive white and middle-class black flight that left it with a smaller tax base and chronic money shortages. Lower state taxes and generally poorer populations meant that the system was never quite able to right itself. Missouri parents who could afford to do so sent their kids to private school—in full disclosure, mine included—or moved elsewhere.[4]

Kansas became a frequent landing place for white flight. Its stronger tax base and significant state investments in education yielded significant results for student outcomes. Through the late 1990s, Kansas consistently ranked in the top ten states in the percentage of persons twenty-five years of age or older with high school diplomas, and in the top tier of midwestern states in percentages of persons with reading and writing proficiency, and with college degrees. Reading and math skills for Kansas fourth graders peaked in 2007 and 2008 at levels well above the national average. Kansas also boasted markedly low dropout rates.[5]

Nostalgia very often arises from false memory. What we see as homesickness or a desire to return to the old ways represents a state that psychologists might deem a post-childhood longing for an idealized time when things felt coherent; a time that may or may not ever have existed. Yet when I returned to Kansas over the summer and early fall of 2017 to research the final section of this book, life felt tangibly different from the Kansas I imagined from my youth. The roads were splattered with potholes. The collaborative, can-do attitude that propelled people across the flat land seemed replaced by resentment.[6]

I crossed the state or conducted phone interviews to speak with people from cities, including Goddard, Wichita, Olathe, Topeka, and Kansas City,

Kansas, about the effects of massive tax cuts and dramatic reductions to state services and school funding enacted by the conservative GOP governor and legislature. I sent queries to politicians, school boards, PTAs, and administrative leadership teams of public school systems and posted requests on education chat boards. I then interviewed parents, teachers, everyday citizens, and politicians in well-to-do enclaves like Prairie Village, a wealthy suburb of Kansas City. I also met with administrators in places like Wichita that had become "minority dominant" or moved toward greater racial and ethnic diversity because of the influx of immigrant families. For a week in the fall, I drove through rural parts of the state to speak with school board members in key districts. Thus my research in Kansas was spent not so much in support or focus groups but talking to people in offices, in their homes, or in cafés. I also spent ample time driving past successions of farms, strip malls, nouveau mansions flying the Stars and Stripes, and any number of cars with the same "Elect Jesus" bumper stickers.[7]

I wished to learn about the everyday experiences of living in a state in which backlash GOP-style austerity politics and steep budget cuts to state budgets, about which much more appears below, came to dominate daily life. Did Kansans experience affirmation of their political beliefs when they saw cuts play out? Or did ideology begin to change when cuts took aim at core issues that impacted schools and children?

Any number of people I met supported the budget cuts and did so with intonations of the ideologies I encountered in other states. "I'm so tired of the unnecessary spending from liberals, of the fake news," a Topeka politician told me. "I've heard that minority districts rent luxury party buses for football games, and there's tons of money they don't use." "I have concerns with how money is spent in these wasteful government ventures to support immigrants," one Olathe parent told me. "One of the main foundations of the Tea Party is less intrusion from government, more local control, local decisions. That's always something I've championed," added another. "Why should we pay for immigrants or for educating their kids when they take our jobs and don't even pay taxes?" was another familiar refrain— mirroring the language of increasingly vocal anti-immigrant politicians in the state.

Yet more than in any other state on my research quest, I found deep layers of buyer's remorse. "Kansas used to have such cachet," an architect from Shawnee Mission told me. "People wanted to live here because our state was progressive, highly educated, and clean. But now, I feel nothing but angry most of the time, angry for what's been done to our home."

"They are stealing money from everywhere they can," a retired postal worker from Prairie Village told me. "From kids. From our pensions. From our health care. From things we need. It's ridiculous."

"I don't know where the money is going," said an engineer from Kansas City, Kansas. "They said businesses would flock to Kansas, but clearly that hasn't happened. They said that more money in rich people's pockets would flow down—but those people are just keeping it and we are getting screwed."

"They never clean our streets anymore," was the refrain of a housewife from Goddard. "People are definitely feeling a change in the mood. We used to say, 'Move to Kansas, it's the greatest, it has all this great stuff.' Now . . . people have lost faith."

I particularly encountered these kinds of sentiments when I spoke to people about schools. "At first, I thought it must have been a mistake, like who would want to harm our great Kansas school system, right?" a parent from Topeka explained. "I even called the governor's office and said, 'Hey, this can't be right.' Boy, was I naive."

The more I spoke to people, researched the history, and dug into the data, the more I realized that these forms of inquietude were far from happenstance and anything but random. Rather—as was the case with gun expansion in Missouri and health care rejection in Tennessee—they reflected policies conceived, passed, and enacted by politicians that many of these same Kansans once supported.

THE KANSAS EXPERIMENT

THE SUMMER AND fall of 2017 felt like a particularly spirited time to do research about public education and budget cuts in Kansas. The state went hard for Trump in the 2016 presidential election, and many administration policies and priorities had begun to take shape. Key among these agenda items were the stirrings of tax reform that led to the so-called Tax Cuts and Jobs Act of 2017, which President Trump signed into law in December of that year. Among other actions, the 2017 GOP bill slashed tax rates for many types of businesses, limited deductions, eliminated alternative minimum taxes paid by corporations, cut estate taxes—and also repealed the individual mandate of the ACA. The bill gifted permanent tax cuts to the wealthiest Americans and provided temporary relief for everyone else.

Though jarring to much of the country, these kinds of actions were far from unfamiliar in the Sunflower State. In large part thanks to the controversial leadership of Governor Sam Brownback and his rightist GOP administration, Kansas was in many ways the godfather of governance via tax cutting, pro-corporate, austerity economics. Kansas became the object lesson in the broad effects of massive-tax-cut governance as a result.

Kansans inaugurated Brownback as the state's forty-sixth governor in January 2011. A onetime member of the House of Representatives and the Senate, Brownback gained a reputation as a social and fiscal conservative who was willing to reach across the aisle. Between 2001 and 2003, he joined forces with California senator Dianne Feinstein to support bipartisan legislation aimed at improving the treatment of unaccompanied immigrant and alien minors. And in 2005, Brownback cosponsored a bill authored by Senators Ted Kennedy and John McCain that aimed to create a path to citizenship for illegal immigrants already living in the United States.

However, as a gubernatorial candidate, Brownback played to resentment of government overreach that had simmered in Kansas for decades before bubbling over after the election of President Barack Obama in 2008. Brownback based his candidacy on a sense of frustration that government had gone too far in regulating, taxing, and ultimately limiting people's abilities to get ahead. As governor, Brownback then became the front man for a backlash conservative takeover unlike any other. With the backing of wealthy benefactors in the state, including the billionaire libertarian Koch brothers of Wichita and their far-reaching networks of influence, along with the support of the Tea Party, Brownback launched an agenda that aimed to prove, once and for all, that the best way to achieve prosperity was by eliminating government from people's lives. At its core lay a philosophy of supply-side economics that argued that tax cuts on wealthy people and corporations paid for themselves by boosting economic growth for everyone.[1]

What followed was a state of affairs that would later derisively be called *austerity fever*. As the *New Republic* described it, "Brownback established an Office of the Repealer to take a scythe to regulations on business, he slashed spending on the poor by tightening welfare requirements . . . and he dissolved four state agencies and eliminated 2,000 state jobs." The administration also rolled back anti-discrimination laws, signed three anti-abortion bills, and tried to eliminate the Kansas Arts Commission by executive order—all in the first year in office.[2]

Brownback next vetoed the expansion of Medicaid coverage under the Affordable Care Act, even after state lawmakers in his own party voted to support the expansion. In August 2011, Brownback announced he was "sending back" a $31.5 million grant from the US Department of Health and Human Services to set up an insurance exchange as part of ACA. Governor Brownback also received an A-plus rating from the NRA after signing a series of "pro-gun" bills into law, including legislation that allowed Kansans to carry concealed firearms in public without permits and entitled students, staff, and professors to carry firearms into classrooms, meetings, fraternity parties, and other sites in colleges and universities. In other words, the Brownback administration put Kansas on trajectories similar to those seen in Tennessee and Missouri. But Brownback did much, much more.[3]

To considerable fanfare, Brownback touted Kansas as a "real live experiment" in the everyday effects of austerity politics—language starkly reminiscent of questions about whether more guns led to less crime in Missouri or whether the health of people in Tennessee improved with health insurance. Recall, for instance, that the *New York Times* described Missouri as a "natural experiment in what happens when a state relaxes its gun control laws," while the *Wall Street Journal* once called TennCare the "Tennessee Experiment."[4]

Brownback's Kansas experiment involved an epic defunding of state government. In 2012, he signed Kansas Senate Bill Substitute HB 2117 into law, enacting one of the largest income tax cuts in state history. The cuts particularly eased the tax burden on wealthy Kansans: the rate for the top bracket fell from 6.45 percent to 3.9 percent, and Brownback promised to eventually reduce it to zero. In real terms, HB 2117 reduced taxes on top brackets by 25 percent. The bill also eliminated income taxes for nearly 200,000 businesses and landowners.

The Brownback administration argued that HB 2117 would provide tax "relief"—to the tune of $231 million after one year, and $934 million after six—as stimulus for flourishing. The administration frequently boasted that the "march to zero income taxes" would catalyze entrepreneurship and job creation at the rate of "25,000 new jobs per year," while at the same time lowering unemployment and increasing construction and development.[5]

Next, Brownback signed a controversial school finance bill, HB 2506, which created tax breaks for corporations that donated to private school scholarship funds, allowed public school districts to hire unlicensed teachers for science and math classes, cut support for at-risk students, and made it easier for schools to fire experienced teachers. HB 2506 further defunded government by supplementing these changes with significant cuts to property taxes. "This is a win for Kansas students," Brownback said at the time. "This is a win for parents. . . . And it's a win for property taxpayers."[6]

The governor couched these developments in lofty terms. In an op-ed penned for the *Wall Street Journal*, Brownback described the Kansas brand of austerity as "a choice between dependence and self-reliance, between intrusion and freedom," while claiming that "economic policy in Kansas . . . means the American Midwest is fulfilling the dream of a Midwest renaissance in America."[7]

But reality turned out to be less than dreamy for many Kansans. It turned out that, contrary to hyperbolic reports of government waste, the state had frequently used tax revenue to pay for roads, bridges, traffic lights, aqueducts, conduits, and causeways—structures often supported by communal governance, and for which wealthy persons who receive tax breaks do not often clamor to invest their surplus funds. Tax revenue also secured the fiscal reputation of the state, enabling the various lending and borrowing vital to a functioning economy.

Cuts to infrastructure became increasingly apparent. Kansas fell below national averages on a wide range of public services, including public transit, housing, and police and fire protection. The American Society of Civil Engineers gave Kansas an overall grade of C-minus on its 2013 infrastructure report card. The report further detailed that "bridges were awarded a D-plus, in part due to Kansas's nearly 3,000 structurally deficient bridges. Only five states have more structurally deficient bridges than Kansas" and that "dams earned the lowest grade of a D-minus. . . . With 6,087 dams, Kansas has the second most dams in the United States next only to Texas. Of the state's dams, 230 are classified as high hazard, meaning failure would likely lead to loss of life and significant property damage." According to the report, these and other low grades resulted primarily from "funding gaps" that delayed upkeep and repair.[8]

Brownback raided Kansas Department of Transportation (KDOT) funding to shore up sagging budgets in the state general fund and other state agencies. In 2015, road repairs fell from 1,200 miles of road per year to a paltry 200—meaning that only the most badly damaged stretches of highway saw attention and that the state hired fewer road workers. "Kansas Will Pay the Price for Diverting Money from Highway Fund," warned a headline in the *Kansas City Star*. *Slate* reported that

since 2011 . . . the state has diverted more than $1 billion in "extraordinary" transfers from KDOT. If you include "routine" transfers, from 2011

through the 2017 budget year the total diversion from the Bank of KDOT
will amount to more than $2 billion. That's more than KDOT's annual
expenditures. It's as if the state, which has the fourth largest number
of public road miles in the nation, had taken away a full year of road
funding.

In response to the increasing shortfalls, KDOT issued a record-setting
$400 million highway construction bond issue. In other words, austerity
forced Kansas to borrow ever-more money from itself.[9]

Meanwhile, the state economy imploded. Tax cuts seemed to bring
out the worst in people, often by placing individual wealth management
ahead of communal good. Growing numbers of people declared themselves
"businesses" in order to pay zero income tax. Rates on the wealthiest citizens fell ever lower, and the wealthy in any case found new ways to game
the system. Several small-business owners told me how large corporations bought up hundreds of "small businesses" in order to lower their tax
obligations.

Growing evidence suggested that these and other actions opened a
staggering loss in revenue. Kansas lost $687 million, or nearly 11 percent
of the state budget, in the first year after the cuts began. By June 2014, the
Kansas treasury fell nearly $300 million short of its projected tax collec-
tions. Moody's downgraded the state's bond rating from AA1 to AA2. Standard & Poor's followed suit and downgraded the state credit rating from
AA+ to AA due to a budget that analysts described as "not structurally
balanced." These developments increased the state's borrowing costs and
further enlarged its deficit. Fiscal year 2015 ended with a budget shortfall
of nearly $800 million. The state began to draw down on its general funds.
Fiscal year 2016 alone saw a budget gap of over $60 million, and the defi-
cit hit $280 million in 2017.[10]

All the while, the benefits of austerity for middle- and lower-income
Kansans grew ever-more difficult to discern. Some small-business owners
decried the ways that Brownback's tax cuts yielded no real relief because
their untaxed profits simply reduced the deductions they were allowed to
take, thus increasing the amounts they owed on federal returns. Many lo-
calities raised sales taxes to offset cuts in state funding. Critics claimed
that the only tax cuts with real effect were those that relieved burdens on
the wealthiest Kansans.[11]

The promised hiring boom never materialized either. Brownback claimed in 2012 that the tax cuts would act as a "shot of adrenaline" for the Kansas economy, spurring job growth in ways that allowed business owners to reinvest their tax savings into their companies. But the cuts acted more like a shot of barbiturate. Kansas added only 29,000 "non-farm" jobs in the two years after the tax cuts took effect—by contrast, Nebraska, an economically similar state with a much smaller labor force, saw a net increase of 35,000 jobs. Kansas began to actually lose jobs in mid-2015; in 2016, Kansas ranked forty-sixth among all states in private sector job growth.[12]

Brownback's support plummeted. According to a survey by the Morning Consult polling firm, Brownback was the single most unpopular governor in the entire United States in 2016, with a 65 percent disapproval rating. A Topeka food server named Chloe Hough, who was serving the governor and his family in a local restaurant, made international news when she crossed out the tip section of his bill and penned in "Tip the schools" instead.[13]

So it was with a bit of irony that, after the presidential election of 2016, conservative politicians touted the "Kansas model" of massive tax and spending cuts as a preview of Trump's economic plans for the nation. It seemed more likely that Kansas warned the nation, ominously, of what was to come. Kansas, the land of Oz, had become a national parable warning of the downside of American austerity economics. *Bloomberg News* summarized: "The Kansas supply-side experiment unravels . . . tax cuts were supposed to spur growth, boost revenue and create jobs. The results were the exact opposite." *Forbes* detailed how "the great Kansas tax cut experiment crashes and burns."[14]

In other words, Kansas more likely presaged fiscal realities that would slowly beset the nation after enactment of the GOP tax bill of 2017 as promises of gold-paved roads for everyone led instead to enhanced income disparity that benefited only a select few. "Taxpayers, You've Been Scammed," read a *Times* headline in 2018, above an op-ed detailing how "the wealthy are giving themselves a big gift, and sending the bill to the middle class."[15]

Then there were the schools. Once the state's pride and joy, Kansas schools were beacons of promise for which my friends' parents uprooted their families, moved, and paid more taxes so that their children would have the chance to get ahead. While running for office in 2010, then candidate Brownback positioned himself as a pro-education centrist who emphasized investing in schools across the state while assuring that "education funding goes to the classroom, not to the administration or the courtrooms." This language mirrored bipartisan initiatives that aimed to assure that sixty-five cents of every education dollar were spent on students and teachers.[16]

Yet education quickly became a target when Governor Brownback took office. The first rounds of tax cuts eliminated about $200 million in education spending—the largest reduction in the state's history. Brownback also changed the school financing formula at the expense of poorer, urban districts. The National Education Association produced a report showing how base state aid per pupil (BSAPP) in Kansas dropped from $4,400 to $3,800, even as enrollment and the costs of health insurance increased for many districts. Further gutting followed subsequent cuts, which led to larger class sizes, rising fees for kindergarten, the elimination of arts programs, and layoffs in every corner of the education system. Procrustean reductions also hit state colleges and universities.[17]

Brownback was not done. In early 2015, he signed a new law that replaced the state's education funding formula with two years of block grants—a strategy later championed by controversial US secretary of education Betsy DeVos. A report in the *Guardian* detailed how budget shortfalls led Brownback to take the highly unusual step of cutting funding to education budgets midyear, thereby pushing Kansas schools to eliminate education programs and shorten school years. "Twin Valley schools, which serves 590 students, is shutting down on Friday, 12 days before it was supposed to end the school year," the *Guardian* detailed. "McClouth, which serves about 500 students, and Concordia schools, which serves about 1,000 students, will close on 15 May instead of 21 May."[18]

In 2016, the Kansas school system again made national headlines when the state Supreme Court set a June 30 deadline to fix its system of financing public schools or face a court-ordered shutdown before the next school year began. The court ruled that the Republican-dominated legislature had not abided by its constitutional mandate to finance public schools equitably: "The legislature's unsuccessful attempts to equitably, i.e., fairly, allocate resources among the school districts not only creates uncertainty in planning the 2016–2017 school year but also has the potential to interrupt the operation of Kansas' public schools."[19]

Many Kansas schools fought to maintain prior levels of excellence for the first years of the austerity famine. A report by the Kansas Association of School Boards (KASB) found that, while "educational spending is a strong predictor of student achievement" and "the amount of spending is more important than the percent spent on instruction," Kansas schools nonetheless defied predictions. "Kansas spends below the national average," the report concluded, "but has outcomes well above the national average. Kansas has better student outcomes than predicted based on the total revenue per pupil, current spending per pupil, and spending on instruction per pupil."[20]

Budget cuts forced school administrators to go beyond belt-tightening into dismantling education programming. "My district has been forced to cut one million dollars a year," the superintendent of a district in southern Kansas told me. "One million dollars. At first, we cut lunch options; but now we're cutting teachers, after-school programs, even whole topics from our curriculum."

By 2015, according to KASB reports, "Kansas graduation rates have generally been rising at a slower pace than the national average and peer states," while fourth- and eighth-grade reading and math skills fell to the extent that "Kansas could expect further declines in national achievement rankings if corrective action is not taken."[21]

Then things got really bad.

INTERVIEW:

A DOWNWARD CYCLE

Interview excerpts, August 17, 2017, Topeka, public high school finance officer

JMM: It seems like the budget cuts have had different effects on students and families depending on where they started out, financially.

AD14: Yeah, well, maybe at first. We did away with a lot of deductions and credits for poor families over the past two years. And then we came back in 2015, and we didn't have the money to pay the bills in the state. So then we raised the sales tax, we raised the cigarette tax, we did away with itemized deductions.

We look at the cumulative impact of those three tax changes . . . chunks of tax changes. And the poorest 40 percent of Kansans saw an average net tax increase. The poorest 40 percent. They saw their taxes go *up* as a result of this. Whereas the wealthiest 5, 10, 15 percent saw just overwhelming reductions as a result. . . . The wealthiest in Kansas saw [tax] reductions, and that was all fine and good up until the point where their schools started sucking, they were having their children shoved into classrooms with thirty other kids. Tuition is going up pretty substantially in the state for all kinds of ed.

Also, projects are no longer getting funded for key infrastructure pieces throughout the state. And so those things started to mount up. Where overwhelmingly you had these small-business owners from around the state march to the capitol last year saying, "Put us back on the payroll. This is absurd. Our schools matter. Our quality of life matters. We can't afford to go down this path."

JMM: What do you think this might all mean, long-term?

AD14: You know, it's . . . you think of where Kansas growth has occurred, it needs an educated workforce. You know, the old farming days, or go work at Delco Battery for a couple generations—those types of jobs are gone. The aviation industry is really struggling . . . [the] single largest employer in the state of Kansas [is facing a] huge bubble of retirements, and there's nobody to backfill those jobs. So it's, you know, it's a little bit of that downward cycle, and unless we do something to yank ourselves up out of it pretty quick, it's going to be hard for Kansas.

AUSTERITY

OW DID POLITICIANS convince citizens to go along with a financial plan that benefited so few people and caused so much pain? After all, the recession of 2008 represented the economic nadir for many Americans—and indeed, for many school systems. Four years later, stimulus packages and an array of important regulations stemmed the tide of panic in many—though certainly not all—sectors of the economy and parts of the country. Federal stimulus offered money for new transit projects, job opportunities, and health, education, and energy infrastructures. Things were looking up.[1]

In response to these seemingly encouraging developments, Kansans empowered a governor and a legislature whose agendas sat in direct opposition to the Obama administration's plans for economic recovery. The new governor oversaw disinvestment in his state's support networks, while at the same time rejecting federal stimulus funds. And he implemented a series of austerity measures that would seem to make more sense, politics aside, in times of crisis or scarcity, but not when the economy was on the upswing.

During the dark days of World War II, for instance, the British government enacted austerity policies that limited use of nonessential resources. Self-denial emerged in this context as a communal form of patriotism. When the war ended, so did the austerity: by the mid-1950s, wine flowed, shelves were restocked, and people ate, drank, and loved to their hearts' content. Similarly, modern-day austerity efforts emerge in the wake of financial turmoil and attempts to reduce structural budget deficits in places like Greece, where government debt and obligations grew beyond control.[2]

All of which makes modern-day American tax cutting and austerity politics a bit harder to figure out. To be sure, economists and citizens voice valid concerns about governmental debt and national overspending (though these concerns seem to have evaporated for GOP politicians during the debate around the 2017 tax bill). Yet US austerity politics often emerge when money remains in people's bank accounts and resources flow through the system, as if preaching a starvation diet when the stores are full of grain. In this sense, US austerity arguments do not so much ask citizens to buckle down in the name of national unity as to reallocate resources from the many to the few.

After the GOP tax bill passed in 2017, sociologist Isaac Martin penned a column in the *New York Times* titled "How Republicans Learned to Sell Tax Cuts for the Rich," in which he lay the answer in good marketing, a rejection of expertise, and the corrupted populism of Andrew Mellon. Mellon found a way to convince the American masses of the faulty proposition that "cutting income tax rates would actually increase tax revenues. In particular, he said, cutting the top income tax rates would encourage rich people to pull their money out of tax shelters and invest in creating jobs."[3]

This idiosyncratic notion of austerity also emerged from dogmatic and largely debunked economic theory. In the 1930s, influential British economist John Maynard Keynes famously argued "the boom, not the slump, is the right time for austerity at the Treasury." This logic took hold in conservative US economic circles along with an unswerving belief that the best way to enact austerity was to shrink government. Economist Arthur Laffer and political advocate Grover Norquist became chief proponents—Laffer sold Ronald Reagan on the notion that tax cuts led to economic prosperity and became a key advisor for Brownback. But as economist Paul Krugman bluntly puts it, data shows that this argument is "manifestly not true."[4]

Among other problems, taking away resources during boom times can lead people to notice the absence of feelings of security during what should otherwise be times of flourishing. Convincing people to "do more with less" when there is otherwise more sometimes also depends on suggesting that groups other than one's own are getting free rides while your group toils in the fields.[5]

This leads to another tension driving American austerity politics: its connections to, and implications for, race and racism. A long literature details relationships between tax cuts, austerity, and race. In the US context, much of this work highlights how tax cuts disproportionately benefit rich white males at the expense of other groups of people in society. Tax cuts also lead to shortfalls in government services and programs that frequently assist women and minorities. Persons on government assistance, undocumented immigrants, and single mothers receiving child support are just a few of the groups who live and work in economies where income is largely fixed and thus unaffected by reduced tax rates.[6]

Cuts to social programs affect many working-class white populations as well and in ways that have long vexed liberals and Democratic politicians—since many poor white populations continue to support GOP tax cuts. In a brilliant analysis of this phenomenon, journalist Gary Younge details a complex dynamic in which poor white populations vote for politicians who enact cuts to government spending out of a combination of anger that the government is wasting money on "people who do not deserve it," alongside guilt that they themselves need help. For Younge, this leads to any number of contradictory interactions reflective of ones I've described in this book:

> In Las Vegas shortly before the 2010 mid-terms I met a woman protesting illegal immigration outside an Obama event who was voting for the tea party candidate Sharon Angle. When it turned out she didn't have health care I asked her if that wouldn't be a reason for her to support Obama. "I haven't really gotten into the whole Obamacare thing," she said. "To be honest I can't even think about that right now. I'm so concentrated on the illegals."

Similarly, writer J. D. Vance, author of the widely acclaimed book *Hillbilly Elegy*, wrote a column after the 2016 presidential election titled "How Donald Trump Seduced America's White Working Class," detailing how GOP tax cuts often come packaged in messages of restored "greatness" and "learned helplessness" whose emotional content supersedes any fiscal details.[7]

Similar dynamics played out in Kansas. The austerity experiment tilted the economic hierarchy further in favor of already-wealthy persons. Disadvantaged populations, such as minority groups, low-income persons, and the elderly, carried more of the burden. The racial and socioeconomic divisions that emerged from this manipulation could not have been clearer.

For instance, a nonprofit group called the Kansas Center for Economic Growth culled data from multiple sources for the first four years after the 2012 tax cuts. The group's report, "Kansas' Tax Plan Makes Racial Economic Disparities Worse," illustrated the extent to which the cuts exacerbated racial wealth disparities. The data showed that the 2012 tax cuts deceptively increased taxes on the bottom 40 percent of earners in Kansas, or those earning $42,000 a year or less, by hiking sales taxes and eliminating tax credits that benefited low-income families. Such trends disproportionately affected minority communities, including 75 percent of African American and 83 percent of Latino households in the state. By contrast, according to the report, "Kansans who saw the biggest tax cut are mostly white. Indeed, the rate of white Kansans in the top tier of earners is two to three times that of black and Latinos in the highest earning tier." Laid out visually, the findings looked like this:[8]

Kansans of Color are More Likely to be in Income Groups Negatively Affected by Tax Plan

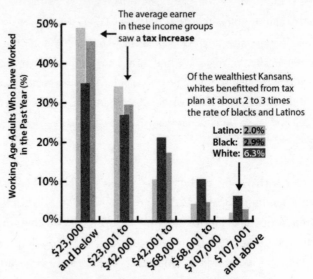

Source: 2014 American Community Survey Public Use Microdata (PUMS), total individual earnings for working age adults (ages 18-64) who have worked in the past year.

Source: "Kansas' Tax Plan Makes Racial Economic Disparities Worse," Kansas Center for Economic Growth, October 14, 2016, retrieved from http://realprosperityks.com /kansas-tax-plan-makes-racial-economic-disparities-worse. Reproduced with permission.

The Kansas Center for Economic Growth report was just one example of an emerging body of evidence suggesting that the Brownback tax cut experiment did little to raise the fortunes of all Kansans or model a new approach to egalitarianism and distributive justice. Rather, the Kansas experiment reinforced existing racial inequities under the cover of economic progress.[9]

Nowhere were problems of inequity more apparent than in public schools. Education budgets became prime targets for agendas that saw starving government functions as the path to prosperity. Partisan agendas promoted attacks on school funding that often centered on emotionally resonant claims of fiscal waste, claimed that public schools mishandled funds, or argued that tax dollars went into the pockets of administrators rather than into classrooms.

In both blatant and invisible ways, the Brownback school budget formulas then exacerbated divides between well-off and poor districts and classrooms. Prior to Brownback, Kansas funded K–12 public schools through formulas that combined payments based on the number of pupils in a district's schools with what were called *weightings*, or extra monies sent to schools that taught immigrant, poor, and at-risk students. This system was set up to fulfill a mandate in the state constitution guaranteeing adequate education for all school-aged children.

The Brownback regime upended this emphasis on fair distribution through a block-grant system that froze funding levels and rewarded investment in private schools. Aid dropped by over $600 per pupil statewide, and the shift hit poorer school systems the hardest. Budget cuts further devastated programs that helped minority, immigrant, and low-income children catch up. "Because of the budget cuts, frozen budgets, we've had to eliminate almost all of our extended learning time," Alan Cunningham, superintendent of Dodge City Public Schools, a district where the first language of a majority of students was not English, told the *New York Times*. "Those kids are not able to get the time they need to learn the things that they need to learn to be successful."[10]

Educational disparities became so extreme that the Kansas Supreme Court intervened. Five years into the tax-cut experiment, the court ruled that the state failed to adequately fund public schools by hundreds of millions of dollars per year and that the cuts and revised formulas disproportionately harmed minority, low-income, and immigrant children the most. "We conclude the state's public financing system, through its structure and implementation, is not reasonably calculated to have all Kansas public education students meet or exceed the minimum constitutional standards of adequacy," the court opined. The ruling explicitly highlighted how the state system failed to prepare over 25 percent of students in basic reading and math skills and shortchanged half of the state's African American students and one-third of its Hispanic students.[11]

The Kansas Supreme Court ruling highlighted just how methodically the Kansas experiment amplified and exacerbated racial and economic disparities. Minority and low-income families regressively payed more taxes and sent their children to worsening schools. All the while, the tax cuts bestowed savings to the well-off—including to lawmakers themselves. Reports later revealed that "nearly 70 percent of Kansas lawmakers or their spouses" owned a business or property that allowed them to benefit from paying no state tax on business income. Beneficiaries included Brownback and his wife, who, as it turned out, owned for-profit farmlands and shares in investment portfolio companies that managed the accounts of some of the wealthiest families in Kansas.[12]

Were the yawning racial and economic disparities that resulted from the Brownback legislation intended outcomes of the Kansas experiment? In 2015, Brownback's office supported a plan to upend a long-standing formula that helped assure equal funding for minority and low-income schools and classrooms by taking a swipe at the state's growing immigrant population. Brownback's deputy communications director wrote in an e-mail sent to supporters that replacing "equalization payments" ensured that "our educational system is not held hostage by a formula that punishes school districts for things that are out of their control, including *changing demographics* [emphasis added]."[13]

Meanwhile, every so often, politicians in the GOP orbit would utter racist comments in official settings. In 2013, a county commissioner in Saline County, Kansas, named Jim Gile told a meeting of local officials that the county should hire an architect to fix its Road and Bridge Department building instead of "n—rigging it." When asked by an attendee to clarify, Gile was exceptionally clear about his meaning: "Afro-Americanized." (The furor that erupted presaged a controversy from 2018, when Representative Steve Alford, a lawmaker from Ulysses, Kansas, told legislators that blacks had worse responses to marijuana than did whites because of their "character makeup, their genetics.")[14]

The Kansas GOP often denounced these types of instances (although this did not stop Gile from being reelected). But racial animus has a long history in Kansas politics. For instance, the Koch family, Brownback's main benefactors, once supported the right-wing John Birch Society during its active campaigns against the civil rights movement. Among myriad other actions, "Birchers" attacked Martin Luther King Jr. and Rosa Parks (and countless others) as communists. In the 1960s, the Birch Society sponsored billboards across Kansas calling for the impeachment of Earl Warren, the chief justice of the US Supreme Court, who had ordered the desegregation of the public schools. Critics saw echoes of Bircherism in Brownback's school legislation. Marcel Harmon, vice president of the board of education in Lawrence, wrote in *Salon* that Brownback's push toward block grants rested on the "ultraconservative" notion that, as Harmon sarcastically put it, schools could then "afford the opportunity to avoid wasting everyone's time teaching things like evolution, climate change, social justice, institutional racism or sex education."[15]

The Brownback era also provided cover for emerging anti-government, anti-immigrant politicians who would push Kansas ever-further rightward. In 2011, Brownback signed anti-Muslim legislation that prohibited local courts from "relying on Sharia law"—even though there was no evidence that a single Kansas court had ever done so. The legislation passed after Robert Spencer and Pamela Geller, cofounders of a hate group called Stop Islamization of America, urged their supporters to flood Brownback's Twitter and "jam his phones" with strong support for the bill.[16]

In 2015, Brownback issued an executive order preventing any state department or agency from assisting the relocation of refugees from other countries in Kansas. In support of the order, the governor cited alleged arrests of refugees with ties to terrorism, as well as alleged terror plots aimed at the state of Kansas. But the 2015 order also conveniently provided a way to ease the spending burdens of the state, mainly by displacing the spending away from the most vulnerable populations. Meanwhile, Kansas Tea Party congressman Tim Huelskamp, who represented the First Congressional District during much of Brownback's tenure in office, emerged as a leader of the so-called House Freedom Caucus, whose initial priorities included ending programs that aided immigrants—such as the Deferred Action for Childhood Arrivals (DACA) program and the Deferred Action for Parents of Americans and Lawful Permanent Residents (DAPA).[17]

The Brownback era also brought to power a secretary of state named Kris Kobach, who would gain national prominence for his hard-line views on immigration, voter ID laws, and the need for a so-called Muslim registry. Kobach rode a wave of white resentment against the state's changing demographics—the percentage of white citizens of the state grew in aggregate numbers but declined by percentage between 2010 and 2014, while the state's Hispanic population increased by almost two-tenths of a percent each year over this same time period. Kobach ran on a platform that promised to crack down on voter fraud in Kansas, specifically through creating a voter ID law and purging ineligible voters from electoral lists. He then followed up on these promises by crafting a law that prohibited 18,000 Kansans from using their ballots. Claims of voter intimidation then followed when it was revealed that in Kansas in 2014, 78 percent of white residents, 67 percent of black residents, 52 percent of Asian residents, but only 38 percent of Hispanic/Latino residents in Kansas were registered to vote. Reports also later revealed that Kobach worked as a lawyer for the Federation for American Immigration Reform (FAIR)—an organization categorized by the Southern Poverty Law Center (SPLC) as a hate group—and was criticized by SPLC for attending a conference sponsored by a white nationalist organization. Kobach denied the characterization, calling the SPLC "unethical smear artists."[18]

None of this is to suggest that all GOP politicians were driven solely by racial concerns or even that racism or xenophobia were the main drivers of the Brownback agenda. Many leaders with whom I spoke seemed genuinely to wish for less government in people's lives and believed this to be the best way to jump-start the economy. At the same time, tax cuts and the school-funding overhaul allowed Kansas GOP politicians to enact an agenda with significant racial implications without expressly needing to talk about race. Instead, the discourse favored by conservatives used seemingly neutral, action-oriented descriptors such as economic "empowerment" and parental "choice." In an ominous preview of policies that would soon be promoted at the national level by Betsy DeVos, the block-grant funding limited the state's ability to shore up schools serving historically vulnerable populations.

So, too, overt concerns about whiteness under attack seemed to come up less frequently in my discussions about tax cuts and schools with every-day Kansans than they did in my interviews about guns and health care in Missouri and Tennessee. In part, this reflected a sampling issue—I came to Kansas six years after Brownback's election and the start of the ill-fated experiment, while the health care debate was ongoing when I visited Tennessee. Further, racial anxieties did not seem to be the main ways that many people talked about economic issues. Many Kansans with whom I spoke supported policies that they believed would make their lives easier, better, and more prosperous—in other words, the same messages that Brownback promoted with his visions of a midwestern renaissance. This branding was particularly resonant in the wake of the 2008 recession that hit small-business owners in Kansas particularly hard.

Yet, here as well, the motivations of voters were ultimately less important than the actual consequences of their votes. The conservative white voters who comprised the majority of Brownback's base elected a politician who implemented a series of policies that, at their core, limited social mobility. Brownback's version of backlash austerity concentrated wealth at the top of the social pyramid while starving the main conduits through which immigrant, minority, and poor communities mobilized upward. This form of anything-but-experimental austerity ensured that people at the top remained there and people at the bottom were forever looking up. Austerity codified hierarchy: the rich got richer, and instead of promoting largesse, tax "relief" made sure that the system that assured their dominance remained ever-more inevitably in place.[19]

As we now turn to explore, it thus makes sense why schools became central battlegrounds and symbols for the Brownback agenda. Schools represented the promise of future betterment and upward mobility for minority and low-income Kansans. Kansas schools also symbolized far larger, national debates about American equality and investment. Much like guns conveyed particular meanings about security in Missouri and health care networks connoted anxieties about cost in Tennessee, schools and infrastructure tapped into particular historical tensions about equal opportunity in Kansas. Defunding public schools in Kansas, the home of

Brown v. Board, thus carried profound unspoken resonance. This history suggests another reason why white Kansans supported economic and fiscal agendas that offered most of them little in the way of material returns.

In another similarity to Missouri and Tennessee, the Kansas brand of backlash austerity soon revealed itself as a Faustian bargain. Well-off white populations may have gained a sense of privilege along with unimaginable financial gain within a rapidly changing world, but spending so much capital on a system that limited mobility and integration boomeranged for middle- and lower-income white populations, and particularly for white families who sent their kids to public schools.

The lens of schools makes it ever-more clear just how much backlash austerity came at a cost paid by everyday Kansans—and often middle- and lower-income white Kansans—who saw communal resources once spent bettering their lives now invested in the communal project of assuring upstream concentrations of wealth and downstream concentrations of despair. Ultimately, the recoil affected Kansas children, including children of many parents who supported the austerity agenda in the first place. These children grew up never fully realizing the extent to which an economic famine voted in by their parents famished their own skill sets and future prospects as well.

INTERVIEW:

A BAD RAP

PA 29: Well, I'll tell you what. Brownback and the cuts have gotten a bad rap because of fake news and the liberal media. And also, what's happened here just reaffirmed what I've always thought about small government being better. And you know, I will add local control to that. Yet there's issues with local control too, but we do the best we can. But yes, absolutely. That's one of the main foundations of the Republican Party is less intrusion from government, more local control, local decisions.

    I have met the Brownback family, and I know some of them personally. And they're a lovely family, and I know most people would probably agree with me on that. They are good to the core. . . . I know Brownback has been in prayer before votes and before important decisions that he's had to make, and you know, he tries to do what he believes is the best thing.

JMM: When you say small government, I think I know what that means as a platform, but what does small government mean in real life?

PA 29: That's a good question. Let me just give you an example. I know that Kansas devotes over 50 percent of its budget to K–12 education. That ranks as one of the highest states that give the highest amount of our general fund to K–12 education in the nation. And I think the more that is demanded

219

from taxpayers and our government to present more and more
funds, and more and more funds, and then it just seems like
they have more, I don't know, the more government is funding something, the more hands and fingers that go into that
money. And it's not always the best way, in my opinion. The
other player is we have a very strong liberal media, the *Kansas City Star*, namely. I think I have seen one positive article
published about Brownback in his, what, seven years in office now? And lots of fake news. I've actually been kind of
shocked by the influence of the media.

JMM: Why do you think schools are such a charged issue?

PA 29: Well, we absolutely want to make sure that our kids get the
best education they can. We absolutely want our schools to
succeed. And you look at that and wonder, is throwing more
money at education really making our test scores go up, really
making the value of our education better? What we're seeing and it's reporting of administrator salaries skyrocketing,
there's even a report of several custodians making more. And
you know what? Honestly, it makes you wonder now, does our
local government know how to disperse these funds?

Honestly right now, the only thing you'll hear: "More
money, more money, more money." That's kind of all the solutions that have been put out there. More money, more money,
more money.

And when you get down to the details and you talk to these
legislators and say, "Really, is this what we need?" Their answers are very interesting. I had one of my favorite Kansas
senators who told me, "You know, we're actually paying for
students who cross the border from Missouri to Kansas to be
in our excellent Kansas schools. We're paying for them to go
to school as well." They have all these little issues that the
public doesn't have a clue about. You know what I'm saying?

JMM: I'm also thinking about what you said about unheard voices—
what about minority populations who feel left out?

PA 29: Okay. Well, as far as the minority populations, you know what,
you are right. We are from western Kansas. Which is funny
because it's an oil town area over there, and they had these

elaborate luxury buses that they would buy and had a lot of private money poured into their school districts. But you're right, there are some areas where, I just don't know enough about to comment on, that I'm sure that tax cuts hurt them.

This is almost a bad word to say, school consolidations out there, there are a lot of schools that depend on the school for jobs in their small town, it's their main economy is their education system out there. And the unpopular idea of consolidating some of those kinds of schools, the problem is they're already traveling an hour on bus to pick up these kids and get them to school. There's all kinds of problems and issues they have.

So honestly, I would say the voices of the immigrants are super important, the voices of the people in western Kansas are super important. And I think that the equity problem is definitely something that continues to need to be looked at.

THE SCHOOLS

THEN THERE WERE the schools.

In the early twentieth century, Kansas schools functioned as symbols of forward-thinking modernity in the Midwest. Through the 1910s and 1920s, education journals highlighted innovations in Kansas schools and praised their efforts to diversify a workforce based largely on farming into one that supported robust multilevel skills and businesses. Kansas also pioneered junior high school education, a new kind of school that changed what had been a direct path from elementary school to farmwork. "Kansas is the leading junior high school state in the Middle West," educator R. L. Lyman wrote in 1928. "In 1925–26 eleven Kansas cities of the first class had twenty-six junior high schools. . . . In no other state in the Mississippi Valley has the movement gained such headway, spreading so regularly and uniformly among communities located evenly throughout the commonwealth."[1]

Kansas was also at the fore of early twentieth-century liberal arts education, supervised study, and a number of teacher training programs. A 1916 article in *The School Review* described innovations in teacher training in Kansas as the result of new standards of excellence that came about because "Kansas laws giv[e] special encouragement and financial aid to high schools." A 1914 article called teacher training in Kansas a vital investment in the "citizens" of the future. Meanwhile, a 1923 article characterized the state's junior college movement as "integral to the workforce, to educate middle and lower income citizens."[2]

For much of the early parts of the twentieth century, Kansas also led the Midwest in educational advancement for minority populations. Kansas teacher training schools represented stepping-stones toward what education historian Kim Cary Warren calls the "quest for citizenship" for African American and Native American communities in the state.[3]

Kansas schools became contested ground in the 1950s, when tensions around access to and integration of public schools emerged as charged national topics. In 1951, Oliver L. Brown, a pastor and welder from Topeka, brought a class action suit on behalf of himself and twelve other African American parents from Topeka, whose children were not allowed to attend white schools. Brown's daughter Linda, a third grader, was forced to walk six blocks to her school bus stop and then ride to a segregated black school one mile away because she was refused entry to a white school seven blocks from her house. The resulting lawsuit, which eventually made its way to the US Supreme Court as *Brown v. Board of Education of Topeka* (1954), led to a ruling that declared state laws establishing separate public schools for black and white students to be unconstitutional, and overturned *Plessy v. Ferguson*'s notion of separate but equal, in place since 1896. The Supreme Court's unanimous decision that "separate educational facilities are inherently unequal" became a landmark for future civil rights cases across the United States.

The historic *Brown* case was neither the beginning nor the end of racial tensions in Kansas education. Many Kansans remained proud of their history as a free state and deemed school segregation as a Southern practice rather than a more-enlightened midwestern one. Yet the state continued to wrestle with questions of equity and advancement through heated debates and policies regarding public schools. Over the latter half of the twentieth and beginning of the twenty-first centuries, Kansas courts intervened repeatedly after conservative legislators promoted vouchers, parental choice formulas that shunted higher funding per pupil toward rural districts and capped the growth of urban ones, and other ostensibly race-neutral policies with racially discriminatory effects.[4]

Brownback cut deeply into these historic fault lines in metaphoric and real-world ways. Most directly, budget cuts upended much of the financial structure put in place to assure that poorer, inner-city schools did not fall behind wealthy suburban ones. Brownback eliminated the formula for state contributions to these schools and replaced it with fixed payments that were frozen at set levels. Soon, any number of inner-city districts were forced to close early, cancel summer classes, and cut an array of programs.

Critics derisively called the tax cuts *Brownback v. Boards of Education.* Lawyers sued the state on grounds that it failed to meet constitutional requirements for equity in school funding. A lengthy 2015 exposé in the *Boston Globe* titled "Old Battle Lines Drawn Anew in Kansas" detailed how, in the state where "separate but equal" died, "governor's bet on supply-side economics imperils school gains," and explained ways that "the themes of the *Brown* case—of race and equality—were again in play." Cynthia Lane, the Kansas City schools superintendent, called the fight over Kansas school funding "the civil rights issue of our time."[5]

Somewhat ironically from a present-day perspective, Kansas public schools thrived in the first place because of Republican governance. In *Red State Religion*, sociologist Robert Wuthnow describes how in the late nineteenth and early twentieth centuries, powerful Republican traditions in Kansas mixed religion, pragmatism, and social action to bolster relationships among neighbors, friends, and fellow churchgoers. Public education was central to these efforts. Centrist, pragmatist voices then continued to defend public schools as community resources for everyone, even in the face of religious extremism. (Though beyond my analysis, this tradition also extended to public universities, which remained in the top tier of national rankings through the early twenty-first century in large part thanks to a collaborative environment in which centrist Democrats and Republicans worked together.)[6]

The Kansas tradition of pragmatism and compromise helps explain why schools in the state often served as symbols of communal investment and civic pride. And it also helps explain why undercurrents of resistance began to form among Brownback's base when he expanded his backlash austerity agenda ever further into the state school system. At a particular moment in time, extensive cuts to schools and infrastructure might have taken backlash governance too far.

"If I have to go to another bake sale, I'm going to scream," a parent from Prairie Village told me. "At first we sold brownies to raise some extra money for school supplies for the district. But now, well, we're being forced to hold a bake sale *every month*, and if we don't raise the funds, they're going to fire the Spanish and French teachers. Can you imagine? We have to bake brownies all the time so that they don't cut classes!"

For an increasingly vocal cohort of Kansans, the downside of austerity hit home when it affected their children. Events on the ground began to

upend the belief that the consequences of tax cuts were happening somewhere else, to someone else. "School cuts definitely started out as something that people thought were only geared toward inner-city, black, and
Hispanic schools and districts," one administrator explained. "That's how
they were sold at first."

Over time, however, the radius extended. Annie McKay, the director
of Kansas Action for Children, explained to me that, "while some communities were better insulated at first, the fires were eventually getting to the
edges of those communities as well, metaphorically speaking, and the sort
of very radical extreme tax policy changes were destroying the way of life
throughout the state."

By 2016, Kansas fell to forty-fourth in the nation in per-pupil spending in public elementary and high schools. Educational attainment results
for students at all levels dropped as well, and for the first time, Kansas
students fell into the lower 25 percent of all states on a number of key education benchmarks. Kansas students plunged to dead last in the United
States in student scores on some sections of national proficiency exams
and into the bottom five in terms of the percentage of students who took the
ACT exam. The state also fell into the bottom ten states in the percentage
of high school graduates who pursued college education.[7]

Meanwhile, Brownback's promise of school "choice"—a catchphrase
for a private-school voucher program that would further undermine the
public school system—remained mired in controversy when it became
clear that the main beneficiaries would be schools linked to churches.
School choice thereby threatened to upend a mandate in the state constitution stating that "no religious sect or sects shall control any part of the
public educational funds."[8]

People across the state began to rethink the Kansas experiment. Not
just Democrats or advocates who had been in opposition all along but moderate Republicans and even onetime Brownback supporters as well.

Some conservatives with whom I spoke kept their concerns to themselves. "My husband and I are both teachers," a woman in Olathe explained, "and we are strong Brownback supporters, or rather we were.
When we saw what was happening in schools, we started to question
the hype about tax cuts and the renaissance . . . but we never spoke
out because of the negative attention we would have received in our
community."

Others became more vocal and voiced their objections in ways that extended well beyond self-interest. Republican LeEtta Felter, a small-business owner and Olathe school board member, was an early backer of Brownback's successful run for governor—even holding a GOP rally for Brownback and conservative senators Rick Santorum and Pat Roberts at a car dealership she and her husband owned. As Felter told it to me, she supported these politicians because they represented her "white, middle-of-the-road, Christian values"—or so she first thought.

Felter ran for the board because "I love our public schools and see them as drivers of prosperity in our state." Yet during her time on the school board, Felter began to recognize the inherent inequality of the policies she was being asked to support. As she put it,

> I see myself as a Republican just because I do believe in constrained growth of government. If you can pull yourself up by your bootstraps, please do. But these Brownback policies . . . I saw them hit the most when I learned about race and poverty in our state. I've become a little bit more broadened by my experience dealing with impoverished folks, the systemic cycle of multigeneration poverty, those living in poverty. I've seen, they don't even have bootstraps to pull themselves up by. It's quite different than what my white, middle-class upbringing led me to believe.
>
> When you are naïve, you don't understand that there is a chronic disparity in the system in the United States. We've got the systemic poverty, and a lot of time generational poverty issues coming to us. The Brownback policies . . . just make that worse.

Felter began to speak out, quietly in social gatherings among friends and neighbors at first, and then publicly and powerfully. As one act of seeming heresy, Felter even spoke critically about her own party, . . . to the *New York Times*.[9]

A May 2016 *New York Times* article titled "Kansas Parents Worry Schools Are Slipping Amid Budget Battles" told the story of Dinah Sykes, a concerned parent who was running for state senate (and would subsequently win). The PTA president at a school in the Kansas City suburbs, Sykes once supported Brownback, but growing class sizes and aging resources prompted her to speak out against the school budget cuts. "We're getting a bad reputation: that our state doesn't care about public education. We live in Kansas because of the great quality of life, the great schools, the great amenities. I want my boys to have the opportunity to have the same." The article also quoted a number of disaffected administrators and politicians who openly denounced the cuts that kept schools from buying new books, threatened their ability to pay utility bills, forced school districts to fire staff and shutter entire buildings . . . and the politicians who ordained those cuts. Mike Rodee, the vice president of the Wichita School Board, was emphatic: "We need to look at all the people that are doing it to us. Our legislators, our government, our governor—we are the ones who are fighting to keep the schools alive, and they are fighting to close them."[10]

Disbelief emerged as something of a refrain in my conversations with centrist GOP state politicians. Republican state representative Melissa Rooker told me that she found it "hard to believe what we've done to our great Kansas public school system, which made Kansas such a great place to live and also gave our state such a competitive advantage because of our educated workforce." Physician and GOP state representative Barbara Bollier worried about the long-term health effects of tax and budget cuts:[11]

> We're made the mistake of starting to cut early childhood education. If you're behind, you basically are never catching up, because you haven't really done work early in childhood and set it up properly. Then you don't end up with the educational capacity, and you don't move on.
>
> We've also cut programs for drug treatment and smoking cessation. Then, the other one is the whole mental health. By not funding proper mental health, we are in a catastrophe in this state because we haven't spent the money and we don't have proper care.

Annie McKay, CEO of Kansas Action for Children, worried about the ways that school cuts had profound negative effects on a number of state quality-of-life indicators:

> I think what's alarming is in some cases how far we've fallen. The issue of schools just scratches the surface of the fall that we are going to see in a lot of other indicators. . . . When the state stopped offering support for public libraries and county health departments and schools, those counties didn't have a reserve, didn't have a cushion. And so, either they were

raising property taxes, or they were cutting back in other investments like parks and recreation, childcare, and other support services.

Meanwhile, public school teachers, administrators, and superintendents from across the state—whose names are redacted given the political sensitivity of their positions—told incredible stories about the effects of austerity policies on daily lives. Here's one superintendent:

> SE 7: They've cut us by a million dollars a year. A million. Can you imagine? And these block grants, we were experiencing not tens of dollars per pupil cut but hundreds of dollars per pupil cut. Right now, it's even hard to know what the base state aid is. It's allegedly $3,852 after they locked us into the block grant . . . I can't even put a number on what the base aid is because the two years that we were locked in at $3,852, we grew about 250 kids. Those kids counted for nothing in any type of formula because there wasn't one, so the base for us is probably theoretically closer to about $3,600 per pupil. Knowing that just ten years ago, it was over $4,400 per pupil.
>
> Seven years ago, if we went in front of elementary parents and said, "You're going to have elementary class sizes of twenty-eight to thirty . . . and maybe some fifth- and sixth-grade and seventh- and eighth-grade classes are going to be above thirty," our parents would've went crazy. But you kind of run into the perfect storm, and politically, I think it plays out well for those making the cuts. As the parents change, unless they had older siblings and were really engaged in the process, they don't really know what they did have.
>
> So the everyday life thing, I think people have, not consciously but subconsciously or [due to] not knowing any better, they've lowered their expectations. The quality education that districts were giving and providing eight or ten years ago, it's gone. Not anybody saying I don't want this for my kids, but they just don't know what we had.

Another longtime administrator saw a hypocrisy in the cuts that made him question his own political leanings:

AD 17: I mean in my own family, we've been lifelong Kansas Republicans. My great-grandfather on down. Didn't matter how
qualified the Democrat was, we could not vote for a Democrat,
just wouldn't do it.

But then working in the schools has changed what I think.
I've been to public school board meetings and seen a parent
who was actually on oxygen screaming out against Medicaid
expansion or money to the schools.

One very wealthy family really believed that there should
be no public education, that each child ought to receive what
the state is going to apply toward education, and then the free
market will take care of it. At the same time, they had a significant high-needs child that we were educating that no one
else in that type of model would have ever educated, and they
were really upset because that child aged out, was going to
turn twenty-two, and no longer receive any of the services provided by our school, and they just couldn't understand why we
would not continue, and I'm like, "What?" It's crazy.

Certainly not everyone agreed. Conservative bloggers attacked articles
suggesting anti-Brownback pushback as "liberalist bile." Rightist organizations such as the Kansas Policy Institute put out head-scratching calculations that, they claimed, showed that school funding was not linked to
student and school outcomes. Brownback himself cast blame not on the
cuts but on a bloated and antiquated finance system. "For decades," he
asserted in a State of the State Address, "the children of Kansas suffered
under an overly complicated education finance formula that lacked accountability for results, handcuffed local school boards, and spent money
unrelated to student achievement. . . . We need to measure success not
by dollars spent but by the achievement of our students." A number of
conservatives dismissed the accounts of school decline as fake news, while
conservative provocateur Dave Trabert defended the tax cuts as a "good
idea" undone by free-spending liberals.[12]

But then something remarkable happened. For a brief moment at
least, conservative arguments about the benefits of austerity failed to hold
sway. The notion that *less was more*, or that "dollars spent" had no correlation with student achievement, elicited increasing disbelief among

the populace. It was as if schools, and their connections to the prosperity of future generations, represented a space in which it was acceptable for otherwise conservative voters to critique backlash governance. Recall, for instance, that voicing reservations about guns or ACA rejection was tantamount to treason in Missouri and Tennessee.

LeEtta Felter explained the change in her own powerful way:

> A number of us, well, we were raised in the Republican Party, it was our home, it was all we knew. But for our Republican governor to dig his heels in and say we are not participating in health care, or taking pension money away, or raiding the road funds, or hurting kids and schools with no real plan for how to make things better. I mean, it's our state right, but it sure screwed us up. We are financially not as strong as we were before we elected Brownback; we just aren't. We voted for him. Shame on us.

By early summer 2017, a coup was brewing in the state legislature. After four years of below-average growth, deepening budget deficits, and steep spending reductions, the GOP-dominated Kansas legislature repealed many of the tax cuts at the heart of the Brownback fiscal agenda. In a dramatic rebuke, Kansas legislators—including a number of Republicans—voted to override Brownback's veto and reverse many of the tax cuts. The result, called Kansas Senate Bill 30, effectively raised the top income tax rate from 4.6 percent to 5.7 percent and eliminated certain exemptions for pass-through businesses. Metrics suggested that these actions would raise up to $1.2 billion in new revenue over two years, which would then go toward closing budget shortfalls and propping up the public school system.[13]

Austerity, for a moment, bred anti-austerity—or at least returned communal tax responsibilities to pre-Brownback levels. As a lead editorial in the *Kansas City Star* would later put it, "The state's budget is closer to balance because members of the Kansas House and Senate found the courage to raise taxes over the governor's veto. The decision not only restored some balance and fairness to the Kansas tax code, it also provided revenue to pay for needed state services such as education and safety."[14]

The question then arose: *What exactly had happened?*

For some people, the legislative action represented a potential Rubicon moment in which common sense and neighborliness turned back the forces of Tea Party–style conservatism. As the Kansas Center for Economic Growth put it, the legislative actions signaled "an end to the most disastrous parts of the Brownback tax experiment" and represented "a crucial first step on Kansas' road to financial recovery."[15]

For others, the legislative action signaled a momentary bump on an otherwise smooth road to Rightsville. Indeed, hard-line anti-immigrant conservative secretary of state Kris Kobach announced his candidacy for the governorship in the same month that legislators overrode Brownback's veto of the tax-cut repeal. Kobach derisively called Kansas the "sanctuary state of the Midwest" that took money from citizens to protect illegal immigrants and, as the *Star* described it, "lambasted Kansas lawmakers for raising taxes 'on hard-working Kansans' by repealing Gov. Sam Brownback's tax cuts Tuesday to fill the state's budget hole and contended that the state could have saved dollars by restricting immigration."[16]

From the perspective of schools, two realities emerged in the aftermath of the legislative vote. First, Kansas public schools were about to receive badly needed infusions of funds. SB 30 phased in a $293 million increase in annual K–12 school spending, a first step toward addressing many of the structural shortfalls and imbalances that resulted from the tax cuts.[17]

But a second reality became clear to me as I spoke with people across the state: the problems caused by cutting school funds would not be wholly rectified simply by returning cash into the coffers. Pulling money out was not fixed simply by putting money back in. Rather, cutting money from schools cut off perfusion and oxygen as if by heart disease, leading to silent ischemia. Part of the reason why this was the case was because reducing funding and eliminating programs did more than simply reduce school capacities. Budget cuts also narrowed people's expectations for what was possible from school in the first place and of what it cost to get there. As one superintendent put it to me:

> It's really hard to see the changes unless you've been a superintendent that whole time, because I don't even think principals who change schools really fully grasp what's going on. And it's rare to have a board member that's been on for ten or twelve years, and it's even more rare to have a board member that's been on that time that's so engaged. It's not anybody saying, "I don't want this for my kids," but they just don't know what we had or what might be possible from great schools.

Fees are one example. Today, we had our budget closeout meeting, and we adopted, for the first time in six years since we started all-day kindergarten, there will be a $205-a-month fee to parents to get all-day K. But then next year, parents won't know that we used to cover it. It's not like they'll say, "What do you mean we don't have to pay for kindergarten?" because they won't have any frame of reference that, well, you really should never have been having to pay for the option of all-day kindergarten.

This narrowing of expectations makes sense. Parents and students are often the main catalysts of school change. But their awareness of a school's environment plays out over a fixed period of time—the first day of middle school, for instance, until the day of graduation to high school. Parents and students rarely know how things worked before they became stakeholders. From this perspective, parents and children might readily identify buildings in need of repair or decrepit playgrounds but not the absence of particular language programs, AP courses, or extracurricular activities. Recognizing the negative impact of large class sizes and high student-to-teacher ratios can only happen if parents and students know what the class sizes were before they got there. A decline in a state's national education rankings is often invisible to people on the ground. By the time parents and students become cognizant of the issues that drive such a fall, it's often too late. Even the most active parents rarely remain connected to a school after their children graduate.

Teachers, of course, often remain in place and experience these kinds of changes firsthand. However, a number of teachers told me that attempts to make parents and students aware of the impacts of reduced funding were often met with derision. Some teachers—who asked to remain anonymous for fear of repercussions—worried that parents interpreted their concerns about funding as "excuses" or "complaints." A number of teachers felt that bringing up concerns about school funding could potentially sow discord between teachers and parents. "How am I going to bring up the need to raise taxes to pay for better schooling," one teacher asked, "when parents come to parent-teacher conferences wearing 'Make America Great Again' hats? It's really, do I want to keep my job?" Such feelings of uncertainty were heightened because Brownback legislation undercut long-term job security for many teachers.

Another complication in recovery from school budget cuts: the long-term effects on student performance and achievement are often difficult to discern. Though many of Brownback's supporters argued otherwise, a great deal of evidence supports the notion that better-funded schools generally outperform poorly funded ones. In part, this is a matter of simple resource allocation. For example, in 2014, Kansas state aid per pupil was less than half of the amount in other parts of the country. When averaged across the state, total per-pupil spending in Kansas schools averaged between $8,000 and $12,000. That same year, by comparison, per-student funding in the Scarsdale Union Free School District schools in New York averaged $24,607. This meant Scarsdale schools could spend dramatically more on teachers, learning technologies, support services, classrooms, and pretty much everything else. It's not surprising, then, that students in Scarsdale averaged higher scores on pretty much every national competency exam than students across the state of Kansas.[18]

But such generalizations about rich versus poor districts, states, and outcomes don't hold across the board. Some schools and districts spend money more wisely than others. Some districts invest in classrooms and teachers, others in administrator salaries or football stadiums. In 2014, the left-leaning Center for American Progress released an extensive evaluation of educational spending versus outcomes across the United States. Among their findings:[19]

- **Some of the nation's most affluent school systems show a worrying lack of productivity.** Our analysis showed that after accounting for factors outside of a district's control, many high-spending districts posted middling productivity results. For example, only slightly more than one-third of the districts in the top third in spending were also in the top third in achievement.
- **In some districts, spending priorities are clearly misplaced.** Texas is one of the few states that report athletic spending at the district level, and the state's data suggest that more than one hundred districts in Texas spend upward of $500 per student on athletics. A few districts in Texas spend more than $1,000 per student annually on athletics. To keep

these numbers in perspective, the average unadjusted per-pupil operating expenditure in the state in 2013 was around $10,000.

- **State budget practices are often inconsistent and opaque.**

Educators and superintendents across Kansas assured me that these kinds of findings echoed and affirmed their views that money did not automatically determine results when it came to education. Yet neither was money wholly unrelated to educational experiences or outcomes—not by a long shot. At the most basic levels, money pays for the stuff on which schools run: books, chalkboards, playgrounds, teacher salaries, buses, lunches. On a less basic level, money represents an investment in future generations. Spending cuts, as we will see, often threaten—and directly impact—both of these modes of currency.

Put it all together, and the Kansas experiment suggests that backlash governance was wearing out its welcome, at least for some people in a previously moderate middle-American state. At some point, among school closings, lackluster responses to natural disasters, and roads and bridges in need of repair, pockets of residents began to reconsider ideologies that shunted funds from communal utilities into the bank accounts of private individuals.

This is not to suggest that right-leaning Kansans suddenly became socialists in droves or woke to the terrible effects of budget cuts in minority-dominant districts. Clearly in many instances, as Annie McKay rightly put it, residents woke to the fires they set in the fields only when the smoke got too close to their homes. And yet, seeing the effects of austerity spurred moments of reflection, for at least some people, about what kind of communities and polities they wanted to live in.

At the same time, Kansas also suggests that turning white voters away from policy preferences that harm their own well-beings won't be easy, or sufficient in itself, if not tied to deep awareness of what cuts actually *do*. In the case of Kansas schools, these awakenings lay in uneasy repose with a very real and uncomfortable follow-up question: *After five years of funding cuts, what damage was already done?*

INTERVIEW:

THE RACE CARD

Interview excerpts, September 12, 2017, Wyandotte, administrator

JMM: You don't have to answer this next question if you don't want to, but I guess I'm wondering about race, about how race plays out in relation to the cuts and the politics overall.

AD 3: Where are you from in Kansas City?

JMM: I grew up near the Plaza.

AD 3: Oh, and where'd you go to school?

JMM: I went to the Hebrew Academy, then I went to Pembroke. I went to UMKC [University of Missouri–Kansas City] for college and med school, so I've been in the area, and I've kind of seen different kinds of education over time.

AD 3: The school-age population in Kansas is definitely more diverse than the general population of Kansas. I think when you look at the legislature, for example, and some of the education committees, you have education committees where only one or two of the people on those committees who have school-age children actually have those children in public schools. People make all kinds of decisions about public versus private and why, and they do it for religious reasons and all kinds of reasons, but there can sometimes seem to be a lack of understanding or empathy for kids that must use the public school system and who depend upon that system.

I never want to—I'm always careful as an African American, I'm careful and cautious about when I call out issues of
race, because when you do, people frequently react, "Oh, he's
just pulling out the race card." So I'm always hesitant. I was
raised that race is going to be an issue, and you as an African
American male are going to have to work harder to get the
same thing as the boy next to you, simply because of the color
of your skin. That's just the way it is. Get over it. Keep moving
forward, because life is like that. So I tend not to call it out.
On the other hand, it's hard to ignore the degree to which it
seems to be okay to put in place policies that impact kids in
negative ways, and I don't think it's a coincidence that those
kids tend to be blacker and browner than the children of the
people who are putting those policies in place.

One of the conservative arguments you hear all the time
from some legislators: "We've got to hold schools more accountable. Schools aren't being held accountable." So I ask
of them, how many of them had changed a school within one
level, went from one elementary school to another. Nobody
had, which is pretty common for middle-class and upper-
middle-class people. But I said, "Our students, we have
schools where 50 percent of the kids who take the state exam
in the spring weren't in that building in August when we
started school."

So even the notion of a school population can mean something very different in a poor community than it might in a
more resourced community. When you say we ought to hold
somebody accountable for that kid's scores, well, who? The
school where they started the year? The school where they
were in December? The school where they were when they
took the test in April? Whom do you hold accountable for
that? It's a tough one, and there isn't any easy answer for it.

But we have these notions of accountability that are based
on assumptions that don't necessarily hold for every community. Some of the things that we have to do as a school district because of who we serve are quite different than what you
might do in a situation where you are going to see the same

kids and the same families for six years of elementary school, or three years of middle school, or four years of high school.

JMM: You mentioned before you feel like even though people have probably the best interests at heart, you said that there might be policies that impact black and brown kids more. What are the policies you think that are disproportionate?

AD 3: We sometimes talk about schools as if the reason kids are not successful is simply because the people in that school just don't care and aren't willing to work to be successful. That ignores a lot of the reality that kids face. That then leads people to want to push for what is called school choice. That's the Trump position now. "Well, if we could introduce competition, then those people would have to work harder."

But they're targeted at the lowest-performing schools in the state, which disproportionately are centered in urban areas and serve more kids of color because of the historic connections in our country between race, class, and achievement. We lose kids and the resources associated with those kids to untested charter schools. In fact, it's interesting, in Missouri you have charter schools in St. Louis and Kansas City. Kansas City probably has more than twenty charter schools. I think that you're getting close to half the population of the city that's in a charter school paid for with public funds. That's had a devastating effect on that district, and that's a district that serves mostly black and brown kids. There are things like that, that the legislature puts in place that disproportionately impacts certain communities, certain kids. You can track some of that by race.

CONGESTIVE
HEART FAILURE

W HAT'S THE VALUE of an education?

The notion that education provides lifelong skills, enables civic participation, and fosters advancement on individual levels and societal gain on communal ones unites people of vastly different backgrounds and ideologies.

"When you educate a man, you liberate a man," then neurosurgeon Ben Carson wrote in his campaign book *One Nation*. Carson's fellow 2016 GOP presidential hopeful Jeb Bush called education "the great equalizer," arguing that "every child must have access to a great school and to great teachers." Not to be outdone, fellow candidate and former Hewlett-Packard CEO Carly Fiorina cited education as the bedrock of American "competitiveness," "fundamental" to national character, and a necessary step that prepared "our children's hearts and minds to lead."[1]

Decades earlier and an ideological world away, Malcolm X once used similar language. Speaking at the founding rally of the Organization of Afro-American Unity in 1964, he asserted that "education is an important element in the struggle for human rights. It is the means to help our children and our people rediscover their identity and thereby increase their self-respect. Education is our passport to the future, for tomorrow belongs only to the people who prepare for it today."[2]

Immense philosophical and contextual differences separate these speakers and their differing expectations about what education is and what

241

it does. But these otherwise divergent voices join in the assumption, supported by a great deal of research, that education represents a present-day investment that sows intellectual, financial, communal, and political rewards in the future.

Social science research demonstrates another benefit of education: a correlation with well-being and longevity. For instance, in 2015, education experts sponsored by the Agency for Healthcare Research and Quality (a government agency under the Department of Health and Human Services) conducted an extensive review of research surrounding the relationships between education and population-level health. The group, led by epidemiologist Emily Zimmerman, found educational attainment to be "a major predictor of health outcomes" and uncovered a growing "gap in health status between Americans with high and low education." All-cause death rates declined steadily for highly educated Americans through the early parts of the twenty-first century. Meanwhile, according to the report

- US adults without a high school diploma can expect to die nine years sooner than college graduates.
- According to one study, college graduates with only a bachelor's degree were 26 percent more likely to die during a five-year study follow-up period than those with a professional degree. Americans with less than a high school education were almost twice as likely to die in the next five years compared to those with a professional degree.
- Among whites with less than twelve years of education, life expectancy at age twenty-five fell by more than three years for men and by more than five years for women between 1990 and 2008.
- By 2011, the prevalence of diabetes had reached 15 percent for adults without a high school education, compared with 7 percent for college graduates.[3]

Zimmerman and her colleagues considered several theories for the growing health disadvantages affecting persons with lower educational attainment. Did people learn how to live healthy lifestyles while in school? Did more education grant them higher income later in life, which then bestowed better health care, lower rates of smoking, healthier foods, and other socioeconomic advantages? Or were both answers correct? The experts also theorized that the "cross-sectional association between education and health" depended on structural factors such as social relationships, access to healthy food, genetics, living conditions, neighborhood effects, stress, social and economic policies, and other "nuanced contextual covariables."[4]

A series of related studies link these trends with geography. Public health scholars Jennifer Montez and Lisa Berkman found that the negative health effects of low educational attainment varied by region and that people living in the northeastern United States "did not experience a significant increase in mortality like their counterparts in other regions." Similarly, political scientists Jacob Hacker and Paul Pierson found that the states with the highest life expectancies were also the states with the highest educational levels (bachelor's degree or higher). States with the highest education levels also tended to collect progressive state and local taxes and invest more readily in "education, infrastructure, urban quality of life and human services." By contrast, states that cut taxes for corporations and wealthy persons and reduced government services saw worse health outcomes.[5]

These kinds of studies provided openings for our data team to think statistically about the potential health effects of the Brownback tax cuts. No doubt, the relationships would likely have been more direct had we studied cuts that directly affected health care delivery or treatment programs. Yet the health effects of cuts to education seemed an untold part of the story, one with potentially devastating, if oft-silent, long-term consequences.

Choosing education as a health indicator made the work speculative. For one thing, there is no consensus regarding which specific educational indicators link to poor health. Does a lack of science training make students sick, as sciences like biology and physiology convey health information? Is poor reading proficiency to blame, as reading fluency helps people navigate the world? Do school attendance or large class sizes play a role? Or, once again, is it none or all of the above?

Complicating the issue, any connections between education and later-life health or illness are indirect at best. Health effects often follow in predictable ways when states invest in, or divest from, communal services such as roads, bridges, or public transit. Less money for Superfund cleanup sites or radon mitigation leads to more cancer, while delayed repairs to roads and bridges result in more car accidents. Conversely, people in Salt Lake City, Utah, saw steady improvements in body mass index after the city built new public transportation infrastructures, and cardiovascular health improved in New Orleans after certain neighborhoods introduced bike lanes.[6]

Education-related health effects take years to develop, by which point it becomes difficult to pin negative health results to any one cause. One person who emerges from a failing educational system might make poor health choices as a result, while another might prosper. Linearity remains difficult to track.

Furthermore, many core benchmarks of educational competence remain mired in politics, and particularly so in Brownback-era Kansas. Like gun data in Missouri or census data in the nation as a whole, education data in Kansas reflects ideological battles about power, wealth, and influence. Many Kansas school administrators I interviewed believed that the Brownback administration lowered testing benchmarks for science and reading proficiency to lessen the perceived effects of budget cuts. Far-right think tanks such as the Kansas Policy Institute, a group with ties to the Koch brothers, produced their own shaky statistical support for the value of "free market" education systems while centrist organizations such as Kansas Action for Children refuted those claims and produced analyses showing devastating effects of cuts.[7]

All of which is to say that, belying their promise of certainty, numbers remain charged, illusive, and circumspect and that, as a result, findings typically suggest general associations between education and health rather than hard-and-fast causes and effects.

However, several reliable data archives do exist. In the fall of 2017, our statistical team systematically searched, organized, and analyzed findings from these sources to understand public education trends in Kansas over the course of the Brownback era. We pulled, stretched, and crunched numbers as if making homemade pasta. Lines and shapes began to emerge from what had previously been formless masses of statistical dough.

For instance, the Kansas Association of School Boards (KASB) compiles student test results and other outcome measures by year using multiple large data sources. KASB also publishes a yearly report card that tracks trends in Kansas school performance and ranks school outcome data relative to outcomes in other states. Our statistical team reviewed its 2016 report and an advance copy of the 2017 report and supplemental data tables.

One key finding that emerged up front: Kansas students performed relatively well on a number of key indicators between 2008 and 2015, undoubtedly due to the tremendous efforts of educators in the face of declining resources and support. At the same time, the Kansas education system had a hard time keeping up with gains seen in other states, which eventually leapfrogged Kansas in national rankings. All states that ranked higher than Kansas in achievement had higher per-pupil funding between 2008 and 2015, and all increased total revenue by at least 9 percent, compared to a mere 4.8 percent increase in Kansas during this time. Kansas's percentage change in per-pupil funding during this time frame was thirty-ninth in the nation. States comparable in population and per-capita income increased funding by more than four times as much.[8]

To see if the data would support media and KASB claims that funding cuts affected student performance, we examined fourth- and eighth-grade Kansas student results from the National Assessment of Educational Progress (NAEP), the largest nationally representative, ongoing assessment of what American students know in various subject areas. Overall, we found support for the 2017 KASB report card's claims of growing gaps between higher- and lower-income students. KASB uses eligibility for the National School Lunch Program as a proxy for socioeconomic status, and the 2017 results show a more than 20 percentage-point difference in "basic level" attainment between higher- and lower-income students. By 2015, only 22 percent of low-income Kansas students scored at the "proficient" level of higher, while 51 percent of non-low-income students did.[9]

These trends also had a significant effect on rankings. As the KASB report put it, "Over the past eight years, the percent of Kansas students scoring at the basic and proficient benchmarks have generally declined, while peer states and the U.S. average have generally improved." Once a regular presence in top-ten rankings—the state ranked sixth in the nation in 2007—student performance in reading and math fell into the midtwenties in a remarkably short period.

We augmented our findings by referencing an interactive database of test results by state compiled by the National Center for Education Statistics (NCES), as well as *Kansas K–12 Education Reports* produced by the Kansas Department of Education. The NCES provided data from national exams every two years, allowing for a more nuanced analysis of trends (2009, 2011, 2013, and 2015, rather than just two years). The NCES data also provided a comprehensive breakdown based on race.[10]

Eye-opening trends emerged in fourth- and eighth-grade math proficiencies, which are frequently held up as indicators of high school graduation down the road. Progress generally improved over the early reporting periods, following trends that began in the prior decade. But the lines flattened out starting in 2011 and then declined considerably in all major demographic groups. Here's an instructive example: gains in math proficiency scores for fourth-grade students in Kansas slowed in 2011 and then began to slip between 2013 and 2015:[11]

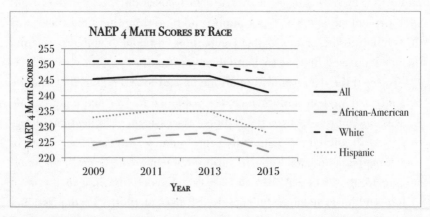

Source: "KASB State-Level Database," Tableau Public, retrieved from https://public .tableau.com/profile/retrac.ted#!/vizhome/State-LevelData/Select.

Increasing numbers of fourth-grade students across the state and in multiple demographic categories fell below basic proficiency levels. This decline was particularly notable among minority students: 28 percent of African American fourth-grade students in Kansas scored below "basic" on the NAEP math exam in 2011, before the cuts took effect. That number rocketed to 43 percent by 2015.

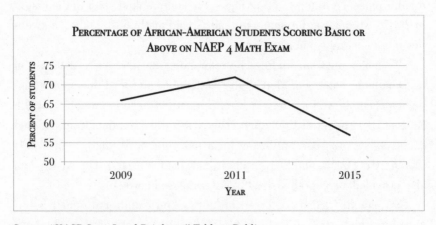

Source: "KASB State-Level Database," Tableau Public.

Hispanic/Latino student performance showed the same general trends, reaching an all-time low of 29 percent "below basic" in 2015.

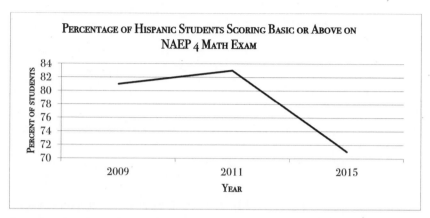

Source: "KASB State-Level Database," Tableau Public.

White student performance, already sliding in the years prior to funding cuts, fell dramatically as well, with an all-time low of 11 percent "below basic" in 2015:

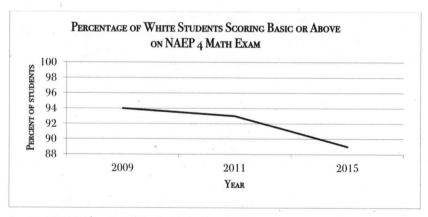

Source: "KASB State-Level Database," Tableau Public.

Similar trends appeared in results for eighth-grade students. Scores generally rose or remained stable on the NAEP 8 math exam until 2013, when drops appeared across most student demographic groups, as seen on the graph on the next page.

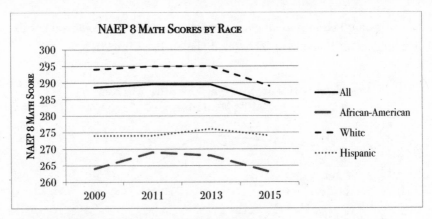

Source: "KASB State-Level Database," Tableau Public.

As a result, the aggregate percentage of Kansas eighth graders scoring basic or above on the national math exam plummeted to an all-time low of 75.5 percent in 2015 as shown below and on the opposite page.

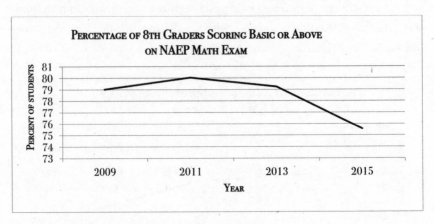

Source: "KASB State-Level Database," Tableau Public.

These exam results illustrate just how badly Kansas failed its students in helping them reach bare minimum achievement levels in math and how that failure disproportionately impacted minority populations by percentage but—in a state whose main demographic was white—overwhelmingly impacted white populations by overall effect.

Parallel stories played out across the education spectrum. Previously stellar scores of Kansas high school students on national college prep exams fell even as national averages rose. Educational attainment rankings

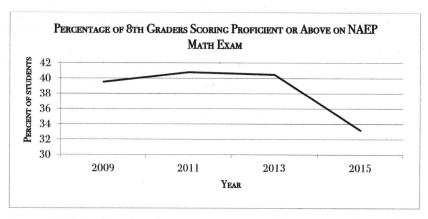

PERCENTAGE OF 8TH GRADERS SCORING PROFICIENT OR ABOVE ON NAEP MATH EXAM

Source: "KASB State-Level Database," Tableau Public.

for students after high school also dropped at historic rates. The percentages of students with high school diplomas, some college, or BA degrees fell steadily, and Kansas plunged from near the top of the nation to near the bottom in many indicators of an educated workforce. By 2015, Kansas also fell into the bottom of states in college completion by young adults ages eighteen to twenty-four and in rates of improvement in addressing higher education attainment. Summarizing the data, the 2017 KASB report warned that

> alarmingly, Kansas ranked in the bottom 10 states in improvement in postsecondary attainment by young adults . . . suggesting that the Kansas workforce is in danger of becoming less competitive with other states. This decline has occurred as Kansas school funding has also declined compared to other states.[12]

Zimmerman and her colleagues theorized that instruction in health-related knowledge and skills might be one reason why education correlated with better health outcomes. Using a database on "national health education standards" produced by the US Centers for Disease Control and Prevention (CDC), we uncovered sharp cuts to grades six through twelve health education courses in Kansas over the Brownback era, including reductions in statewide instruction in emotional and mental health (86.9 percent to 77.8 percent), alcohol and drug use prevention (32 percent to 22 percent), tobacco-use prevention (69 percent to 60.2 percent), and violence prevention (73.3 percent to 64 percent). The percentage of Kansas schools that taught health education classes fell across the state, from 48 percent to 41 percent. Startling reductions particularly appeared in high school instruction related to health and sexuality, including instruction in sexually transmitted disease (STD) prevention, safe sex practices, and HIV:

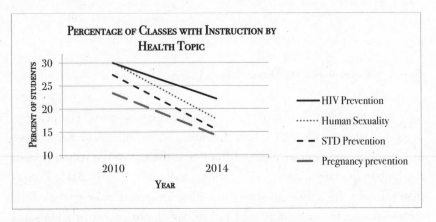

Percentage of Kansas Public Schools with instruction in human sexuality, 2010–2014;
Source, CDC National Health Education Standards[i]

Source: "National Health Education Standards," Centers for Disease Control and Prevention, 2016, accessed April 25, 2017, https://www.cdc.gov/healthyschools/sher/standards/index.htm.

The final way we assessed potential health effects of the tax cuts was by imagining what education trends might have looked like had Brownback never taken office. Our statistical research team dove into the data on high school graduation and dropout rates (these rates are related but not the same, since dropout rates apply to students across the high school years while graduation rates assess seniors). Recall that research suggested that a high school diploma led to improved mortality. On average, US adults without a high school diploma can expect to die nine years sooner than college graduates. Research also directly correlates low graduation rates to low levels of school funding.[13]

Graduation and dropout rates are relatively straightforward statistics. We pulled data from the Kansas Department of Education and looked at graduation and dropout rates between 2009 and 2016, broken down by race, ethnicity, and gender. This involved a somewhat painstaking process of selecting each academic year separately, culling the graduation data, then calculating graduation rates as a percentage of total "head-count enrollment" for each class in each year.[14]

As we did when researching the loosening gun laws in Missouri and health trends in Tennessee, we plotted two types of lines, one set that showed *actual* rates in Kansas public schools and another that showed what rates *would* have looked like had they followed trends set prior to the Brownback tax cuts. In statistical terms, we derived this second theoretical line ("projected") by extrapolating the available graduation and dropout rates prior to cuts from pre-Brownback years; calculating a regression equation based on that data; using that equation to build a trendline; and plotting it on the same graph as the actual data in order to show probable values that we then compared to the actual trends.

Overall, we found that high school graduation rates fell and dropout rates rose. Dropout rates across the state had fallen to all-time lows in 2010, before the cuts, but started rising in 2012. Graduation rates rose steadily in the state until 2011, then slowed until 2012, and then began to show sharp decline in comparison with the projected rate:

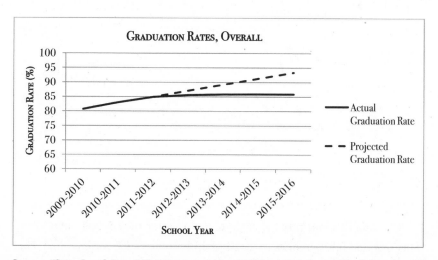

Source: "State-Level Data," Kansas Association of School Boards, retrieved from https://kasb.org/research/national-data/#1494251157868-15c8d733-78e9.

We then charted the dropout and graduation rates for the state's three largest demographic groups—white, African American, and Hispanic/Latino—and further divided by gender.

It became obvious rather quickly that graduation rates fell and dropout rates rose for most minority populations in tandem with falling school-funding levels, with vast gaps between what actually happened compared to what might have been. For instance, graduation rates for Hispanic/Latino (again, using imperfect US Census categories) students in Kansas rose steadily over much of the first part of the twenty-first century. The combined Latino/a student graduation hit a high of 70 percent in 2009, and then kept rising. Eighty percent of Latino/a students graduated in the 2012/2013 school year, and projections yielded a theoretical rate of 90 percent by 2016, including 96 percent for girls and 86 percent for boys, absent the budget cuts. Just like fourth- and eighth-grade exam results, graduation rates stalled and then fell well below projections once the budget cuts were enacted:[15]

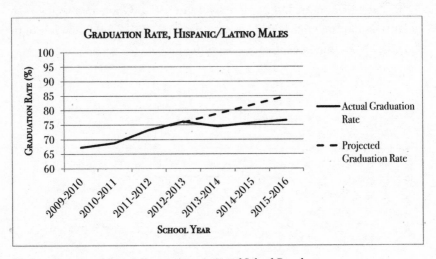

Source: "State-Level Data," Kansas Association of School Boards.

Latino/a dropout rates also skyrocketed after the budget cuts. These rates reached historic lows in 2010 (2.25 for males, 1.5 for females). Had these trends continued, dropout rates would have fallen to 1.5 for males and 1.0 for females. But instead, the actual rates were 3.0 and 2.0 by 2016.

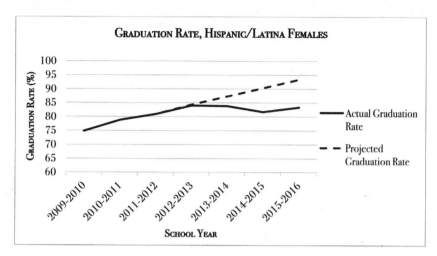

Source: "State-Level Data," Kansas Association of School Boards.

African American student graduation rates also fell well below projections in every year after the cuts. In an ideal world, one projected by data prior to the cuts, black male graduation rates might have approached 88 percent by 2016. Black women had shown such strong improvements in

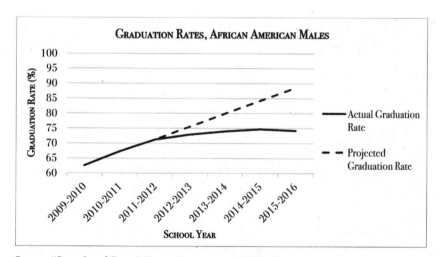

Source: "State-Level Data," Kansas Association of School Boards.

graduation rates in the pre-Brownback era that, had these trends continued, statistical modeling showed a nearly 100 percent rate by 2016. However, in reality, the trends appeared as shown on the next page.

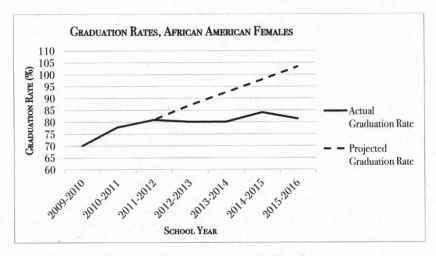

Source: "State-Level Data," Kansas Association of School Boards.

Again, these figures are projections of what *could have been* had prior trends held to form. In this case, the prospect of Kansas graduating every non-dropout African American female in its public schools was statistically within grasp in 2012. Then the budget cuts took hold, and the trends reversed.

Dropout rates for black males were high to begin with—black male students dropped out at rates nearly double those of other students in 2010. This trend improved annually in the years leading up the cuts, spiked dramatically in the year after, and then returned to trajectories found prior to the cuts by 2016. Meanwhile, in a show of resilience, African American women were the lone group whose dropout rates remained largely the same between 2010 and 2016.

A cynical observer of these trends might contend that these trajectories represented inevitable outcomes of funding cuts that, if not overtly racist in intent, targeted minority schools and populations in effect, thereby jeopardizing the educations and futures of the most vulnerable students and communities. And, of course, race correlates with differing levels of disadvantage or opportunity in the United States more broadly.

But here once again, policies that redistributed wealth and resources away from minority populations had tremendously negative effects for white populations as well. As Booker T. Washington once put it, "You can't hold a man down without staying down with him." In some instances, white populations saw the most dramatic cumulative negative effects of any subgrouping. For instance, stagnant white graduation rates had shown steady improvements until 2012, when the rates began to flatten out and fall 5–8 percent below projections:[16]

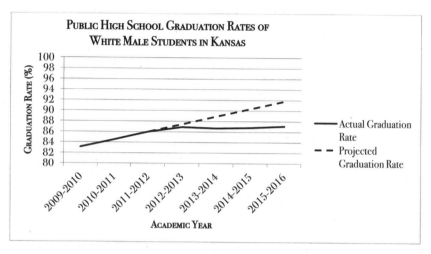

Source: "State-Level Data," Kansas Association of School Boards.

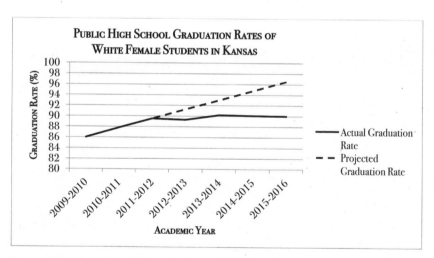

Source: "State-Level Data," Kansas Association of School Boards.

Meanwhile, the graph on the next page shows dropout rates for white public high school students reversed decades-long improvements in the years after the cuts began to take effect, rising from lows of 1.3 percent to highs that approached 1.6 percent for males, and variable but rising rates for females.

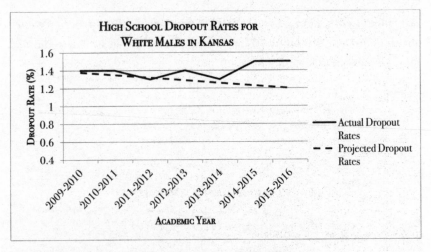

Source: "State-Level Data," Kansas Association of School Boards.

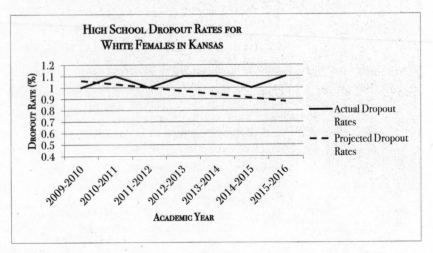

Source: "State-Level Data," Kansas Association of School Boards.

Taken as a whole, the KASB data shows increasing numbers of Kansas high school students dropping out of school or failing to graduate over the first four years after the Brownback cuts took effect. Like gun data in Missouri and health data in Tennessee, trends that impacted minority populations broadened to impact white populations as well. Students of all backgrounds and foregrounds, with lives and futures ahead of them, thereby became cannon fodder in the fight to redistribute wealth upward.

The data trends also highlighted particular issues or questions for specific groups of students. Latino and Latina graduation rates fell far below what they were projected to be absent the Brownback cuts. Meanwhile, dropout rates for both Latino males and females—rates that had shown tremendous improvement pre-Brownback—jumped markedly. Did cuts to ESL and other support programs put these students at an inherent disadvantage?[17]

African American students saw flatlined graduation rates and failed to hold gains that emerged in the pre-Brownback years. Schools in minority districts struggled to hold on to prior gains and often slipped back without ongoing support. Sixty years after *Brown*, was the system becoming inherently *separate and unequal* once again?

White graduation rates plateaued and dropout rates rose. While these percentages were lower than for other groups, they were devastating on an aggregate level simply because there were far more white students in public schools across the state. Over 80 percent of the state's population identified as non-Hispanic white, and just 6 percent as African American. From 10 percent to 20 percent of the population identified as Hispanic origin. Simply put, white Americans dominated most population categories in Kansas—including that of students in the state's public schools. What were the effects of falling educational attainment in white-dominated parts of the state?[18]

As a final analysis, we plugged dropout rate data into the frameworks laid out by Zimmerman and colleagues to estimate their potential effects on future health. We calculated the difference between the actual and the projected rates, quantifying the space between the two lines in each graph—one that charted what might have, or should have been, while the other showed what actually took place. We then multiplied the difference between the two numbers by some of the main findings uncovered by Zimmerman and colleagues—namely, that *failure to attain a high school diploma correlated with nine years of life lost*, in conjunction with rising rates of smoking, illnesses such as diabetes, and missed doctor visits.

The results were grim.

Rising dropout rates in the four years after the cuts meant that 801.97 more Latino and Latina high school students dropped out than would have otherwise (2,193.12 students dropped out, when the number could have been 1,391.15 if trends prior to the cuts continued, for a difference of 801.97 students). When filtered through the future health effects numbers cited by Zimmerman, this suggested *7,217.73 additional lost Latino/a life years*.

Dropout data was somewhat more complicated for African American students, who fell back to dropout levels that were high to begin with, then improved dramatically in the years before Brownback, then fell back to where they had once been after the cuts erased hard-earned progress. On the aggregate level, this meant that our pre- and post-method yielded little difference: 1,089.04 students dropped out, when the number could have been 1,078.8. We felt that these numbers did not quite capture the enormity of the problem of rising African American dropouts and falling graduations. As a thought exercise, we calculated what the health effects might have been had they approached even the worst post-Brownback year for white students—which, as it turned out, would have represented a dramatic improvement over the rates seen in black student populations. We found that if the dropout rate for black students had equaled trends for actual white dropouts, there would have been only 508.1 dropouts—meaning a difference of 570.7. This potentially meant *5,136.3 additional lost African American life years.*

Meanwhile, 5,069.11 white students dropped out between 2012 and 2016, when the number could have been 4,400.716. Those 688.39 additional dropouts over four years amounted to *6,195.51 additional lost white life years.*[19]

Even one avoidable dropout is one too many. Yet when we started to add it all up, a new aggregate price tag for tax cuts began to emerge. More smokers, diabetes, and missed doctor visits. More people in menial jobs. *Eighteen thousand, five hundred fifty* lost years of life after only four years of budget cuts—and using data that conservatively addressed rising dropout rates and not the larger figures of falling graduations.

The correlational effects—as graph after graph showed flatlined gains followed by steep drops—felt immense, overwhelming, and ultimately damning of the argument that massive tax cuts would bring prosperity to all citizens of Kansas. Instead, the cuts made the rich richer. Meanwhile, even just four years of school budget cuts set in motion systemic changes across public education that reversed progress on multiple levels, from fourth-grade test results to health classes to high school graduation rates and postsecondary career options.

Were the causes of the subsequent health effects anything but politically induced, they would have been the subject of any number of public health campaigns. *Beware Budget Cuts: The Silent Killer.* But because austerity tied to political ideologies, its pernicious effects were far harder to discern for people on the ground. All the while, the amount of money people saved on their taxes was rendered moot by all kinds of hidden costs. Tax cuts provided moderately lower bills at the end of the year, but at the expense of underfunding key elements of the state's infrastructure—and at the expense of long-term well-being.

What might the graphs look like in ten, twenty, or fifty years if the cuts continued? Would the results even be quantifiable? Or would education-related morbidity and mortality seep into the soil like toxins; and when the crops grew more sparse and anemic with each year, famine would just seem the new norm?

Ultimately, the decision to elect a governor whose central platform depended on continued cutting, shifting burdens, and amplifying wealth disparities between rich and poor led to a subsequent series of choices. Hard choices about the types of investments that societies make to bolster the common good, versus the enablement of monies stashed away in the portfolios of people who may or may not have had any intention of letting it trickle down.

As it turned out, the Kansas experiment presaged arguments that would soon emerge among white conservatives on the national level—namely, that education itself was not worth the investment. In 2017, an annual survey conducted by the Pew Research Center showed plummeting support for higher education among Republican voters. For generations, voters of all stripes had voiced positive views of higher education and its overall effects on the future prosperity of the nation. But for the first time, a majority (58 percent) of Republicans felt that colleges had a negative overall effect on the country, compared to 36 percent saying they had a positive effect.[20]

Next came a national survey that found falling support for higher education among the white working class as well. "Losing the White Working Class, Too," read a title in *Inside Higher Education* introducing how a "survey of the voting bloc that favored Trump finds skepticism about value of higher education." Among the survey's many findings was that growing numbers of Southern and midwestern working-class whites (72 percent) said they preferred factory jobs over office jobs (28 percent) and that "when these voters hear people tell them that the answer to their concerns is college, their reaction is to essentially say—don't force your version of the American Dream on me."[21]

Since 2015, Republicans' views of the impact of colleges have turned much more negative

*% who say **colleges and universities** have a ____ effect on the way things are going in the country*

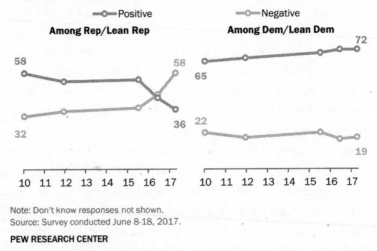

Note: Don't know responses not shown.
Source: Survey conducted June 8-18, 2017.

PEW RESEARCH CENTER

Source: "Sharp Partisan Divisions in Views of National Institutions," Pew Research Center, July 10, 2017, retrieved from www.people-press.org/2017/07/10/sharp-partisan -divisions-in-views-of-national-institutions. Reproduced with permission.

Such sentiments likely reflect material realities of people's lives. The cost of higher education rocketed ahead of inflation; working-class people became saddled with student debt as a result of seeking better lives for future generations. Meanwhile, overblown press reports about liberal bias in colleges and universities made higher education seem like an effete Democratic way to spend the formative years of one's life.

Yet our data highlighted problems with a GOP turn against public education that began in states like Kansas and then spread nationally. For one thing, the problems with education did not result from rising costs or inherent evils with education per se. Rather, public education became less efficient, and often more expensive, because of policies that Brownback and then Trump supporters *voted for*. Subsequent policies and legislative efforts that increased class sizes and reduced the quality of instruction chipped away at the overall value of what education was and what it did. Conservative rhetoric blamed the objects of tax cuts (schools) while often giving the subjects that implemented the cuts (politicians and policies) a free pass.

And as support for Brownback gave way to support for Trump, Kansas rallied around politicians who gave coded messages about fighting for the forgotten man and the middle class, only to see their state's education system—the pride of the Sunflower State, "the great equalizer" that could improve their lives and their children's lives—gutted, while the funds that may have saved the system funneled upward instead.

Defunding education also deeply impacted minority and immigrant populations who, as the Pew poll suggested, remained strongly in support of education as a way up and out. Blocking these pathways was, in many subtle and historical ways, part of the overall aim of the Kansas budget cuts. But once again, austerity proved a poison pill for *everyone*.

In these ways, modern-day trickle-down theories seem to fail on their titular promise. Nothing trickles down. Wealth condenses, and the system repays the shareholders rather than the consumers of services.

Over time, monumental tax cuts diminish far more than near-term budgets. The cuts diminish services, change expectations, and impede development in ways that impact the health and well-being of citizens for generations to come. As an Olathe administrator put it when we spoke in his office,

> I just think, as a society, not just Olathe or Johnson County, we're all running fast, lives are more complicated, and we don't really see anything. And we think, *Wow, I don't want to pay taxes, and my kids seem to be getting a good education*. But taxpayers and parents don't understand how close we are to the cliff, that that won't be true any longer. Not that it happens all at once; it takes so long to play out. And suddenly, we don't have a very good workforce in twenty years, and we don't have doctors, or we don't have lawyers or teachers. And all we have is a divided upper and lower class.

Some of the downstream fissures started to show sooner than expected, if in subtle ways. In late 2017, Kansas and Missouri aggressively pitched a joint proposal to become the home of Amazon's second headquarters (HQ2). Kansas City mayor Sly James garnered attention by purchasing one thousand items from amazon.com and posting pro–Kansas City comments in the product review sections of the website. And the Kansas City Area Development Council promised numerous tax credits and abatements to sweeten the potential deal. Yet among the reasons why the Kansas City proposal came up short: the region had too few skilled workers in science and math. As the *Kansas City Star* put it,

> Some involved in the Amazon effort say they're most worried about the area's relative lack of highly-skilled, highly-trained employees. This process reinforced those concerns.
>
> "The region has a well-educated workforce," a 2014 study concluded. But it "does not produce enough educated or STEM-qualified workers (science, technology, engineering and math) to keep pace with employer demand." Yet this week, Kansas State University may announce a $10 million cut to its operating budget. And *The Atlantic* recently wrote about the worrisome decline of Midwestern research universities.[22]

Yet for the most part, the dynamic was difficult to discern from the outside. Even as I drove for interviews at a number of public schools, I could not help but notice the tranquility that the schools projected to the outside world. School buildings seemed immaculate and well maintained. Football teams practiced on well-mowed fields. Students strolled through the grounds laughing with each other on the way to class, their futures but a light weight in their backpacks. Much like global warming, the threats of educational disaster seemed, at the individual level, almost impossible to discern. The day was bright, the sun was warm; all seemed well.

The data told a different story, one of invisibly slipping skills and invisibly crumbling communities. Of ever-more students falling through the cracks, only to later appear, as if weeds from the underground, working at menial jobs or walking the streets. Or wheeled, short of breath, into emergency rooms.

In this sense, the Kansas education experiment during the Brownback years warned of even larger declines at the national level as Kansas became a model for the GOP tax cuts signed into law by President Trump in 2017.

INTERVIEW:

NO MATTER
WHAT HE DOES

Interview excerpts, September 14, 2017, Kansas City, parent

JMM: We were talking about Governor Brownback a moment ago. I'm wondering, what are your thoughts on his appointment as an ambassador for religious freedom in DC?

PA 48: Honestly, it's great that we are finally getting him out of Kansas—he's just been an absolute disaster on all levels. Raided money from the highways. Raided money from old people and the pensions. Worst of all, he destroyed our public schools. They used to be so great . . . now all we do is worry about them. Total disaster. It's a good thing he's gone.

JMM: Yes, looks like he's landed on his feet in the Trump administration.

PA 48: Maybe he'll do better there. I'm sure Trump will straighten him out.

JMM: You're supportive.

PA 48: I'm a huge Trump supporter.

JMM: Many people are. But from the perspective of Kansas . . . it just seems interesting that many of the same policies that seem to have failed so miserably in Kansas now form the basis for what Trump's trying to do. Like huge tax cuts for wealthy people and corporations, or defunding schools and proposing

block grants. These were the very policies that got Brownback
into trouble, no?

PA 48: Who knows? Maybe you're right. You probably are, come to
think of it. I just know that it's not just me. My husband and
his brother, and my nephew and all of his friends, are gonna
support Trump no matter what he does. It's not all that much
about his policies or anything. They just feel like, as white
men in America, their voice wasn't being heard. Trump gave
them their voice back.

MILLIONS OF
MILLIONS

A ND JUST LIKE that, it was back to the beginning. After the final interview, I considered my Kansas research complete. But Kansas instead
showed the extent to which American polarization thrives by resisting compromise or closure. Issues of common good pull to the right and then jump
jarringly back to the center or left, only to pull rightward once again. Such
is the nature of our current American atmosphere in which politics vac-
illate endlessly, exhaustingly, between ever-shifting poles. Victories and
defeats then never represent ends in themselves but rather open spaces for
further points of contention. All the while, the American political system
finds new ways to upend the kinds of calm that people might want so that
they can worry about other things—and replaces it with new versions of
old forms of conflict.

As the ink dried on the final section of the book, controversial secretary of state Kris Kobach emerged as a leading contender for state governor. Kobach relentlessly attacked Kansas public schools as excessive
and wasteful and laid out a plan for budget cuts and fiscal regulations
that exceeded those enacted during the Brownback years. Chiding high-
functioning public school administrations as "crystal palaces," Kobach
promoted rolling back centrist tax increases, spending fewer dollars on
public education, and severely mandating how school districts were allowed to use public funds. Kobach also championed widespread standard-
ized testing and promoted school vouchers.[1]

These calls went hand in hand with overt and implied appeals to white backlash and, in its worst moments, white ethnonationalism. Kobach touted a constitutional amendment that took away the Kansas Supreme Court's power to rule on adequate funding of public education, thus limiting its ability to rectify spending disparities to minority and low-income districts. He upped the volume on anti-immigrant rhetoric and decried nonexistent cases of voter fraud—to the point where a restrictive voting law he championed was forcefully struck down by a federal district judge. President Trump endorsed Kobach even after it was revealed that the Kobach campaign employed three members of a white nationalist group called Identity Evropa. Kobach meanwhile made national news when he ridiculously paraded through Kansas towns in a jeep painted like an American flag with a replica of a .50-caliber machine gun attached to the back.[2]

Following my research, and after Kobach won the tightly contested GOP primary in August, I reached out to ten Kansans I had interviewed the year before to ask what this return to educational austerity and cutting might mean. As with seemingly everything else in state politics, I found that these potential developments exposed and expanded rifts among friends and neighbors.

Kobach supporters seemed hardened in their positions. Education was a waste. Kobach promised to restore order. Brownback had not gone far enough—"Brownback's experiment went wrong because he didn't make enough cuts to follow the lowering taxes." The language they used to describe agreement with Kobach's education proposals often emphasized individual protection and gain in much the same way as gun supporters in Missouri justified carrying their firearms in public spaces. Individual gain, they believed, was under attack: "It feels like the world is against the conservatives and all they're trying to do is give you more money in your paycheck." Responses frequently flowed, unprompted, from the wastefulness of public schools to the drains on the system posed by immigrants. Another parent told me that "it costs us so much money, taking care of these undocumented and even just people who are here temporarily, and medical bills and incarceration . . . all Kobach is saying is one place we're spending millions of millions of millions of dollars is on these illegal immigrants. That's part of the problem with our budget."

Democrats and Republican centrists, meanwhile, seemed in a state of disbelief. "This is like Brownback on steroids," one educator told me.

"We just started to turn things around," said another. Or, "If Brownback was the common cold to public education, Kobach will be heart disease." When I asked critics why they thought Kansas might vote for Kobach after the state's experiences with Brownback, every respondent answered by describing Kobach supporters with language of misinformation, amnesia, and lack of education. "People just forget how bad things were," was a familiar refrain. Or, "They just believe everything they hear on Fox."

Everyone with whom I spoke hinged their expectations on the coming gubernatorial election, which pitted Kobach against a moderate Democrat and an upstart independent. And to be sure, the election would dictate any number of real-world decisions about the future of the state.

But it also seemed clear that no matter the outcome, the divisions that the coming election represented were not going away any time soon—and that, without at some point addressing deeper biases and ideologies, arguments like those championed by Kobach and Trump would keep returning if from the collective repressed. There was no end to funds or resources—"millions of millions of millions of dollars"—that could be hoarded or social programs that could be cut. American whiteness itself and its ever-perilous, doubly unconscious hold on power remained the condition that always, always needed to be defended.

CONCLUSION

THE CASTLE DOCTRINE

O N THE NIGHT of November 21, 2014, Becca Campbell, a twenty-six-year-old woman from Florissant, Missouri, died of whiteness.

Campbell was a white, lower-middle-class, single mother of two who worked as a server at Tigín Irish Pub in downtown St. Louis. According to media and police reports, Campbell and her thirty-three-year-old boyfriend had a few drinks at the pub after her shift ended. The pair then drove off in a 2006 Toyota Highlander.[1]

November 2014 was a particularly fraught time in St. Louis. Earlier that year in nearby Ferguson, Darren Wilson, a twenty-eight-year-old white police officer, shot and killed an unarmed African American teenager named Michael Brown. The disputed circumstances of Brown's death in August spurred protests that intensified through October and November as a grand jury met to decide whether to indict Wilson for manslaughter.

On October 3, street protests in Ferguson grew so large that the town police department ceded its jurisdiction to the St. Louis County Police Department. On October 6, largely white supporters of Wilson clashed with largely African American protestors outside a St. Louis Cardinals baseball game. Later that week, Ferguson protesters launched a week of resistance throughout greater St. Louis, marching to such gentrified locales as the Powell Symphony Hall. On November 17, as images of unrest in the St. Louis area played on television screens across the country, Missouri governor Jay Nixon declared a state of emergency in Ferguson and signed an executive order activating the National Guard.[2]

In this charged environment, Becca Campbell and her male friend left work and drove into the night. What happened next is in some respects a matter of dispute. Either he drove or she drove. Either the gun she pulled from her purse was one that she owned for several years or, as seems more likely, was one that she purchased several days prior. Either she bought the gun as protection for her children or for personal safety in anticipation of rioting after the grand jury verdict.[3]

According to police reports and subsequent media accounts, Campbell waved the gun around her head while in the moving vehicle as if an urban desperado. While waving the gun, Campbell joked that she was getting "ready for Ferguson." At that moment, with the couple's attention transfixed on the orbiting pistol, their vehicle rear-ended the car in front of them. As the cars collided, Campbell's hand did what hands tend to do in moments of impact: it clenched, including the finger on the trigger of the gun. Then the gun did what it was built to do in response to a clenched finger. It killed.[4]

Becca Campbell died of a gunshot wound to the temple fired by her own hand from her own gun.

I thought frequently about Becca Campbell over the course of writing this book. I did not know Campbell or interview her. What I learned about her case came from media reports. Yet for me, Campbell's tragic story became emblematic of the larger narrative I've tracked in this book, regarding the kinds of mortal trade-offs white Americans make in order to defend an imagined sense of whiteness. It's a narrative about how "whiteness" becomes a formation worth living and dying for, and how, in myriad ways and on multiple levels, white Americans bet their lives on particular sets of meanings associated with whiteness, even in the face of clear threats to mortality or to common sense. A central political script then emerges in ways that, in its worst moments, defines the boundaries of white America in relation to real or imagined others who want to take what it has or be what it is. The story of Becca Campbell—and, indeed, of *Dying of Whiteness*—asks us to consider what white Americans give up when they invest so heavily in remaining at the top of social hierarchies or, more often, in defending a notion of status or privilege that appears under attack. In many instances, we give up days and months and years of life, as well as skills that might lead to better, more nonhierarchical, and less lethal solutions to the anxieties brought about by living in an ever-more integrated world.[5]

The Becca Campbell story seemed important because it highlighted a central point of this book—namely, that the mortal risks of whiteness extend beyond questions of whether or not any one person holds any one set of biases or beliefs. Risk evolves from politics or policies that surround identities and give shape to interactions among people and communities.

I say this in large part because Campbell's death became a kind of Rorschach test in which different people interpreted her intentions and actions in politically distinct ways. Media, the police, and Campbell's family members engaged in a protracted and painful public debate about whether the shooting resulted from Campbell's own, deep-seated racism and was motivated by animus toward black protesters or whether she rallied in support of the protests and wanted to see Ferguson police officer Darren Wilson behind bars. Left-leaning commentators on websites like *Huffington Post* voiced sentiments such as "sounds like they were going to troll the streets of Ferguson with a gun looking for trouble" and "she was worried about black people," while right-wing sites such as an outlet called Weaselzippers asserted that "Becca Campbell was [herself] a #Ferguson protester." Campbell's mother later claimed that Becca "got involved in Ferguson protests to fight for racial equality."[6]

Becca Campbell may or may not have acted because of her own beliefs about African Americans—we may never know her true intentions. And to be sure, any number of individual-level factors undoubtedly fueled the events that played out on Campbell's final, fateful night. Campbell's own finger rested on the trigger—a finger being a voluntary digit linked by striated muscle and controllable nerve to a voluntary part of the brain. The trigger released the firing mechanism of the gun Campbell chose to own. The events took place in Campbell's own car.[7]

Yet what everyone seemed to overlook in their interpretation of Campbell's death is the point I've made throughout this book: we lose perspective when we explain racially charged encounters in the United States solely on the basis of what exists in people's minds or on their individual actions. Doing so blocks recognition of the ways racial anxieties manifest themselves in laws, policies, and infrastructures—in ways that carry negative implications for everyone. These latter forms of bias result not just from personal attitudes or choices but from the investments and disinvestments that we as a society vote on, implement, and live with in the day to day. In an increasingly polarized country, such structures silently shape larger American interactions surrounding race, as well as intimate encounters that impact how we live, work, think, feel, and die.[8]

For instance, any number of policies and political formations similar to ones I've described in this book surrounded Campbell on that fateful night. Consider as one example the possibility that Campbell's concerns about safety reflected not simply a concern about black protesters but also a sense that she was responsible for her own security—within a city that had long been divided by race and class in ways that created an often-untenable divide among communities. St. Louis is described as one of the most segregated cities in America, a city with a massive racial split in which high crime, poor health, and low economic mobility reside mainly on the black side of town and privilege and opulence on the white side. The tensions around this split heightened in the years leading up to Ferguson due to a series of draconian tax and budget cuts enacted by the increasingly conservative Missouri legislature. Among other effects, the cuts reduced the size of police forces throughout the state and slashed funding for victims' advocacy programs, drug treatment centers, and a number of social services.[9]

Reductions to police funding and infrastructure carried lethal implications for minority populations in places like Ferguson, where, to make up for lost revenues, police shifted from protective models of public engagement to oppressive and financially predatory ones. Department and government analyses later found that Missouri police were "being pushed into the role of revenue generators" when dealing with minority populations, leading to "aggressive actions that reflect and exacerbate racial bias." In an entirely different register, cuts to police impacted white communities as well, inasmuch as a smaller police presence left many white communities feeling less protected. White Missouri residents voiced concern about slowed police response times and long delays for 911 calls. Reductions in hiring new police and training classes for officers led concerned citizens to hold urgent town hall meetings—at one, Tammy Dickinson, the US attorney for the District of Western Missouri, called police budget cuts "crime-fighting kryptonite."[10]

After the accidental shooting, emergency workers rushed Campbell to a hospital, where she would be declared dead. If that ambulance jolted over potholes on the way, it was quite possibly a result of extensive cuts to infrastructure spending that negatively impacted maintenance and construction of Missouri's roads and bridges. An infrastructure report card produced by the American Society of Civil Engineers graded Missouri roads with a C because of "significant funding shortfalls" that forced state administrators to funnel dollars into failing bridges and highways at the expense of city roads.[11]

Even the hospital system that attended to Becca Campbell in her dying moments reflected policy decisions that worked against the well-being of lower- and middle-income white citizens of Missouri. St. Louis is a city that boasts an important history of medical innovation in trauma care, thanks in large part to pioneering work done at level-one medical facilities such as Washington University School of Medicine, Barnes-Jewish Hospital, and the Saint Louis University Hospital. The state's rejection of Medicaid expansion under the Affordable Care Act led to "tough and uncertain times," manifested by service cuts and massive layoffs at area hospitals and reductions to emergency services. To be sure, no intervention would have saved Becca Campbell, who arrived at the hospital with a bullet lodged deep in her brain. But the system that she entered in the waning moments of her life was also itself hemorrhaging vitality due in part to a host of self-inflicted legislative and economic wounds.[12]

Then there was the gun. Even ten years earlier, it would have been exceedingly difficult for a Missourian to purchase, conceal, and transport a handgun due to state and federal regulations. However, in the years and months leading up to Campbell's death, a steady stream of pro-gun laws made it easier for citizens to own firearms and carry them in public. Two months before Campbell's death, Missouri lawmakers passed a law that allowed citizens to carry concealed handguns at schools, annulled most city and regional gun restrictions, and allowed just about anyone over the age of nineteen and not in jail to carry a concealed weapon without a permit. Among Missouri's pro-gun laws were so-called Castle Doctrine statutes that permitted gun owners to shoot perceived intruders in their homes, "free from legal prosecution for the consequences of the force used." Gun sales spiked in St. Louis in anticipation of the Darren Wilson verdict, and particularly among "new, inexperienced gun owners." In the months after Campbell died, legislation would extend Castle Doctrine protections to . . . a person's car.[13]

As the first section of this book details, beyond the headlines about black Missourians shooting each other in droves, white residents of Missouri increasingly died from gun-related accidents and suicides that took place with nary a person of color in sight. Indeed, between 2008 and 2013, white persons from Missouri unintentionally shot and killed themselves, their friends, and their family members ten times more frequently than did other groups of persons. In 2014, the list of white Missourians who died by self-inflicted gunshot included a notable name: Becca Campbell.[14]

None of this context detracts from the individual-level tragedy of Becca Campbell's death. Two children lost their mother, a mother who herself was someone's daughter. The loss was as preventable as it was nonsensical. But in a broader sense, the death of Becca Campbell embodied the larger tensions and politics regarding what it means to be a white American, and particularly white and lower- or middle-income in a conservative state in the era of Ferguson, the Tea Party, and Donald Trump.

Regardless of her intentions, then, Becca Campbell's final actions suggest a woman whose decisions were buoyed by privileges, laws, policies, and institutions that enabled her to buy a gun and ride around one of the most segregated cities in America. But when read through a larger perspective, it becomes clear that Becca Campbell paid dearly for these privileges—in fact, she paid with her life. By this latter reading, the same laws, policies, and institutions that seemingly supported Campbell worked against her own existential self-interests. Fewer police officers drove the streets, and fewer medical personnel worked the hospitals. Roads potholed. Tax-cutting politics that bolstered upper-income white people and their property also yielded a growing unease among lower- and middle-income white people who didn't quite have enough. The laws that allowed Campbell to purchase, conceal, and carry a handgun with neither training nor a permit quite literally put self-inflicted death within her car and within her reach.[15]

In the years following Campbell's death, political decisions to slash taxes, defund health care reform, or spread guns became ever-more vocally tied to promises to "restore" an imagined sense of lost white privilege. Yet much as with the case with Campbell, when read through the lens of health, these decisions often boomeranged back at population levels to deliver the opposite.

Graphs showing rising morbidity and mortality, or illness and death, which follow these decisions complicate common assumptions about injury or death. We usually define mortality as linked to biology, genetics, fate, accident, or illness. Or we think about death from unwanted intruders, pathogens that invade through the water or the air. Yet the kinds of data I've tracked in this book raise the specter that American human frailty is in part man-made, rendered all the more tenuous not by invasions of *them*, the immigrants or pathogens, but by political choices made by *us*, the white electorate.

Sometimes, the risks that emerge from these political choices often come from direct effects, such as more shootings from more guns or fewer doctors in times of need. At other times, the effects are far less obvious—such as when picking up a gun in the face of Ferguson protests seems the only option because the environment forecloses other ways of addressing societal problems, or of imagining avenues for equitable societies in which guns and protests are not needed.

It is also important to note, one final time, that policies that carry negative mortal consequences for everyday people are not the sole domain of any one political party or ideological persuasion. Closing this book with an example from St. Louis, a city that upheld decades of segregation and injustice through a series of policies authored by both Democrats and Republicans, suggests one example of how seemingly "liberal" initiatives can also have disastrous consequences for the people they claim to help. The history of Missouri cities shows how liberal desegregation efforts can lead to worsening economic and racial segregation. More broadly, anthropologist Adam D. Kiš, in a book titled *The Development Trap: How Big Thinking Fails the Poor*, explains how grand attempts by organizations such as the World Bank to eradicate poverty can end up making life all the worse for people at the lower ends of the economic spectrum.[16]

Yet liberal initiatives in the United States often fail because they try to do too much at once, such as trying to provide health care or education for wide swaths of the population, without addressing the underlying social or economic systems that produce poor health or low educational attainment in the first place. Liberals also frequently fail to explain adequately the every day benefits of their initiatives for everyday people in ways that resonate or that address historically based tensions or concerns.[17]

Meanwhile, the kinds of legislation I track in this book, and that have become more prevalent under the Trump administration, exact their negative health effects by cutting programs or services, or by privileging the rights of particular subsets of Americans—such as gun owners or exceedingly wealthy persons—above those of everyone else. These latter approaches open the door to the types of racial anxiety, xenophobia, and misguided nationalism amplified in the United States of late because they divisively suggest that minorities and immigrants are hoarding resources or that people need to protect themselves from one another.

It does not have to be this way. We know from American history that our communal, electoral power allows us to build vibrant social networks, safer communities, and better education systems—when we decide to do so. If impoverished structures lead to negative outcomes, then a renewed focus on restoring equitable structures and infrastructures will improve individual and communal health. In obvious and counterintuitive ways, fixing the electoral and economic structures that sustain structural racism and oppression will then better life, not just for racial and ethnic minority communities who are the objects of oppression, but, indeed, for *everyone*. Beyond the clear benefits of better roads, wages, schools, hospitals, or gun laws, a renewed focus on structure might also silently promote more healthy and self-reflective frameworks . . . of structural whiteness.

Every so often while researching and writing this book, I came upon other ways forward, other models, in unforeseen places. In Kansas, for instance, I met centrist GOP politicians who bucked their party's orthodoxy and pushed to raise taxes to address budget holes created by the Brownback cuts. Their efforts showed almost immediate benefit for state finances. As the *Kansas City Star* put it in early 2018, the decision "not only restored some balance and fairness to the Kansas tax code, it also provided revenue to pay for needed state services such as education and safety."[18]

When I spoke with officials who helped bring about these changes (many of which were later targeted by the Kobach campaign), I was struck by the extent to which they described their actions using language of social justice in addition to rhetoric about finance and budgets. Melissa Rooker, a GOP Kansas state representative, told me that raising taxes helped address some of the "inherent institutional racism" brought about by tax cuts that punished minority and low-income communities disproportionally. For Barbara Bollier, a GOP state senator, reversing the Brownback fiscal damage involved combating white racial attitudes that justified tax cuts through a logic that "minorities don't deserve my money in any way, shape, or form . . . blacks are just lazy SOBs who don't want to work." Bollier, a physician, saw these kinds of attitudes as targets that government needed to address if it was to create better lives for "all Kansans."

LeEtta Felter, the Olathe school board representative, detailed how becoming involved in politics changed her deepest understandings of race and equity. "I was raised middle-of-the-road evangelistic Christian," she explained. "We love the Lord and believe he's in the fiber of our being." Yet as she toured her district and met people, her understandings of compassion evolved:

> When you are naive, you don't understand that there is a chronic dispar-ity in the system, a chronic disparity that, specifically with education, impacts achievement gaps. All of us don't have the level playing ground that just a middle-of-the-road, middle-class white student has. It's not just about race, it's context of any of these indicators that put a child at risk. I have learned so much more about it that, it's not just one or two kids, in Olathe, that's 28 percent of our children. Those social inequities make a more complicated student coming to us, and it's our responsibil-ity to make sure that we invest in them at all levels so that their educa-tion that is afforded to them gets rooted, they learn how to learn, they are lifelong learners, they're contributing to society, and the state is not just a pipeline to prison.

I encountered similar opinions expressed in conversations about health care and guns. For instance, Beth Roth, director of a nonpartisan gun violence prevention organization in Tennessee (of which I then be-came a member), told me that she grew up in a "traditional" Republican home and became a supporter of George W. Bush. Her political organizing around gun violence brought her into minority neighborhoods where she encountered "African American families who were as concerned about vi-olence as I was" and who worked to create safe communities for their fam-ilies. She describes slowly waking up to a "*shaming* realization . . . that the stereotypes I held about gun violence being an inner-city problem were simply untrue and that I was going to need to examine my own privilege and that of my own community if I wanted to make any dent in this issue."

Ultimately, "it dawned on me, and now seems so obvious, that white politicians were the ones pushing for all the guns, and gun violence was a societal issue that reflected mainstream white values and problems too."

Toward the end of my writing, a brave group of student survivors emerged from the carnage of a mass shooting in their high school in Parkland, Florida, shouting #NeverAgain, and by so doing raised new opposition, not just to the NRA but to the underlying myths of armed white militancy it promoted. These efforts opened the door for new avenues of protest. "I'm not afraid of you," gun-owning journalist Linda Tirado wrote in an open letter to Dana Loesch and the NRA that would have been unimaginable before Parkland. "Or your single percent of the population, or the money of the people who pay you, or your clenched fists."[19]

These kinds of sentiments might seem par for the course in some parts of the country, but they felt remarkable coming from the mouths of red-state Republican politicians and activists or gun owners, even if centrist ones. This language suggested more than an awareness of social issues; it also described challenges to underlying biases and assumptions about self and community—as Roth put it, a "*shaming* realization" of one's own privilege—that then impacted what these people sought to achieve politically. It was in many ways a language of humility and compromise rather than of domination.

I come from a family of Democrats, but I found myself secretly tapping along as I listened to Rooker, Felter, and other GOP politicians, not so much because I agreed with their every sentiment but because their self-reflection and seeming willingness to compromise made it easier to think about new coalitions and avenues for alliance.

As I thought about what these politicians and activists were doing to move political rhetoric away from humiliation and blame and toward actually getting things done, I often found myself wondering: What might American politics look like if white humility was seen not as a sellout or a capitulation but as an honest effort to address seemingly intractable social issues?

For instance, what would it mean to talk honestly about the relationships of guns and gun violence with notions of American whiteness? Such associations are sometimes mentioned in the aftermath of mass shootings but rarely appear in conversations that might unify rather than divide. Imagine gun suicide–prevention programs in "Gun Country" that ask people to talk not just about their symptoms of depression but about the meanings or powerful historical fantasies they associate with guns. Or community gatherings where people of color could talk to white Americans about the feelings and anxieties engendered by *white* gun ownership. Or a gun lobby that, even as it protects Second Amendment rights, engages with its members about a larger question: *Why do we feel we need so many guns in the first place?*

What might it mean to create community health initiatives that reward collaboration among racially and economically disparate communities? Or merge small-government, pro-business rhetoric with genuine attempts to build causeways, greenways, and other points of connection among neighborhoods? Or reenvision health or business models that welcome immigrants to the American collective, rather than casting them as rivals?

In the current charged historical moment, drives toward inclusion can feel utopian. *New York Times* articles detail how Democrats suffer at the ballot box by emphasizing "pluralistic" issues such as immigration rather than "practical ones" of greater interest to working-class white voters. Meanwhile, once again, *diversity* was one of the words allegedly forbidden from research proposals at the CDC. Yet alliances that result from attempted cooperation, rather than attempted domination, are often shown to be healthier than nondiverse ones, all things being equal. Research has repeatedly demonstrated that socially diverse groups are more innovative than homogeneous groups and that diversity encourages people to become more creative, diligent, and hardworking. Scholars who study this phenomenon often attribute these differences to ways that people with different backgrounds bring new information and alternative viewpoints to workplaces or communities, leading to collaborative processes for reaching consensus.[20]

It makes sense when you think about it. People start to see one another not so much as competitors but as collaborators. The breakdown of automatic negative assumptions then promotes the kinds of unity that W. E. B. Du Bois argued American racism (and the so-called *wages* paid for joining the category of whiteness) works to prevent. Neighbors begin to form alliances based on common interest. Society, as the African American men in our focus groups succinctly put it, begins to work better for "everyone."

In this regard, the tragedy of purple- and red-state whiteness became ever-more clear to me over my years of talking with people for this book. Many persons with whom I spoke genuinely sought safety and security for themselves and their families. Expressions of overt racism or xenophobia remained the exception rather than the norm. It was not as if the people I encountered—at least the ones willing to speak with me—could not form out-group alliances under different circumstances.

Tensions upholding whiteness were not the only factors blocking collaboration. Any number of larger factors seemed to work to make sure that compromise never took place. For instance, after an eleven-year-old Tennessee boy shot and killed an eight-year-old neighbor using his father's unlocked shotgun, Beth Roth's Safe Tennessee organization helped sponsor a bill called MaKayla's Law that would put the onus on adults to safely store their weapons when kids are around. The bill received bipartisan support until an NRA lobbyist flew to Nashville to warn GOP politicians about forging consensus of any type. "She was disappointed I voted the other way," a GOP politician recalled the lobbyist telling him after a first round of voting. "You want your NRA score to be as high as you can get it." A week later, the bill was effectively dead.[21]

Similarly, efforts to incorporate immigrants into communities or promote trust across racial or ethnic lines become ever-more difficult when politicians repeatedly cast immigrants as threats to working-class white interests, African Americans as thugs or criminals, or even football players who kneel for justice as American traitors. Before the 2018 Super Bowl, an event around which Americans come together across racial and class lines, President Trump refused the traditional presidential pregame interview and divisively sent tweets reigniting racial tensions about kneeling, patriotism, and protest. Here and elsewhere, the superstructure worked overtime to subvert compromise among the base.[22]

We live in a country built by various types of immigrants, and our distinctiveness emerged by at least attempting to build community despite various traumatic or privileged pasts. People descend from slaves, peasants, landowners, refugees, and stowaways and try to make it work as best they can. Diversity provides strength and the promise of a better life, even as racial tensions hover not far beneath the surface. Increasingly, though, forces from above play to white Americans' worst demons to assure that they don't trust or work with others. In the absence of such collaboration, large sections of white America then come to identify these larger forces (NRA, Tea Party, Trump) as ones that keep them safe, powerful, and better off than people of other racial or ethnic groups. What follows, as this book has shown, is the promise of greatness, coupled with a biology of demise.

On stepping down from the US presidency in 1809, Thomas Jefferson famously wrote to his republican supporters that a primary lesson he learned as head of state was how "the care of human life and happiness, and not their destruction, is the first and only legitimate object of good government." Somewhere along the road from then to now, a politics that spreads guns, blocks health care, and defunds schools seems to have forgotten Jefferson's basic principle. Behind these agendas are core assumptions that the happiness of a select few persons takes precedence over the care of a great many others. Human life has suffered as a result, as has the notion that good government protects and promotes well-being in the first place.[23]

Backlash governance leads to states of denial, displacement, or amnesia, even in moments that demand accountability and self-reflection. In the aftermath of horrific mass shootings, including ones in his own state, Kentucky governor Matt Bevin took to claiming that laws and governments were no match for "evil"—overlooking the ways that this particular form of evil amassed arsenals under the protection of gun laws that conservatives like Bevin created or supported. On leaving the Kansas governor's office for an esteemed position in the Trump administration, Sam Brownback lambasted a decaying state psychiatric facility as "a pit" and decried the underfunding of state hospitals, prisons, and schools—conveniently forgetting that he more than anyone else created the problem in the first place.[24]

Over time, people begin to lose hope that someone in power might work to avert the next mass shooting or school closure. Leaders who offer zero solutions for the problems their own policies help create undermine core assumptions behind Jefferson's notion of good governance: that government serves people rather than dividing them or making them sick.[25]

This is in no way to suggest that external threats don't exist or that diversity is the answer to every problem. Sometimes it's good to remain in your group—and indeed, sometimes, in moments of danger, it's good to have a gun. Becca Campbell may have faced real peril on that November night, and she had every right to defend herself as best she knew how. We might imagine that, from her perspective, the prospect of confrontation by any number of forms of lawlessness likely felt salient and real, and a gun may well have appeased this sense of mortal danger as she rode, armed and dangerous, on the lookout for external threats.[26]

But in a larger sense, the connection of her actions to Ferguson, the NRA, and the racial politics of white protection and black protest cast Campbell's attempts at self-defense to something larger than herself. She protected a castle.

Despite the uncertainty regarding her intensions, Becca Campbell then joined a group of persons whose rights and privileges render life ever-more perilous for everyone—including persons in the supposedly privileged groups. Sometimes, the perilous nature of these privileges appears obvious, even absurd. In Oktaha, Oklahoma, a self-proclaimed armed "patriot" defending a gun store that posted a sign declaring itself a "Muslim-free" establishment dropped his own gun and shot himself in the arm. An employee at the NRA's National Firearms Museum in Fairfax, Virginia, shot himself in the leg during a firearms training session at the organization's headquarters. In Fort Worth, Texas, a man shot himself in the head while standing in the infield of the NRA 500 NASCAR Sprint Cup Series stock car race at Texas Motor Speedway. At other times, the dangers are tragic and spectacular, such as when increasing numbers of white Americans—schoolchildren, churchgoers, country music fans—perish after being shot by white male mass shooters.[27]

In these cases and others, injury and death result from the barrels of weapons raised not by invading armies but by the card-carrying mainstream. After these weapons lead to various forms of self- or self-group-harm, a concerted effort emerges that tries to isolate the wayward individual or weapon from the dominant group and to blame untoward effects on outliers. As but one example, pro-gun politicians and the NRA go into overdrive after mass shootings in order to fault "mental illness" as the culprit while shifting focus away from guns or gun policies. The approach probably works: a national survey taken in May 2018 after a succession of school shootings at Parkland High School in Florida and Santa Fe High School in Texas found that Americans were more than twice as likely to blame "illegal gun dealers" and "mental illness" than politicians, policies, or the NRA for mass shootings.[28]

From a practical standpoint, these beliefs rarely hold up to scrutiny. Not a single high-profile mass shooting in 2018 had to that point been carried out using an illegally obtained weapon. As is often the case in mass shootings, the guns were legally obtained—this is in part what makes them so hard to prevent. The same holds true for accidental shootings. Meanwhile, mental illness is rarely the main causal factor in mass shootings—people who are the most severely disordered lack the capacity to plan complex crimes or are already barred from obtaining firearms.[29]

But logic makes sense in the context of rhetorical strategies that reiterate, over and again, that guns are *us*, and that *we* live in (or are) castles in need of defense. Even mass shootings or tragic accidents lead back to a need to fortify the walls and guard the gates from the barbarians amassed just beyond the moat.

As I've shown, the construction of whiteness as a castle under siege, and the policies that sustain it, comes with certain benefits—such as the ability to carry guns in public without automatically being seen as suspect. But this construction works overtime to obscure the plagues that arise from within the castle walls. Ever-more guns, or ever-more tax cuts or health care system rejections, promise to make the citizenry great again or to afford protection but in reality only weaken the foundation and heighten the calculus of risk. Threat then emerges not from shady gun dealers, insane persons, immigrants, or protesters but from the far more existential threats to well-being posed by the king, the queen, the prince, the subjects, and perhaps most important, from the royal self.

This stronghold of rights and privileges thereby crafts the ellipsis of its own undoing. And the threats to life then rise, invisibly, when white America is otherwise protected by laws and policies, loaded handguns, and, in the case of Becca Campbell, the security locks and safety bags of a Toyota Highlander.

ACKNOWLEDGMENTS

This book began as an undertone.

In 2010, I moved to Nashville to take a position at Vanderbilt. One of my first research projects involved talking to patients at the Vanderbilt Medical Center about their feelings regarding health care reform. Many of the persons with whom I spoke struggled medically or financially in ways that had potentially dire consequences for themselves or their families. Recent diagnoses for chronic conditions, medical bankruptcies, or repeat emergency room visits were commonplace. The interviews took place against a backdrop of growing national momentum for state and federal legislative actions that would address many of the medical and financial pressures that these persons experienced. The Affordable Care Act, though not yet implemented, promised to reform atomized and often unjust health care delivery and insurance systems in ways that would provide much-needed support for lower-income patients and their families.

These conversations occurred largely before *Obamacare* became a Southern invective. Yet a subset of the people with whom I interacted, and most often white Southerners, would have none of it. They eschewed the notion of health care reform, even after it became clear that the improvements might help them in their times of crisis. The reasons they provided had relatively little to do with their own situations or even with misinformation—many of the people were well informed about the potential benefits of the legislation. But the notion that a large-scale social program might disperse their social capital, or would benefit people like Mexicans, welfare queens, or immigrants who they believed were gaming the system, provided greater pull in shaping their negative opinions about the ACA than did the pressures of their own circumstances.

At the time, these seemed like opinions that were prone to change, if not for specific individuals than for the region. The ACA was primed to become the law of the land, and people are generally loath to give up benefits or entitlements once they get used to the assistances they provide. However, there was something jarringly powerful about a rationale that pushed people to focus on the encroachments of others, even at moments when they were so mortally concerned with their own well-being. In many ways, the power of these projections seemed to redirect what might otherwise be assumed core human drives, like self-preservation, while channeling uncertainty or fear outward. Even though I profoundly disagreed with their sentiments, it felt impossible to wholly discount the ways in which people voiced willingness to risk their bodies, even die, in defense of their sense of whiteness.

I watched—and began to chronicle—as undertones of this logic expanded in the region over subsequent years. Voters and politicians fought to reject health care reform, eviscerate social programs, and allow the ready spread of civilian-owned firearms into

285

communal spaces like parks and schools. The results were often catastrophic at the levels of individual health. Yet larger narratives about the fears of encroachment or change often proved to be more powerful forces that were arguments based in public health.

Then came the 2016 presidential election. Rather than fading away, the logic that I encountered in interviews in Tennessee amplified in a resounding national platform. As Trump progressed from sideshow to candidate to president, the notion that others were out to usurp privilege that was rightfully "ours" gained intensity as if by propulsion. And the types of policy decisions that once seemed limited to red and purple states became increasingly difficult for the rest of the country to ignore. Cutting health care, along with gutting safety nets, social programs, and environmental protections, became justified under a narrative that claimed to protect "our" interests and restore "our" greatness against the encroachments of an ever-growing list of others. Immigrants, gang members, convicts, journalists, women, liberals, longtime trade partners . . . it's hard to imagine just how long the list will grow by the time this book is published.

Again, it might well be argued that the logic I encountered in the Tennessee interviews carried the day for Trump and the GOP—inasmuch as the efforts of foot soldiers who refused even their own treatment and care provided the foundation on which the GOP orchestrated the demise of the ACA and other programs. Had white Southerners instead embraced the ACA, reversing its effects would have been far more difficult. The same might be said for persons who bought guns and left them on their nightstands even though they knew the lethal potential of firearms, or parents who voted for tax cuts that affected even the schools that their own children attended. Yet the central existential questions that seemed to surround and elude the patients with whom I spoke in the hospital grew evermore salient as a result. What was the mortal cost to us, as a communal body or the idea of a nation, of defining our sense of greatness by dehumanizing "other" groups of persons—rather than by building just and confident institutions? What further acts of self-sabotage or self-denial were required to keep the system afloat?

When read as such, the lost days, dollars, and opportunities that I track in this book become object lessons that quantify a larger story about the invisibility of particular forms of expiration. Here, people live shorter lives or have fewer places to turn in times of need as a result of political or policy decisions that they themselves may have supported. But because these decisions are made under the cover of the norm or the mainstream, their downstream effects become all the more difficult to discern. All the while, traditions of compromise that created American greatness in the first place fall by the wayside. And while it has become en vogue to tell the story of this rightward turn through the framework of socioeconomic class—and for good reason—the histories of guns, health care, and education help bring the narrative back to the centrality of race to the rise of Trumpism.

So very much work went into transforming the tensions of these early interviews into a sustained narrative. From the moments of first observation onward, I've been privileged to learn, once again, that what we call single-authored books are in fact reflections of broader networks, support systems, and communities.

First, I give thanks to the brilliant research assistants, students, and statistical collaborators with whom I've worked over the past five years. Sarah Rudasill is a medical student of boundless energy, who is poised to become an important national leader. Vladimir Enlow is a statistical researcher who finds paths of reason among the chaos of numerical blizzards. Adithya Sivakumar is a student researcher and soon-to-be medical student whose genius rests in transforming complex ideas into understandable visual stories. I am also grateful for help along the way from Molly Pahn, Jackie Genow, Mia Keys, and Jennifer Ohnstad, among others.

My remarkable colleagues at Vanderbilt, and particularly in the vibrant Center for Medicine, Health, and Society, provided vital feedback and support along the way. I'm also deeply grateful to the leadership of the university, from the chancellor and provost on down, for creating a community in which complex and oft-conflicting ideas are allowed to thrive and flourish in ways that provide hope that even the most entrenched positions benefit from thoughtful analysis and debate. Vanderbilt also had the foresight to hire the terrific communications coordinator Amy Wolf, who continually shines light on the important work of academic research.

My research benefited immeasurably from the insights provided by colleagues from beyond Vanderbilt. As always, I give thanks to the members of the Oxidate writing group; our yearly immersive retreat is sustained in equal measures by generosity and brilliance. I also thank Eric Klinenberg, Caitlin Zaloom, and the community at the Institute for Public Knowledge (IPK) at New York University, where I worked on early portions of this book. Melissa Harris-Perry, Helena Hansen, Joel Braslow, and Nadav Davidovitch have been important interlocutors. John Carson, Anna Kirkland, Domna Stanton, and Carol Boyd are always on my mind, even when far away. At every step along the way, my research was enriched by the kindness of persons who shared time, resources, access, or contacts. I particularly thank the remarkable Stacey Newman in Missouri, Beth Joslin Roth in Tennessee, and LeEtta Felter, Annie McKay, Joy Koesten, Barbara Bollier, and Melissa Rooker in Kansas for their vital assistance and thoughtful insights. I also thank Bob Milgrim, who shared a trove of stories and materials that helped paint the picture of everyday gun transactions in Missouri in decades before the "new" NRA.

One could not hope for better agents than Zoë Pagnamenta and Alison Lewis, at the Zoë Pagnamenta Agency, or a more attentive and engaged editor than Brian Distelberg at Basic Books. Their insights, advice, and attention to detail remained constant and consistently inspiring. Editorial help along the way from Pete Beatty and Roger Labrie combed, directed, and guided the manuscript into shape.

So many amazing friends provided support along the way. Ian Jones, Liz Feinberg, Beth Roth, Jennifer Lee, JuLeigh Petty, and the lovely Alisa and Nelson Ng are bedrocks of support. Kecia Élan Cole and the team at BRIC provided a space and a sounding board. Sasha, Ida, and Joe Ginnetti were vital parts of my life for the early parts of this project—I feel your absence deeply and wish you all the happiness in the world. I'm also so grateful to my outstanding teammates, all, at the WSL—I experienced some forbidding run-ins with the limits of embodiment over the course of writing this book and at those times felt the power and support of community. Special thanks to the management of Holland Cowger, Gerald Marquez, and Juan Monroy, and also to the amazing Layne Martin. So, too, Sherie M. Randolph and I cooked up many core ideas over the course of a life-changing trip to California.

Finally, to the Metzls of Kansas City, New York, and Denver, who continue to provide foundations of equity, justice, and community engagement that guide me. My father and his parents escaped the horrors of Europe during WWII and survived because of the safe haven that was America during a time of despair. My mother's grandparents were immigrants from Russia who settled in Queens. Each gave back in their own ways. My father joined the air force and then became a physician for generations of children, while my mother became a psychologist, a psychoanalyst, and community leader. Persisting in the face of numerous obstacles and points of strain, my parents built a family that derived strength of purpose through service to others. My amazing brothers work as a sports medicine doctor, a blazing thought leader, and a surgeon, and my sister-in-law is a lawyer. Each works in their own way to build and sustain community through values of service, equity, and the respect for diversity that, to my mind, lie at the core of the American dream.

As I detail at multiple points in this book, the story of the Midwest is in many respects also a story about the communities in which we grew up. In our Midwest, there were certainly tensions about fitting in—as Jews, we were, in many ways, white outsiders. But our family also thrived in Missouri and Kansas because of strong regional traditions of neighborliness, kindness, compromise, and goodwill. These are the very traditions that seem ever more in peril in our current moment of divisiveness. A moment when one "side" of a debate amasses arms, guts social programs that benefit minority and low-income communities, and falls into a narrative in which the viability of certain groups exists only in relation to the despair of others. Part of what I've tried to show in this book is that it was not always this way and that getting back to a place where America is truly great depends on the hard work of talking with and listening to each other and recognizing how much we actually need each other, instead of falling prey to prefabricated and manipulated polarizations. Let us hope, for all of our sakes and for the future of our nation, that the white America of which I am a part can find a politics worth living for, rather than one whose enormity is marked by increasingly autoimmune forms of conflict, disempowerment, and demise.

NOTES

INTRODUCTION: DYING OF WHITENESS

1. Martha White, "Why Trump Voters Will Be Hit the Hardest by His Policies," NBC News, February 6, 2017, accessed April 23, 2018, https://nbcnews.to/2HWDCq7. Editorial Board, "Trumpcare Is Already Hurting Trump Country," *New York Times*, May 19, 2017, accessed April 23, 2018, https://nyti.ms/2jtcRuS. Daniel Malloy, "Obamacare Is Retreating—and It's Hurting Trump Voters, Big Time," *OZY*, July 10, 2017, accessed April 23, 2018, https://bit.ly/2rrvjIx. Also see Adam Behsudi, Ayanna Alexander, John F. Harris, and Will Marshall, "Trump's Trade Pullout Roils Rural America," *Politico*, August 7, 2017, accessed April 23, https://politi.co/2j1yxgO.

2. Leo Shvedsky, "Trump Freely Admits His Biggest Supporters Will Be Hurt Most by Healthcare Plan," *Daily Good*, March 16, 2017, accessed April 23, 2018, https://www.good.is/articles/trump-admits-republicans-suffer-healthcare-bill. Also see Matthew Yglesias, "Trump to Tucker Carlson: 'I Know' Counties That Voted for Me Will Lose Under the Republican Health Plan," *Vox*, March 16, 2017, accessed April 23, 2018, https://www.vox.com/policy-and-politics/2017/3/16/14945030/trump-tucker-carlson-health-care.

3. Katherine Gallagher Robbins, Rejane Frederick, and Rachel West, "10 Ways President Trump's Agenda Will Harm His Supporters in Rural and Small-Town America," Center for American Progress, April 3, 2017, accessed April 23, 2018, https://ampr.gs/2mCDLQL. Also see Chauncey DeVega, "First Installment on the Butcher's Bill: Donald Trump's Supporters Will Be Made to Pay," *Salon*, February 24, 2017, accessed April 23, 2018, https://www.salon.com/2017/02/24/first-installment-on-the-butchers-bill-donald-trumps-supporters-will-be-made-to-pay. Nat Malkus, "How the Republican Tax Plan Uses School Savings to Hurt States," *New York Times*, December 19, 2017, accessed April 23, 2018, https://nyti.ms/2oUh00z.

4. Editorial Board, "The False Premise Behind GOP Tax Cuts," *New York Times*, January 20, 2018, accessed April 23, 2018, https://nyti.ms/2tnGW5h.

5. Jelani Cobb, "In Trump's World, Whites Are the Only Disadvantaged Class," *New Yorker*, August 4, 2017, accessed April 23, 2018, https://www.newyorker.com/news/news-desk/in-trumps-world-whites-are-the-only-disadvantaged-class.

6. Thomas Frank, *What's the Matter with Kansas?: How Conservatives Won the Heart of America* (New York: Holt, 2004). George Yancy, *Backlash: What Happens When We Talk Honestly About Racism in America* (New York: Rowman & Littlefield, 2018).

7. See, for instance, Michael Tesler, "Economic Anxiety Isn't Driving Racial Resentment. Racial Resentment Is Driving Economic Anxiety," *Washington Post*, August 22,

2016, accessed April 23, 2018, https://www.washingtonpost.com/news/monkey-cage
/wp/2016/08/22/economic-anxiety-isnt-driving-racial-resentment-racial-resentment
-is-driving-economic-anxiety. Also see German Lopez, "The Past Year of Research Has
Made It Very Clear: Trump Won Because of Racial Resentment," *Vox*, December 15, 2017,
accessed April 23, 2018, https://bit.ly/2ATCQa4.

8. For the racial underpinnings of the Tea Party, see Devin Burghart and Leonard
Zeskind, "Tea Party Nationalism: A Critical Examination of the Tea Party Movement and
the Size, Scope, and Focus of Its National Factions," Institute for Research & Education on Human Rights, accessed April 23, 2018, https://bit.ly/2FVWq36. Also see Ewen
MacAskill and Ed Pilkington, "Report Links Tea Party Movement to White Supremacist
Groups," *Guardian*, October 20, 2010, accessed April 23, 2018, https://www.theguardian
.com/world/2010/oct/20/report-links-tea-party-to-white-supremacist-groups. David Ferguson, "Missouri 'Tea Party for Trump' Speaker Assures Rally: It Is Not Racist to Hate
Mexicans," *Raw Story*, August 31, 2016, accessed April 23, 2018, https://www.rawstory
.com/2016/08/missouri-tea-party-for-trump-speaker-assures-rally-it-is-not-racist-to-hate
-mexicans. Frances Kai-Hwa Wang, "Missouri Asian-American Community Speaks Out
Against 'Xenophobic' Campaign Ads," NBC News, July 26, 2016, accessed April 23,
2018, https://www.nbcnews.com/news/asian-america/missouri-asian-american-community
-speaks-out-against-seemingly-xenophobic-campaign-n616951. For an excellent analysis of concerns about status, see Diana C. Mutz, "Status Threat, Not Economic Hardship, Explains the 2016 Presidential Vote," *PNAS* (April 2018): 201718155; doi:10.1073
/pnas.1718155115. Writing in response, sociologist Andrew Cherlin importantly points
out that "those who try to distinguish between the explanatory power of stagnant wages
and a declining industrial base on the one hand, and anxieties about the ascent of minority
groups on the other, miss the point: These are not two different factors but two sides of the
same coin." See Andrew J. Cherlin, "You Can't Separate Money from Culture," *New York
Times*, May 6, 2018, accessed May 6, 2018, https://nyti.ms/2KF9PzX.

9. Massive tax cuts for corporations paid for by gutting Medicaid and child tax credits, for instance, contained no strategies whatsoever for ways that corporate funds might
then support elderly care or early-child development. For weakened protections, see, for
instance, Neil Schoenherr, "WashU Expert: Missouri SB 43 Would Weaken Discrimination Protections," *Source*, March 10, 2017, accessed April 23, 2018, https://source.wustl
.edu/2017/03/washu-expert-missouri-sb-43-weaken-discrimination-protections.

10. Robert Leonard, "They're Trump-Strong in Rural Iowa—and Not Changing Their
Minds," *Kansas City Star*, October 27, 2017, accessed April 23, 2018, https://www.kansas
city.com/opinion/readers-opinion/guest-commentary/article181300286.html. Ryan Struyk,
"It Looks Like Tax Reform Is Already Paying Off with the GOP Base," CNN, December 17,
2017, accessed April 23, 2018, http://cnn.it/2kBa2rB.

11. For a terrific historical anatomy of this strategy, see Rick Perlstein, *Nixonland:
The Rise of a President and the Fracturing of America* (New York: Scribner, 2009). Arlie
Russell Hochschild, *Strangers in Their Own Land: Anger and Mourning on the American
Right* (New York: New Press, 2018). Frank, *What's the Matter with Kansas?* Nancy Is-
enberg, *White Trash: The 400-Year Untold History of Class in America* (London: Atlantic
Books, 2017). Though beyond the frame of my analysis in the book, any number of scholars
theorize whiteness in global perspective. See, for instance, Aileen Moreton-Robinson, *The
White Possessive: Property, Power, and Indigenous Sovereignty* (Minneapolis: University of
Minnesota Press, 2015).

12. Sarah Smarsh, "Liberal Blind Spots Are Hiding the Truth About 'Trump Country,'" *New York Times*, July 19, 2019, accessed July 19, 2019, https://www.nytimes.com /2018/07/19/opinion/trump-corporations-white-working-class.html.

13. Steve Coll, "The Distrust That Trump Relies Upon," *New Yorker*, December 22, 2017, accessed April 23, 2018, https://www.newyorker.com/news/daily-comment/the -distrust-that-trump-relies-upon; John Cassidy, "Las Vegas, Gun Violence, and the Failing American State," *New Yorker*, October 4, 2017, accessed April 23, 2018, https://www .newyorker.com/news/john-cassidy/las-vegas-gun-violence-and-the-failing-american -state.

14. An expanding volume of important research tracks the biological effects of racism. Citations of this work often begin with landmark studies of John Henryism: S. A. James, N. L. Keenan, D. S. Strogatz, S. R. Browning, and J. M. Garrett, "Socioeconomic Status, John Henryism, and Blood Pressure in Black Adults. The Pitt County Study," *American Journal of Epidemiology* 135, no. 1 (January 1992): 59–67. For present-day scientific examples, see: Tené T. Lewis, Susan A. Everson-Rose, Lynda H. Powell, Karen A. Matthews, Charlotte Brown, Kelly Karavolos, Kim Sutton-Tyrrell, Elizabeth Jacobs, and Deidre Wesley, "Chronic Exposure to Everyday Discrimination and Coronary Artery Calcification in African-American Women: The SWAN Heart Study," *Psychosomatic Medicine* 68, no. 3 (May 2006): 362–368, doi:10.1097/01.psy.0000221360.94700.16; Naa Oyo A. Kwate, Heiddis B. Valdimarsdottir, Josephine S. Guevarra, and Dana H. Bovbjerg, "Experiences of Racist Events Are Associated with Negative Health Consequences for African American Women," *Journal of the National Medical Association* 95, no. 6 (2003): 450–460; Myra J. Tucker, Cynthia J. Berg, William M. Callaghan, and Jason Hsia, "The Black-White Disparity in Pregnancy-Related Mortality From 5 Conditions: Differences in Prevalence and Case-Fatality Rates," *American Journal of Public Health* 97, no. 2 (February 2007): 247–251, https://doi.org/10.2105/AJPH.2005.072975; "Sleep Problems May Be a Link Between Perceived Racism and Poor Health," *ScienceDaily*, June 14, 2011, accessed April 23, 2018, https://www.sciencedaily.com/releases/2011/06/110614101112.htm; Mario Sims, Ana V. Diez-Roux, Amanda Dudley, Samson Gebreab, Sharon B. Wyatt, Marino A. Bruce, Sherman A. James, Jennifer C. Robinson, David R. Williams, and Herman A. Taylor, "Perceived Discrimination and Hypertension Among African Americans in the Jackson Heart Study," *American Journal of Public Health* 102, no. S2 (May 2012), doi:10.2105/ ajph.2011.300523; Y. C. Cozier, J. Yu, P. F. Coogan, T. N. Bethea, L. Rosenberg, and J. R. Palmer, "Racism, Segregation, and Risk of Obesity in the Black Women's Health Study," *American Journal of Epidemiology* 179, no. 7 (April 2014): 875–883, https://doi .org/10.1093/aje/kwu004. To feel it and understand it, urgently read Claudia Rankine, *Citizen: An American Lyric* (New York: Harper Perennial, 2015).

15. Elizabeth Page-Gould, "The Unhealthy Racist," in *Are We Born Racist? New Insights from Neuroscience and Positive Psychology*, ed. Jason Marsh, Rodolfo Mendoza-Denton, and Jeremy Smith (Boston: Beacon Press, 2010), 41–52.

16. Mark Beaulieu and Tracey Continelli, "Benefits of Segregation for White Communities: A Review of the Literature and Directions for Future Research," *Journal of African American Studies* 15, no. 4 (December 2011): 487–507, doi:10.1007/s12111-011-9158-1.

17. Jim Tankersley, "Kansas Tried a Tax Plan Similar to Trump's. It Failed," *New York Times*, October 24, 2017, accessed April 24, 2018, https://nyti.ms/2yWqkRt.

18. See, for instance, Nadine Cohodas, *Strom Thurmond & the Politics of Southern Change* (Macon, GA: Mercer University Press, 1994). Paul Starr, "The Health Care Legacy

of the Great Society," in *LBJ's Neglected Legacy: The Policy and Management Legacies of the Johnson Years*, ed. Norman J. Glickman, Laurence E. Lynn, and Robert H. Wilson (Austin: University of Texas Press, 2015), 235–258, https://bit.ly/2pZnefe. R. D. Schremmer and J. F. Knapp, "Harry Truman and Health Care Reform: The Debate Started Here," *Pediatrics* 127, no. 3 (March 2011): 399–401, doi:10.1542/peds.2010-2151.

19. W. E. B. Du Bois, *Black Reconstruction in America: An Essay Toward a History of the Part Which Black Folk Played in the Attempt to Reconstruct Democracy in America: 1860–1880* (New York: Atheneum, 1975). David R. Roediger, *The Wages of Whiteness: Race and the Making of the American Working Class* (London: Verso, 2007). "Aftermath: Sixteen Writers on Trump's America," *New Yorker*, November 21, 2016, accessed April 24, 2018, https://www.newyorker.com/magazine/2016/11/21/aftermath-sixteen-writers-on-trumps-america#morrison. Michael Eric Dyson, *Tears We Cannot Stop: A Sermon to White America* (New York: St. Martin's Press, 2017), 44. For James Baldwin in 1963, white invincibility depended on unquestioned belief in a series of destructive "myths . . . that their ancestors were all freedom-loving heroes, that they were born in the greatest country the world has ever seen, or that Americans are invincible in battle and wise in peace." See James Baldwin, *The Fire Next Time* (New York: Dial Press, 1963), 101–102.

20. Jennifer Malat, Sarah Mayorga-Gallo, and David R. Williams, "The Effects of Whiteness on the Health of Whites in the USA," *Social Science & Medicine* 199 (July 2017): 148–156, doi:10.1016/j.socscimed.2017.06.034.

21. Ta-Nehisi Coates, "The First White President," *Atlantic*, October 2017, https://www.theatlantic.com/magazine/archive/2017/10/the-first-white-president-ta-nehisi-coates/537909. Henry A. Giroux, *The Public in Peril: Trump and the Menace of American Authoritarianism* (New Jersey: Routledge, 2017). For the landmark study showing how these trends began before Trump, see A. Case and A. Deaton, "Rising Morbidity and Mortality in Midlife Among White Non-Hispanic Americans in the 21st Century," *Proceedings of the National Academy of Sciences* 112, no. 49 (2016): 15078–15083, doi:10.341 0/f.725940664.793520684.

22. For balkanization, see Amanda Taub, "Why Americans Vote 'Against Their Interest': Partisanship," *New York Times*, April 12, 2017, accessed April 24, 2018, https://nyti.ms/2osaziL. For CDC ban, see Julia Belluz, "The CDC's 'Word Ban' May Be Politics as Usual. But It's Still Concerning," *Vox*, December 20, 2017, accessed April 24, 2018, https://www.vox.com/2017/12/18/16792124/cdc-word-ban-science.

23. I want to again emphasize that I in no way mean to suggest that men like Trevor are duped or uninformed. Logics and strategies of people we might not agree with make sense in context as modes of meaning-making. As the work of linguist George Lakoff shows, conservative voters often support politics that reflect highly developed worldviews, identities, and "moral systems," even at the expense of their material interests. I also note the work of historian Geoffrey Kabaservice, who demonstrates ways that populist conservatives support seemingly illogical positions about matters such as "fake news" not because they necessarily believe them but because these positions convey what are held to be underlying conservative "symbolic truths." See George Lakoff, "Why It Matters How We Frame the Environment," *Environmental Communication* 4, no. 1 (March 2010): 70–81, https://doi.org/10.1080/17524030903529749. Also see Geoffrey Kabaservice, "The Great Performance of Our Failing President," *New York Times*, June 9, 2017, accessed May 1, 2018, https://nyti.ms/2t3Y6S6. As such, I take issue with recent analyses of working-class

populations that frame white lives defined by despair and for which empathy and understanding represent the best ways forward. (See, for instance: Michael Lerner, "Stop Shaming Trump Supporters," *New York Times*, November 9, 2016, accessed May 1, 2017, https://nyti.ms/2k2amBU; Colby Itkowitz, "What Is This Election Missing? Empathy for Trump Voters," *Washington Post*, November 2, 2016, accessed May 1, 2017, http://wapo .st/2faYnx7?tid=ss_mail&utm_term=.e593cf95a6b9.) Such arguments risk treating Trump supporters as unruly children in need of paternalistic love rather than as autonomous subjects who make decisions based on their own calculus of risk versus reward. Liberal empathy can also itself reflect laden assumptions about which persons or groups are deserving of empathy and which groups are not. (See, for instance, Sarah Lerner, "Stop Telling Us to Empathize with Trump Supporters," *Medium*, November 3, 2016, https://medium.com/ @sarahlerner/stop-telling-us-to-empathize-with-trump-supporters-597d21756d54.) Even though I trained as a psychiatrist, my analysis leads not to a call for individual empathy or for attempts to talk anyone out of their votes but for greater awareness of the health implications of particular policies, and for better policies and structural change.

24. Steve Phillips, "Trump Wants to Make America White Again," *New York Times*, February 15, 2018, accessed April 24, 2018, https://nyti.ms/2BvTvQ0.

THE CAPE

1. Jonathan M. Metzl, "Are Looser Gun Laws Changing the Social Fabric of Missouri?," *New Republic*, March 10, 2016, accessed April 30, 2018, https://bit.ly/2wjvURD. "Crack of the Pistol: Dueling in 19th Century Missouri," Crack of the Pistol Political Duels, accessed April 30, 2018, https://bit.ly/2KG188D. Sabrina Tavernise, "In Missouri, Fewer Gun Restrictions and More Gun Killings," *New York Times*, December 21, 2015, accessed April 30, 2018, https://nyti.ms/2JXw42O.

2. "Missouri Right to Bear Arms, Amendment 5," Ballotpedia, August 2014, accessed April 30, 2018, https://ballotpedia.org/Missouri_Right_to_Bear_Arms,_Amendment_5 _(August_2014). Tara Dodrill, "Open Carry Ban Overturned in Missouri," *Inquisitr*, 2014, accessed April 30, 2018, www.inquisitr.com/1602089/open-carry-ban-overturned-in -missouri. Also see: Jill Ornitz, "Mo. Legislators Pass New Gun Laws," CBS St. Louis, 2014, accessed April 30, 2018, http://stlouis.cbslocal.com/2014/09/11/mo-legislators-pass-new -gun-laws; Danny Wicentowski, "Gun Rights Supporters Head to Gateway Arch, Citygarden to Test Missouri's New Gun Laws," *Riverfront Times*, 2014, https://bit.ly/2Id0scz.

3. For information about these measures, see, for instance, "Missouri: Castle Doctrine and Training Bill Passes House," NRA-ILA, accessed April 30, 2018, https://bit.ly /2rpbXnr. Also see: Jason Hancock, "Missouri Republicans Vote to Override Veto of Gun Bill," *Kansas City Star*, September 14, 2016, accessed April 30, 2018, https://bit .ly/2cvnnho; "Missouri Gov. Vetoes Concealed Carry Bill," KMBC, October 6, 2017, accessed April 30, 2018, https://bit.ly/2IjcNvu; Associated Press in Jefferson City, "Missouri Approves Concealed Guns at Schools and Open Carry in Public," *Guardian*, September 11, 2014, accessed April 30, 2018, https://bit.ly/2FNeP1X.

4. As later parts of this section detail, Missouri effectively became a highly contested ground for gun researchers and gun-rights activists. Editorial Board, "Missouri: The Shoot-Me State," *New York Times*, September 16, 2016, accessed April 30, 2018, https:// nyti.ms/2rp8jJA. Laura Bult, "New Missouri Laws Are Good for Gun Owners, Bad for

Voters," *NY Daily News*, September 16, 2016, accessed April 30, 2018, https://nydn.us/2c
f0y3W. Keith Wood, "Best States for Gun Owners," *Guns & Ammo*, 2015, accessed April
30, 2018, https://bit.ly/1LA2P2J. By 2018, even the most basic efforts to curb gun-
related injury and death were being shot down. That year, Missouri representative
DaRon McGee from Kansas City introduced a bill to curb celebratory gunfire. House Bill
2302, or Blair's Law, was named in honor of a young girl killed by celebratory gunfire
in 2011. Soon thereafter, the NRA listed the bill as "anti-gun" and urged members to
"contact your legislators" in opposition. See Editorial Board, "Weapons Down: Missouri
Lawmakers Should Curb Celebratory Gunfire," *Kansas City Star*, March 18, 2018, accessed March 20, 2018, https://www.kansascity.com/opinion/editorials/article204212379
.html. Also see "Missouri: Updates on Pro-Gun and Anti-Gun Legislation," NRA-ILA,
March 8, 2018, accessed March 20, 2018, https://www.nraila.org/articles/20180308
/missouri-updates-on-pro-gun-and-anti-gun-legislation.

5. Daniel Webster, Cassandra Kercher Crifasi, and Jon S. Vernick, "Erratum To: Effects of the Repeal of Missouri's Handgun Purchaser Licensing Law on Homicides," *Journal of Urban Health* 91, no. 3 (2014): 598–601, doi:10.1007/s11524-014-9882-7. This
study is discussed in detail below. Also see: Brian Burnes, "Missouri Gun Deaths Sur-
pass Vehicle Deaths in 2013, Part of National Trend," *Kansas City Star*, accessed April
30, 2018, https://bit.ly/2HUn423; Jesse Bogan, "Behind a Rising Suicide Rate, a Struggle
for Answers," Stltoday.com, October 7, 2012, accessed April 30, 2018, https://bit.ly/2K
FxekX; Christopher Ingraham, "People Are Getting Shot by Toddlers on a Weekly Basis
This Year," *Washington Post*, October 14, 2015, accessed April 30, 2018, https://wapo
.st/2rpcndv; Mary Sanchez, "Why the Gun Lobby Wants to Arm Children," *Kansas City
Star*, accessed April 30, 2018, https://bit.ly/2HT9lZh; Sarah Fenske, "More People in Missouri Died from Guns in 2014 Than Car Accidents," *Riverfront Times*, 2016, accessed
April 30, 2018, https://bit.ly/2I0i341. For a local take on concealed carry, see Will Schmitt,
"Newly Relaxed Concealed-Carry, Deadly-Force Laws Put Missouri in the National Spot-
light," *Springfield News-Leader*, September 18, 2016, accessed April 30, 2018, https://
sgfnow.co/2ro7cK5.

6. I write about this research in brief at Jonathan M. Metzl, "Guns in Donald
Trump's America," *New Republic*, August 30, 2016, accessed April 30, 2018, https://bit
.ly/2HUTucP. Also see "Missouri Election Results 2016: President Live Map by County,
Real-Time Voting Updates," *Politico*, 2016, accessed April 30, 2018, https://politi.co
/2JUI9Ga. For Clinton on gun policy, see "Gun Violence Prevention," Office of Hillary
Rodham Clinton, accessed April 30, 2018, http://hrc.io/2FQhW94.

7. Phill Brooks, "Passing Echoes of Legislative Bipartisanship," *Gladstone Dispatch*,
September 20, 2016, accessed April 30, 2018, https://bit.ly/2jzvDRq.

8. For the thorough DOJ report, see "Investigation of the Ferguson Police Department," United States Department of Justice Civil Rights Division, 2015, accessed April 30,
2018, https://bit.ly/1lV31kb. For the earlier police report, see *Overcoming the Challenges
and Creating a Regional Approach to Policing in St. Louis City and County* (Washington,
DC: Police Executive Research Forum, 2015), www.bettertogetherstl.com/wp-content
/uploads/2015/04/PERF-Report-Overcoming-the-Challenges.pdf.

9. Nick Chabarria, "MSHP: Opioid, Heroin Trafficking up in Southeast MO," KFVS12,
September 19, 2016, accessed April 30, 2018, https://bit.ly/2rob4eK. Charles S. Gascon
and Joseph McGillicuddy, "Some Sectors Are Strong in Cape Girardeau, but Recovery from

Recession Remains Elusive," Federal Reserve Bank of St. Louis, July 15, 2016, accessed April 30, 2018, https://bit.ly/2FQiprQ. For a terrific history of the town, see "History of Cape Girardeau," City of Cape Girardeau, accessed April 30, 2018, https://bit.ly/2I1cQsR.

10. "U.S. Census Bureau QuickFacts: Cape Girardeau County, Missouri," Census Bureau QuickFacts, accessed April 30, 2018, https://bit.ly/2Iiy4pi. See "Missouri Election Results 2016," *Politico*.

11. For airports, see "A Win for Conceal and Carry Permit Holders at Missouri Airports," KFVS12, December 15, 2016, accessed April 30, 2018, https://bit.ly/2rmT5Fs.

RISK

1. Émile Durkheim, John A. Spaulding, and George Simpson, *Suicide: A Study in Sociology* (New York: Snowball Publishing, 2013).

2. Lisa Pan et al., "17.2 Neurometabolic Disorders: Potentially Treatable Abnormalities in Patients with Treatment Refractory Depression and Suicidal Behavior," *Journal of the American Academy of Child & Adolescent Psychiatry* 55, no. 10 (2016), doi:10.1016/j.jaac.2016.07.757. Nigel E. Bush, Derek J. Smolenski, Lauren M. Denneson, Holly B. Williams, Elissa K. Thomas, and Steven K. Dobscha, "A Virtual Hope Box: Randomized Controlled Trial of a Smartphone App for Emotional Regulation and Coping with Distress," *Psychiatric Services* 68, no. 4 (2017): 330–336, doi:10.1176/appi.ps.201600283.

3. Xiulu Ruan, Jin Jun Luo, and Alan David Kaye, "Commentary: Hypnotic Medications and Suicide: Risk, Mechanisms, Mitigation, and the FDA," *Frontiers in Psychiatry* 7 (2017), doi:10.3389/fpsyt.2016.00210.

4. Mary F. Cwik, Lauren Tingey, Alexandra Maschino, Novalene Goklish, Francene Larzelere-Hinton, John Walkup, and Allison Barlow, "Decreases in Suicide Deaths and Attempts Linked to the White Mountain Apache Suicide Surveillance and Prevention System, 2001–2012," *American Journal of Public Health* 106, no. 12 (2016): 2183–2189, doi:10.2105/ajph.2016.303453.

5. For these websites, see "Risk Factors and Warning Signs," American Foundation for Suicide Prevention, https://afsp.org/about-suicide/risk-factors-and-warning-signs, and "Risk of Suicide," National Alliance on Mental Illness, https://www.nami.org/Learn-More/Mental-Health-Conditions/Related-Conditions/Suicide.

6. The overall US suicide rate rose by 24 percent between 1999 and 2014. The rise in suicides was particularly intense starting in 2006–2007, when national rates suddenly doubled. Sabrina Tavernise, "U.S. Suicide Rate Surges to a 30-Year High," *New York Times*, April 22, 2016, accessed April 30, 2018, https://nyti.ms/2wi5e3F. K. A. Hempstead and J. A. Phillips, "Rising Suicide Among Adults Aged 40–64 Years: The Role of Job and Financial Circumstances," *American Journal of Preventive Medicine* 48, no. 5 (May 2015): 491–500, https://bit.ly/2wepJOF. Mike Maciag, "Suicide Rate Highest in Decades but Worst in Rural America," *Governing*, February 7, 2018, accessed April 30, 2018, https://bit.ly/2F3NCsj.

7. For this history, see W. S. F. Pickering and Geoffrey Walford, *Durkheim's Suicide: A Century of Research and Debate. Routledge Studies in Social and Political Thought* (London: Routledge, 2000), 69. Also see: Ronald W. Maris, Alan L. Berman, Morton M. Silverman, and Bruce Michael Bongar, *Comprehensive Textbook of Suicidology* (New York: Guilford Press, 2000); Norman St. John-Stevas, *Life, Death and the Law: Law and Christian*

Morals in England and the United States (Bloomington: Indiana University Press, 1961). For U.S. attitudes, see "Survey Finds That Americans Value Mental Health and Physical Health Equally," Anxiety and Depression Association of America, 2015, accessed April 30, 2018, https://bit.ly/2HTA3Bb.

8. Sally C. Curtin, Margaret Warner, and Holly Hedegaard, "Increase in Suicide in the United States, 1999–2014," Centers for Disease Control and Prevention, April 22, 2016, accessed April 30, 2018, https://bit.ly/2ihEJTP. "Guns and Suicide" Fact Sheet, Violence Policy Center, 2011, www.vpc.org/fact_sht/Guns%20and%20Suicide.pdf. Kate Masters, "New CDC Report Shows America's Gun Suicide Problem Getting Worse," *Trace*, April 26, 2016, accessed April 30, 2018, https://bit.ly/1SxeovO.

9. Omnibus Consolidated Appropriations Act of 1997, Pub. L. No. 104-208 (1996), https://bit.ly/22zCqKD. Michael Hiltzik, "The NRA Has Blocked Gun Violence Research for 20 Years. Let's End Its Stranglehold on Science," *Los Angeles Times*, June 14, 2016, accessed April 30, 2018, www.latimes.com/business/hiltzik/la-fi-hiltzik-gun-research-funding -20160614-snap-story.html.

10. Miguel A. Faria Jr., "The Tainted Public-Health Model of Gun Control," Foundation for Economic Education, April 1, 2001, accessed April 30, 2018, https://bit.ly /2HVEHdO. Paul Hsieh, "Why I Don't Trust Government-Backed 'Gun Violence' Research," *Forbes*, June 22, 2016, accessed April 30, 2018, https://bit.ly/2KEfEO4. "Disarming the Data Doctors: How to Debunk the 'Public Health' Basis for 'Gun Control,'" Gun Owners of America, 2009, accessed April 30, 2018, https://bit.ly/2FOUGIE. Arthur L. Kellerman et al., "Gun Ownership as a Risk Factor for Homicide in the Home," *New England Journal of Medicine* 329, no. 15 (1993): 1084–1091, https://www.nejm.org/doi/full/10.1056 /NEJM199310073291506.

11. Kate Masters, "Read the Letter from 141 Medical Groups Urging Congress to Restore Funding for Gun Violence Research," *Trace*, April 20, 2018, accessed April 30, 2018, https://bit.ly/2jwpghE. Also see: American Association of Pediatrics to the Senate Appropriations Committee, July 10, 2013, https://bit.ly/2JTbYXB; Scott Gale, "Drama at AMA: Anti-Gun Resolution Passes," *MD Magazine*, June 14, 2016, accessed May 1, 2018, https://bit.ly/2roHcy1; "AMA Calls Gun Violence 'A Public Health Crisis,'" American Medical Association, June 14, 2016, accessed May 1, 2018, https://bit.ly/2r6NmCd.

12. H. Bauchner, F. P. Rivara, R. O. Bonow, et al., "Death by Gun Violence—a Public Health Crisis," *JAMA Neurology* 74, no. 12 (2017): 1402–1403, doi:10.1001/ jamaneurol.2017.3533.

13. Jonathan Metzl, *The Protest Psychosis: How Schizophrenia Became a Black Disease* (Boston, MA: Beacon, 2010).

14. Arthur L. Kellermann, Frederick P. Rivara, Grant Somes, Donald T. Reay, Jerry Francisco, Joyce Gillentine Banton, Janice Prodzinski, Corinne Fligner, and Bela B. Hackman, "Suicide in the Home in Relation to Gun Ownership," *New England Journal of Medicine* 327, no. 7 (1992): 467–472, doi:10.1056/nejm199208133270705. Also see Whet Moser, "Doctors' Group Asks Congress to Nix Gun-Violence Research Ban (Again)," *Chicago*, June 15, 2016, accessed May 1, 2018, https://bit.ly/2HZbaA3.

15. David E. Stark and Nigam H. Shah, "Funding and Publication of Research on Gun Violence and Other Leading Causes of Death," *JAMA* 317, no. 1 (2017): 84, doi:10.1001/ jama.2016.16215.

16. Matthew Miller and David Hemenway, "Guns and Suicide in the United States," *New England Journal of Medicine* 359, no. 10 (2008): 989–991, doi:10.1056/

nejmp0805923. Also see: "Homicide," Harvard Injury Control Research Center, June 30, 2016, accessed May 1, 2018, https://www.hsph.harvard.edu/hicrc/firearms-research/guns -and-death; E. J. Kaufman, C. N. Morrison, C. C. Branas, and D. J. Wiebe, "State Firearm Laws and Interstate Firearm Deaths from Homicide and Suicide in the United States: A Cross-Sectional Analysis of Data by County," *JAMA Internal Medicine* (March 2018), doi:10.1001/jamainternmed.2018.0190.

17. "Risk of Suicide," NAMI, accessed May 1, 2018, https://bit.ly/2HRtPS1. Also see: Madeline Drexler, "Guns & Suicide: The Hidden Toll," *Harvard Public Health*, spring 2013, 24–35, accessed May 1, 2018, https://www.hsph.harvard.edu/magazine/magazine _article/guns-suicide; "Lethality of Suicide Methods," Harvard T. H. Chan School of Public Health, January 6, 2017, accessed May 1, 2018, https://bit.ly/2HnKTLK.

18. Thomas R. Simon, Alan C. Swann, Kenneth E. Powell, Lloyd B. Potter, Marcie-Jo Kresnow, and Patrick W. O'Carroll, "Characteristics of Impulsive Suicide Attempts and Attempters," *Suicide and Life-Threatening Behavior* 32, no. S1 (2001): 49–59, doi:10.1521/ suli.32.1.5.49.24212. Also see Eberhard A. Deisenhammer, Chy-Meng Ing, Robert Strauss, Georg Kemmler, Hartmann Hinterhuber, and Elisabeth M. Weiss, "The Duration of the Suicidal Process," *Journal of Clinical Psychiatry* 70, no. 1 (2008): 19–24, doi:10.4088/ jcp.07m03904.

19. R. S. Spicer and T. R. Miller, "Suicide Acts in 8 States: Incidence and Case Fatality Rates by Demographics and Method," *American Journal of Public Health* 90, no. 12 (2000): 1885–1891, doi:10.2105/ajph.90.12.1885; "Lethality of Suicide Methods."

20. Drexler, "Guns & Suicide," 24. Also see Catherine W. Barber and Matthew J. Miller, "Reducing a Suicidal Person's Access to Lethal Means of Suicide," *American Journal of Preventive Medicine* 47, no. 3 (2014), doi:10.1016/j.amepre.2014.05.028. For an important counterpoint, see, for example, Jeffrey W. Swanson, Michael A. Norko, Hsiu-Ju Lin, Kelly Alanis-Hirsch, Linda K. Frisman, Madelon V. Baranoski, Michele M. Easter, Allison G. Robertson, Marvin S. Swartz, and Richard J. Bonnie, "Implementation and Effectiveness of Connecticut's Risk-Based Gun Removal Law: Does It Prevent Suicides?," *Law and Contemporary Problems* 80 (2017): 179–208.

21. See Sigmund Freud, *Beyond the Pleasure Principle*, trans. and ed. James Strachey (New York: Norton, 1975). For ethnicity and suicide, see: "Results from the 2013 National Survey on Drug Use and Health: Mental Health Findings," Center for Behavioral Health Statistics and Quality, 2013, accessed May 2, 2018, https://binged.it/2roavkp; Alex E. Crosby, Beth Han, LaVonne A. G. Ortega, Sharyn E. Parks, and Joseph Gfroerer, "Suicidal Thoughts and Behaviors Among Adults Aged ≥ 18 Years—United States, 2008–2009," Centers for Disease Control and Prevention, October 21, 2011, accessed May 2, 2018, https://bit.ly/2JTPZjl; Ronald C. Kessler, Guilherme Borges, and Ellen E. Walters, "Prevalence of and Risk Factors for Lifetime Suicide Attempts in the National Comorbidity Survey," *Archives of General Psychiatry* 56, no. 7 (1999): 617, doi:10.1001/archpsyc.56.7.617; R. C. Kessler, P. Berglund, G. Borges, M. Nock, and P. S. Wang, "Trends in Suicide Ideation, Plans, Gestures, and Attempts in the United States, 1990–1992 to 2001–2003," *Journal of the American Medical Association* 293, no. 20 (2005): 2487–2495; Mercedes Perez-Rodriguez, Enrique Baca-Garcia, Maria A. Oquendo, and Carlos Blanco, "Ethnic Differences in Suicidal Ideation Attempts," *Primary Psychiatry*, 15, no. 2 (2008): 44–53; Brian K. Ahmedani, Christine Stewart, Gregory E. Simon, Frances Lynch, Christine Y. Lu, Beth E. Waitzfelder, Leif I. Solberg, Ashli A. Owen-Smith, Arne Beck, Laurel A. Copeland, Enid M. Hunkeler, Rebecca C. Rossom, and Keoki Williams, "Racial/Ethnic Differences

in Health Care Visits Made Before Suicide Attempt Across the United States," *Medical Care* 53, no. 5 (2015): 430–435, doi:10.1097/mlr.0000000000000335.

22. See "Suicide Facts at a Glance, 2015," Centers for Disease Control and Prevention, 2015, https://bit.ly/2ipST4k. Also see: "Suicide Statistics," US Suicide Statistics, 2001, accessed May 2, 2018, https://bit.ly/2JVzAuE; *Teen Homicide, Suicide, and Firearm Deaths* (Bethesda, MD: Child Trends, 2015), https://www.childtrends.org/wp-content/uploads/2014/10/70_Homicide_Suicide_Firearms.pdf; Bill Johnson II, "Gone Too Soon: Black Males and Suicide," *Huffington Post*, September 5, 2016, accessed May 2, 2018, https://bit.ly/2JXCAGT; Caroline Jiang, Andreea Mitran, Arialdi Miniño, and Hanyu Ni, "Racial and Gender Disparities in Suicide Among Young Adults Aged 18–24, United States, 2009–2013," National Center for Health Statistics, 2015, https://www.cdc.gov/nchs/data/hestat/suicide/racial_and_gender_2009_2013.htm; Laura Kann et al., "Youth Risk Behavior Surveillance—United States, 2013," Centers for Disease Control and Prevention, June 13, 2014, accessed May 2, 2018, https://bit.ly/2HTBcsb; B. K. Ahmedani et al., "Racial/Ethnic Differences in Health Care Visits Made Before Suicide Attempt Across the United States," Medical Care, May 2015, accessed May 2, 2018, https://bit.ly/2FPGrmS.

23. "A Look at the 1940 Census," United States Census Bureau, https://bit.ly/2nEEIYy. Also see: Frank Hobbs and Nicole Stoops, "Demographic Trends in the 20th Century," US Census, 2002, https://bit.ly/1L2PcKJ; "Historical Racial and Ethnic Demographics of the United States," *Wikipedia*, https://bit.ly/1S7o6nX; Michael Walsh, "US Percentage of Non-Hispanic Whites Hits All-Time Low of 63%," *NY Daily News*, June 13, 2013, accessed May 2, 2018, https://nydn.us/1OX4b9U; the census remains highly political. See Herbert J. Gans, "The Census and Right-Wing Hysteria," *New York Times*, May 11, 2017, accessed May 2, 2018, https://nyti.ms/2HVFjnO.

24. Similar findings appear in multiple studies. An analysis released by the National Center for Health Statistics found that white men experienced a particularly dramatic spike in gun suicides between 2006 and 2014 and used guns to kill themselves more than any other method. A published analysis of WISQARS trends over time showed that the US suicide rate declined "by 18% between 1986 and 1999" but then began to rise dramatically due primarily to an increase in gun suicide among "whites aged 40–64 years." A 2015 report released by the Child Trends Databank found that "among males, suicide rates have been increasing among white teens since 2007, but decreasing or remaining steady among other racial and ethnic groups" because of the differential impact of gun suicides. See: Curtin et al., "Increase in Suicide"; Masters, "New CDC Report"; and G. Hu, H. C. Wilcox, L. Wissow, and S. P. Baker, "Mid-Life Suicide: An Increasing Problem in U.S. Whites, 1999–2005," *American Journal of Preventative Medicine* 37, no. 6 (2009): 579–593. Also see Kerry Shaw, "10 Essential Facts About Guns and Suicide," *Trace*, September 6, 2016, accessed May 2, 2018, https://bit.ly/2HSD6t6.

25. Matthew Frye Jacobson, *Whiteness of a Different Color: European Immigrants and the Alchemy of Race* (Boston, MA: Harvard University Press, 1999).

26. Roberto A. Ferdman, "The Racial Divide in America's Gun Deaths," *Washington Post*, September 19, 2014, accessed May 2, 2018, https://wapo.st/2IlXyCb. Drew DeSilver and Kristen Bialik, "Blacks and Hispanics Face Extra Challenges in Getting Home Loans," Pew Research Center, January 10, 2017, accessed May 2, 2018, https://pewrsr.ch/2j2sf2q.

27. Richard V. Reeves and Sarah Holmes, "Guns and Race: The Different Worlds of Black and White Americans," Brookings Institution, 2015, accessed

May 2, 2018, https://www.brookings.edu/blog/social-mobility-memos/2015/12/15/guns-and-race-the-different-worlds-of-black-and-white-americans.

28. D'Vera Cohn, Paul Taylor, Mark Hugo Lopez, Catherine A. Gallagher, Kim Parker, and Kevin T. Maass, "Gun Homicide Rate Down 49% Since 1993 Peak; Public Unaware," Pew Research Center, May 7, 2013, accessed May 2, 2018, https://pewrsr.ch/1l6vGRe.

29. A. W. R. Hawkins, "2/3rds of Obama's Gun Death Stats Are Suicides," Breitbart, January 5, 2016, accessed May 2, 2018, https://bit.ly/1IPLlkQ.

30. Margot Sanger-Katz, "Gun Deaths Are Mostly Suicides," New York Times, October 8, 2015, https://www.nytimes.com/2015/10/09/upshot/gun-deaths-are-mostly-suicides.html. Andrew Conner, Deborah Azrael, and Matthew Miller, "Public Opinion About the Relationship Between Firearm Availability and Suicide: Results from a National Survey," Annals of Internal Medicine 168, no. 2 (2017): 153, doi:10.7326/m17-2348.

31. Donald Braman and Dan M. Kahan, "More Statistics, Less Persuasion: A Cultural Theory of Gun-Risk Perceptions," University of Pennsylvania Law Review 151, no. 1291 (2002), doi:10.2139/ssrn.286205. Steve Tarzia, J. Kyle White-Sullivan, Rich Gordon, Joe Germuska, Hailey Melville, Alex Sher, Isaac Lee, Patrick Hoy, and Mengyi Jenny Sun, "How Americans Think and Feel About Gun Violence," Northwestern University Knight Lab, September 21, 2016, accessed May 2, 2018, https://bit.ly/2whDzzD. Kerry O'Brien, Walter Forrest, Dermot Lynott, and Michael Daly, "Racism, Gun Ownership and Gun Control: Biased Attitudes in US Whites May Influence Policy Decisions," PLOS ONE 8, no. 10 (2013), doi:10.1371/journal.pone.0077552. Rachel Nuwer, "Americans Who Have Stereotypical Ideas About Race and Violence Are More Likely to Own Guns," Smithsonian.com, November 6, 2013, accessed May 2, 2018, https://bit.ly/2Id8LFh. Cohn et al., "Gun Homicide Rate."

32. "Do the MAOA and CDH13 'Human Warrior Genes' Make Violent Criminals— and What Should Society Do?," Genetic Literacy Project, January 12, 2018, accessed May 2, 2018, https://bit.ly/2BP70qj. "Re: Why Do Black People Commit More Crime?," Alternative Hypothesis, July 19, 2016, accessed May 2, 2018, https://bit.ly/29WriE2. Richard Lynn, "Racial and Ethnic Differences in Psychopathic Personality," Personality and Individual Differences 32, no. 2 (2002): 273–316, https://bit.ly/2rpiFcd. Ishita Aggarwal, "The Role of Antisocial Personality Disorder and Antisocial Behavior in Crime," Inquiries Journal 5, no. 9 (2013): 1–2, https://bit.ly/2jDxKDP. Leonardo F. Andrade and Nancy M. Petry, "White Problem Gamblers Discount Delayed Rewards Less Steeply Than Their African American and Hispanic Counterparts," Psychology of Addictive Behaviors 28, no. 2 (June 2014): 599–606, doi:10.1037/a0036153. Terri E. Moffatt et al., "A Gradient of Childhood Self-Control Predicts Health, Wealth, and Public Safety," PNAS 108, no. 7 (2011): 2693–2698, https://bit.ly/2ro0ogf. Sharon D. Herzberger and Carol S. Dweck, "Attraction and Delay of Gratification," Journal of Personality 46, no. 2 (June 1978): 215–227, doi:10.1111/j.1467-6494.1978.tb00176.x. Jiemin Ma, Elizabeth M. Ward, Rebecca L. Siegel, and Ahmedin Jemal, "Temporal Trends in Mortality in the United States, 1969–2013," JAMA 314, no. 16 (2015): 1731, doi:10.1001/jama.2015.12319.

33. I invite readers to attempt these searches using these databases. For instance, a PubMed search is as follows: https://www.ncbi.nlm.nih.gov/pubmed/?term=%E2%80%9Cwhites%E2%80%9D+are+biologically+or+genetically+prone+to+gun+suicide (search, December 30, 2016); a Psychiatry Online search looks like this: http://ajp.psychiatryonline.org/action/doSearch?field1=AllField&text1=%E2%80%9C

whites%E2%80%9D+biologically+genetically+prone+to+gun+suicide&Ppub=&P
pub=&AfterMonth=&AfterYear=&BeforeMonth=&BeforeYear= (searched December 30,
2016); and a Google search looks like this: https://www.google.com/search?q=%E2%80
%9Cwhites%E2%80%9D+are+biologically+or+genetically+prone+to+gun+suicide&oq
=%E2%80%9Cwhites%E2%80%9D+are+biologically+or+genetically+prone+to+gun
+suicide&aqs=chrome..69i57j69i60.835j0j4&sourceid=chrome&ie=UTF-8 (searched December 30, 2016).

34. Merriam-Webster, s.v. "risk," accessed May 4, 2018, https://bit.ly/2gQtQo7. Sarah
S. Lochlann Jain, *Injury: The Politics of Product Design and Safety Law in the United States*
(Princeton, NJ: Princeton University Press, 2006).

35. Amanda Taub, "Behind 2016's Turmoil, a Crisis of White Identity," *New York
Times*, November 1, 2016, accessed May 4, 2018, https://nyti.ms/2ImmsSo. Phoebe Maltz
Bovy, "In the 'Crisis of Whiteness,' Where Do Jews Fall?," *Forward*, November 3, 2016,
accessed May 4, 2018, https://bit.ly/2HYfqnu. Chauncey DeVega, "Dear White America:
Your Working Class Is Literally Dying—and This Is Your Idea of an Answer?," *Salon*, No-
vember 6, 2015, accessed May 4, 2018, https://bit.ly/1QjDPQf.

36. Émile Durkheim, *The Division of Labor in Society* (New York: MacMillan, 1964).
Also see Pickering and Walford, *Durkheim's Suicide*.

37. Arlie Russell Hochschild, *Strangers in Their Own Land: Anger and Mourning
on the American Right* (New York: New Press, 2018). Sacco Vandal, "White American
Anomie," *Taki's Magazine*, 2016, accessed May 4, 2018, https://bit.ly/2JY0Dp0. Gina
Kolata, "Death Rates Rising for Middle-Aged White Americans, Study Finds," *New
York Times*, November 2, 2015, accessed May 4, 2018, https://nyti.ms/2FO9w20. Anne
Case and Angus Deaton, "Rising Morbidity and Mortality in Midlife Among White Non-
Hispanic Americans in the 21st Century," *PNAS* 112, no. 49 (2015): 15078–15083. Also
see Shannon Monnat, "Study: Communities Most Affected by Opioid Epidemic Also Voted
for Trump," interview with Scott Simon, NPR *Weekend Edition*, December 17, 2016, audio,
4:27, https://n.pr/2FPipbz.

38. "Cardinal Raymond Leo Burke on the Catholic 'Man-Crisis' and What to Do
About It," New Emangelization Project, January 5, 2017, accessed May 1, 2018, https://bit
.ly/1xGn1Kp.

39. Philip Wylie, *A Generation of Vipers* (Champaign, IL: Dalkey Archive Press, 2017).
Sarah E. Chinn, "Tackling the 'Masculinity Crisis': Male Identity in the 1950s," *GLQ:
A Journal of Lesbian and Gay Studies* 12, no. 3 (2006): 507–510, https://muse.jhu.edu
/article/197476. Susan Faludi, *Stiffed: The Betrayal of the American Man* (New York: Wil-
liam Morrow, 1999). Ina Zweiniger-Bargielowska, "Building a British Superman: Physical
Culture in Interwar Britain," *Journal of Contemporary History* 41, no. 4 (2006): 595–610.
James Burkhart Gilbert, *Men in the Middle: Searching for Masculinity in the 1950s* (Chicago, IL: University of Chicago Press, 2005).

40. Harrison Pope, Katharine A. Phillips, and Roberto Olivardia, *The Adonis Complex: How to Identify, Treat, and Prevent Body Obsession in Men and Boys* (New York:
Touchstone, 2002). For a fascinating political perspective, see Claire Cain Miller, "Republican Men Say It's a Better Time to Be a Woman Than a Man," *New York Times*, January 17,
2017, accessed May 4, 2018, https://nyti.ms/2jVBgHu.

41. Cherríe Moraga and Gloria Anzaldua, eds., *This Bridge Called My Back: Writings
by Radical Women of Color*, 4th ed. (New York: State University of New York Press, 2015).

42. Jennifer Carlson, *Citizen-Protectors: The Everyday Politics of Guns in an Age of Decline* (Oxford, UK: Oxford University Press, 2015). Angela Stroud, *Good Guys with Guns: The Appeal and Consequences of Concealed Carry* (Chapel Hill: University of North Carolina Press, 2015).

43. Richard Klein, *Cigarettes Are Sublime* (Durham, NC: Duke University Press, 1995).

THE MAN CARD

1. "Proof of Your Manhood—the Man Card from Bushmaster," AmmoLand.com, May 7, 2010, accessed May 4, 2018, https://bit.ly/2HZ1IMU.

2. Alex Seitz-Wald, "Assault Rifle Company Issues 'Man Cards,'" *Salon*, December 17, 2012, accessed May 4, 2018, https://bit.ly/2IiUYN7. Scott Lamb, "Bushmaster's Shockingly Awful 'Man Card' Campaign," BuzzFeed, 2012, accessed May 4, 2018, https://bzfd.it/2KGaUrl. J. Paul Vance, "Update: State Police Identify Weapons Used in Sandy Hook Investigation," State of Connecticut Department of Emergency Services & Public Protection Connecticut State Police, 2016, https://bit.ly/2HRDGqZ.

3. Emma Gray, "Bushmaster Rifle Ad Reminds Us to Ask More About Masculinity and Gun Violence," *Huffington Post*, December 7, 2017, accessed May 4, 2018, https://bit.ly/2I17TjK. Lamb, "'Man Card' Campaign." Jessica Valenti, "This Is an Ad for the Gun Adam Lanza Used to Murder 20 Children & 6 Adults. We Need to Talk About American Masculinity," Scoopnest, https://www.scoopnest.com/user/Jessica Valenti/280711110485762048. Paul Waldman, "Not Man Enough? Buy a Gun," CNN, December 21, 2012, accessed May 6, 2018, https://cnn.it/2wouXHs. Soon thereafter, *Gawker* posted a piece titled "Bushmaster Firearms, Your Man Card Is Revoked" that asserted "it should not have taken a mass shooting for us all to realize that the connection between guns and masculinity is ridiculous." See Hamilton Nolan, "Bushmaster Firearms, Your Man Card Is Revoked," *Gawker*, December 17, 2012, https://bit.ly/2HUDjw8.

4. For correlations between masculinity, mental illness, and guns that play out after high-profile US mass shootings, see Jonathan M. Metzl and Kenneth T. Macleish, "Mental Illness, Mass Shootings, and the Politics of American Firearms," *American Journal of Public Health* 105, no. 2 (2015): 240–249, doi:10.2105/ajph.2014.302242.

5. *Oxford Dictionary*, s.v. "privilege paper," accessed May 6, 2018, https://bit.ly/2FNrjGw. *Dictionary.com*, s.v. "privilege," accessed May 6, 2018, https://bit.ly/2yoj9lR. For the graph, see Google Ngram Viewer, https://books.google.com/ngrams/graph?content=privileges&year_start=1800&year_end=2008&corpus=15&smoothing=7&share=&direct_url=t1%3B%2Cprivileges%3B%2Cc0.

6. Edmund S. Morgan, "Slavery and Freedom: The American Paradox," in *Colonial America: Essays in Politics and Social Development*, 4th ed., ed. Stanley N. Katz, John M. Murrin, and Douglas Greenberg (New York: McGraw-Hill, 1993). Daniel H. Usner Jr., *Indians, Settlers, & Slaves in a Frontier Exchange Economy: The Lower Mississippi Valley Before 1783* (Chapel Hill: University of North Carolina Press, 1992). Robert J. Cottrol and Raymond T. Diamond, "The Second Amendment: Toward an Afro-Americanist Reconsideration," *Georgetown Law Journal* 80 (1991): 309–361, www.guncite.com/journals/cd-recon.html. Benjamin Quarles, *The Negro in the Making of America*, 3rd ed. (New York: Macmillan, 1987).

7. "A well-regulated Militia, being necessary to the security of a free State, the right of the people to keep and bear Arms, shall not be infringed." For relevant commentary, see Nelson Lund and Adam Winkler, "The 2nd Amendment of the U.S. Constitution," National Constitution Center, accessed May 6, 2018, https://bit.ly/2fuU0Qp. Adam Winkler, "The Secret History of Guns," *Atlantic*, September 2011, accessed May 6, 2018, https://theatln .tc/2I1BOs5. Soon thereafter, the Uniform Militia Act of 1792 then expressly called for arming only "able-bodied white male citizens." See Cottrol and Diamond, "The Second Amendment."

8. Les Adams, *The Second Amendment Primer: A Citizen's Guidebook to the History, Sources, and Authorities for the Constitutional Guarantee of the Right to Keep and Bear Arms* (Birmingham, AL: Palladium Press, 1996). David C. Williams, *The Mythic Meanings of the Second Amendment: Taming Political Violence in a Constitutional Republic* (New Haven, CT: Yale University Press, 2003). Jill Lepore, "Battleground America," *New Yorker*, April 23, 2012, accessed May 6, 2018, https://bit.ly/2ykbjwD. Garry Wills, *A Necessary Evil: A History of American Distrust of Government* (New York: Simon & Schuster, 2002). Saul Cornell, *Whose Right to Bear Arms Did the Second Amendment Protect?* (Boston: Bedford / St. Martin's, 2000).

9. Carl T. Bogus, "The Hidden History of the Second Amendment," *UC Davis Law Review* 31 (1998): 309. Carl T. Bogus and Michael A. Bellesiles. *The Second Amendment in Law and History: Historians and Constitutional Scholars on the Right to Bear Arms* (New York: New Press, 2001). Carl T. Bogus, "Guns/Second Amendment," Carl T. Bogus's website, accessed May 6, 2018, https://bit.ly/2IhDxwI. Cottrol and Diamond, "The Second Amendment," 331.

10. Deborah Gray-White, Mia Bay, and Waldo E. Martin, *Freedom on My Mind: A History of African Americans*, 2nd ed., vol. 1 (Boston: Bedford / St. Martins, 2013). Eric Foner, ed., *Nat Turner* (Englewood Cliffs, NJ: Prentice-Hall, 1971). Francis Newton Thorpe, *The Federal and State Constitutions, Colonial Charters, and Other Organic Laws of the States, Territories, and Colonies: Now or Heretofore Forming the United States of America* (Grosse Pointe, MI:Government Printing Office, 1909).

11. Thorpe, *The Federal and State Constitutions*, 6:3424. "The State v. Elijah Newsom," Guncite, accessed May 6, 2018, https://bit.ly/2rtxH0S. Stefan Tahmassebi, "Gun Control and Racism," *George Mason University Civil Rights Law Journal* 2, no. 1 (1991): 67. Act of Jan. 6, 1847, ch. 87, § 11, 1846 Fla. Laws 42, 44; Act of Dec. 17, 1861, ch. 1291, § 11, 1861 Fla. Laws 38, 40. Cottrol and Diamond, "The Second Amendment," 338.

12. "Equal Protection Clause," *Wikipedia*, https://bit.ly/2HW1jPq. Michael Les Benedict, *The Fruits of Victory: Alternatives to Restoring the Union 1865–1877* (New York: J. B. Lippincott, 1975). Also see: Francis L. Broderick, *Reconstruction and the American Negro, 1865–1900* (London: Macmillan, 1969); Dan T. Carter, *When the War Was Over: The Failure of Self-Reconstruction in the South, 1865–1867* (Baton Rouge: Louisiana State University Press, 1985); Eric Foner, *Reconstruction* (New York: Harper & Row, 1988). Adam Winkler, *Gunfight: The Battle Over the Right to Bear Arms in America* (New York: Norton, 2013).

13. "The black man has never had the right either to keep or bear arms; and the legislatures of the states will still have the power to forbid it," Douglass famously argued in a speech to the American Anti-Slavery Society in 1865. "What I ask for the Negro is not benevolence . . . but simply justice." Frederick Douglass, *The Need for Continuing Anti-Slavery Work Speech in the Life and Writings of Frederick Douglass*, ed. Philip S. Foner (New York: International, 1975).

14. "Negroes with Guns: Robert Williams and Black Power," PBS, accessed May 6, 2018, https://to.pbs.org/29DYgY9.

15. "Malcolm X on the 2nd Amendment," YouTube video, 1:14, posted by "Occupy the Media," February 27, 2018, https://www.youtube.com/watch?v=5g_TxOA3i-g. Winkler, "The Secret History of Guns," 2017. Huey P. Newton, *The Huey P. Newton Reader*, ed. David Hilliard and Donald Wiese (New York: Seven Stories Press, 2002).

16. Lyndon B. Johnson, "Remarks Upon Signing the Gun Control Act of 1968," American Presidency Project, 1968, accessed May 6, 2018, www.presidency.ucsb.edu /ws/?pid=29197. Richard Harris, "If You Love Your Guns," *New Yorker*, April 20, 1968, accessed May 6, 2018, https://www.newyorker.com/magazine/1968/04/20/if-you -love-your-guns.

17. United States Congress, Senate, Committee on the Judiciary, Subcommittee on the Constitution, *The Right to Keep and Bear Arms: Report of the Subcommittee on the Constitution of the Committee on the Judiciary, United States Senate, Ninety-Seventh Congress, Second Session* (Washington, DC: US Government Printing Office, 1982). Lepore, "Battleground America."

18. Lois Beckett, "Gun Inequality: US Study Charts Rise of Hardcore Super Owners," *Guardian*, September 19, 2016, accessed May 6, 2018, https://bit.ly/2FQPXpM.

19. "2014 Political Polarization and Typology Survey, Final Topline," Pew Research Center, 2014, https://pewrsr.ch/2I1Lp25. Also see Rich Morin, "The Demographics and Politics of Gun-Owning Households," Pew Research Center, July 15, 2014, www.pew research.org/fact-tank/2014/07/15/the-demographics-and-politics-of-gun-owning-house holds. Morin, "The Demographics and Politics." Dara Lind, "Who Owns Guns in America? White Men, Mostly," *Vox*, December 4, 2015, www.vox.com/2015/12/4/9849524 /gun-race-statistics.

20. Lind, "Who Owns Guns." Tariro Mzezewa and Jessica DiNapoli, "African--Americans Still Favor Gun Control, but Views Are Shifting," Reuters, https://reut .rs/2FPB9Ia.

21. Tara Dodrill, "Open Carry Ban Overturned in Missouri," *Inquisitr*, 2014, accessed April 30, 2018, www.inquisitr.com/1602089/open-carry-ban-overturned-in-missouri. Also see: "Gun Laws in Missouri," *Wikipedia*, accessed April 29, 2018, http://en.wikipedia.org /wiki/Gun_laws_in_Missouri. Samantha Rinehart, "Open Carrying in Compliance: Some Worry About Changes in Cape Girardeau Ordinance," *Southeast Missourian*, December 16, 2014, accessed May 1, 2018, https://bit.ly/2rpFUDT.

22. Bob Cook, "Georgia's Gun Laws Allow Man to Freak Out Sports Parents at Park," *Forbes*, April 29, 2014, https://bit.ly/2JWzZNn. Carol Kuruvilla, "Georgia Cops Defend Man with Gun Who Scared Parents at Children's Baseball Game," *NY Daily News*, April 26, 2014, https://nydn.us/2Ii82m5.

23. Tom Boggioni, "Miss. Police: Open Carry Laws Kept Us from Arresting Shotgun-Toting Man Who Terrorized Walmart Shoppers," *Raw Story*, June 23, 2015, https://bit .ly/1JgwrD1. Terrence McCoy, "In Jim Cooley's Open-Carry America, Even a Trip to Walmart Can Require an AR-15," *Washington Post*, September 17, 2016, https://wapo.st/2wi8hsz.

24. Jeremy Adam Smith, "Why Are White Men Stockpiling Guns?," *Scientific American*, March 14, 2018, accessed May 2, 2018, https://blogs.scientificamerican.com /observations/why-are-white-men-stockpiling-guns/.

25. Inae Oh, "Black Man Lawfully Carrying Gun Gets Pummeled by White Vigilante at Walmart," *Mother Jones*, June 24, 2017, https://bit.ly/2IiG0Xt.

26. Charles P. Pierce, "The Difference Between a White Man and a Black Man with a Gun," *Esquire*, July 6, 2016, accessed May 6, 2018, https://bit.ly/29k2hQt. Ciara McCarthy, "Florida Deputy Cleared in Killing of Black Man by 'Stand-Your-Ground' Law," *Guardian*, July 28, 2016, accessed May 6, 2018, https://bit.ly/2JYtGZA.

27. Chris Mooney, "The Science of Why Cops Shoot Young Black Men," *Mother Jones*, June 24, 2017, accessed May 6, 2018, https://bit.ly/2HUJgZY.

28. "WVU's Smith Named NRA Gunslinger of the Week," Lindy's Sports, 2012, accessed May 6, 2018, https://bit.ly/2jA7GcI. "Gunslinger at NRA Show, Modern Cowboy Trick Shooter with Both Pistol AND 1911!," YouTube video, 1:09, posted by "Spookybacon," July 23, 2012, accessed May 6, 2018, https://bit.ly/2Ij6S9S. "John Wayne Tribute Schofield Revolver," *American Rifleman*, 2016, accessed May 6, 2018, https://bit.ly/2wf 6Nzj. Francis X. Clines, "The N.R.A. Says, Go Ahead, Make My Fantasy," *New York Times*, April 24, 2017, accessed May 6, 2018, https://nyti.ms/2KH80SX. "John Wayne 1971 'Racist' Playboy Interview (in Full)," YouTube video, 56:09, posted by "Mrmidnightmovie," January 13, 2014, accessed May 6, 2018, https://bit.ly/2HZuFby.

29. Scott Melzer, *Gun Crusaders: The NRAs Culture War* (New York: New York University Press, 2012).

30. Ibid., 30–33.

31. "The Armed Citizen®," *American Rifleman*, accessed May 6, 2018, https://bit .ly/2gj1asz. "Advertisement for the Tavor SAR," *American Rifleman*, July 2013, accessed May 6, 2018, https://bit.ly/2HW9gQu. Gregory Smith, "Glock's "Confidence to Live Your Life" Campaign," Selling the Second Amendment, May 21, 2014, accessed May 6, 2018, https://bit.ly/2jB5lhy.

32. Leonard Steinhorn, "White Men and Their Guns," *Huffington Post*, February 16, 2014, accessed May 6, 2018, https://bit.ly/2KHfR36.

33. Mary Pat Clark, "Why Own a Gun? Protection Is Now Top Reason," Pew Research Center, March 12, 2013, accessed May 6, 2018, https://pewrsr.ch/1kqgvOv. Kim Parker, Juliana Menasce Horowitz, Ruth Igielnik, Baxter Oliphant, and Anna Brown, "America's Complex Relationship with Guns," Pew Research Center, June 22, 2017, accessed May 6, 2018, https://pewrsr.ch/2txQZSP.

34. Ana Marie Cox, "The NRA Way: Celebrate Buying Guns in a City Where 4 People Got Shot Last Night," *Guardian*, April 25, 2014, accessed May 6, 2018, https://bit .ly/2ro6e1a. Ana Marie Cox, "The NRA Has Declared War on America," *Guardian*, April 28, 2014, accessed May 6, 2018, https://bit.ly/2jBgZsT. Agunda Okeyo, "Before Ferguson: America's Disturbing Legacy of White Supremacy and Guns," *Salon*, September 3, 2014, accessed May 6, 2018, https://bit.ly/2jA7Osn. "Join the National Rifle Association," NRA's Facebook page, June 12, 2017, accessed May 6, 2018, https://bit.ly/2HVaaRu. Zack Beauchamp, "This Chilling NRA Ad Calls on Its Members to Save America by Fighting Liberals," *Vox*, June 29, 2017, accessed May 6, 2018, https://bit.ly/2FP5OW6. Jonathan M. Metzl, "Mainstream Anxieties About Race in Antipsychotic Drug Ads," *Virtual Mentor* 14, no. 6 (2012): 494–502, doi:10.1001/virtualmentor.2012.14.6.imhl1-1206.

35. Angela Stroud, *Good Guys with Guns: The Appeal and Consequences of Concealed Carry* (Chapel Hill: University of North Carolina Press, 2015), 88–89. See also 96 and 100–102.

36. Hanna Kozlowska, "This Insane Campaign Ad Shows Missouri's GOP Gubernatorial Candidate Casually Firing a Massive Machine Gun," *Quartz*, August 3, 2016, accessed

May 6, 2018, https://bit.ly/2jCWvQ9. Rob Garver, "Trump: 'I Always Carry a Gun,'" *Business Insider*, February 11, 2016, accessed May 7, 2018, https://read.bi/1o4wn0s.

37. Anthony G. Payne, "Acquisition, Preservation Against Loss, and Perpetuation: The Basic Drives Underlying Biology & Evolution as Expressed in Human Psychology & Culture," HealingCare4U.org, 2002, accessed May 7, 2018, https://bit.ly/2HXgnwf. Stroud, *Good Guys*, 122. Kathy Jackson and Mark Walters, *Lessons from Armed America: True Stories of Men and Women Who Defended Themselves and Their Families* (Washington: Independent Publishing Platform, 2009).

38. Michelle Alexander, "Ta-Nehisi Coates's 'Between the World and Me,'" *New York Times*, 2015, accessed May 7, 2018, https://nyti.ms/2FQHbIG. Joe Pinsker, "Why So Many Rich Kids Come to Enjoy the Taste of Healthier Foods," *Atlantic*, January 28, 2016, accessed May 7, 2018, https://theatln.tc/2kZLhs3. Jon Greenberg, "10 Examples That Prove White Privilege Protects White People in Every Aspect Imaginable," *Everyday Feminism*, November 30, 2015, accessed May 7, 2018, https://bit.ly/2I18sK4.

Preventative Medicine

1. Tim Parker, "Calculating Risk and Reward," *Investopedia*, January 30, 2018, accessed May 7, 2018, https://bit.ly/2HYuYTP. "Evidence at the Point of Care," BMJ Best Practice, accessed May 7, 2018, https://bit.ly/2FSLGSP. "Cochrane Training," Cochrane Handbook for Systematic Reviews of Interventions, accessed May 7, 2018, https://bit.ly/2x Kif4T. "How to Calculate Relative Risk," YouTube video, 3:14, posted by "Terry Shaneyfelt," October 6, 2012, accessed May 7, 2018, https://bit.ly/2jCld3n.

2. Erin Dunkerly, "The Gun Lobby Is Hindering Suicide Prevention," *New York Times*, December 27, 2017, accessed May 7, 2018, https://nyti.ms/2IkYExT. Glenn E. Rice and Joe Robertson, "Kansas City's Terrifying Year of Homicides—the Worst in 24 Years," *Kansas City Star*, January 7, 2018, accessed May 7, 2018, https://bit.ly/2HZg5Rv. Ashley Southall, "Crime in New York City Plunges to a Level Not Seen Since the 1950s," *New York Times*, December 27, 2017, accessed May 7, 2018, https://nyti.ms/2KGssUl. "H.R. 38: Concealed Carry Reciprocity Act of 2017," Congress.gov., 2017, https://bit.ly/2gdvG6N.

3. "SB656—Modifies Provisions Relating to Firearms and Corporate Security Advisors," Missouri Senate, accessed May 7, 2018, https://bit.ly/2K2vxwF. Jeffrey W. Swanson, Michael A. Norko, Hsiu-Ju Lin, Kelly Alanis-Hirsch, Linda K. Frisman, Madelon V. Baronski, Michele M. Easter, Allison G. Robertson, Marvin S. Swartz, and Richard J. Bonnie, "Implementation and Effectiveness of Connecticut's Risk-Based Gun Removal Law: Does It Prevent Suicides?," *Law and Contemporary Problems* 80 (2017).

4. Doug Stanglin, "Connecticut Passes Toughest U.S. Gun Laws," *USA Today*, April 4, 2013, accessed May 7, 2018, https://usat.ly/2JZF8nS.

5. Daniel Webster, Cassandra Kercher Crifasi, and Jon S. Vernick, "Effects of the Repeal of Missouri's Handgun Purchaser Licensing Law on Homicides," *Journal of Urban Health* 91, no. 3 (2014): 598–601, doi:10.1007/s11524-014-9882-7. Daniel W. Webster and Jon S. Vernick, eds., *Reducing Gun Violence in America: Informing Policy with Evidence and Analysis* (Baltimore: Johns Hopkins University Press, 2013).

6. Cassandra K. Crifasi, John Speed Meyers, Jon S. Vernick, and Daniel W. Webster, "Effects of Changes in Permit-to-Purchase Handgun Laws in Connecticut and Missouri on Suicide Rates," *Preventive Medicine* 79 (2015): 43–49, doi:10.1016/j.ypmed.2015.07.013.

7. John Lott Jr., *More Guns Less Crime: Understanding Crime and Gun Control Laws*, 3rd ed. (Chicago: University of Chicago Press, 2010), 135–136.

8. Crifasi et al., "Effects of Changes."

9. "Suicide-by-Firearm Rates Shift in Two States After Changes in State Gun Laws," Johns Hopkins Bloomberg School of Public Health, 2015, https://www.jhsph.edu/news /news-releases/2015/suicide-by-firearm-rates-shift-in-two-states-after-changes-in-state -gun-laws.html.

10. See for instance, John R. Lott, "Opinion: Media Cherry Picks Missouri Gun Data to Make Misleading Case for More Control," Fox News, 2014, accessed May 7, 2018, https://fxn.ws/2chOxWR. "Charles C. W. Cooke," *National Review*, accessed May 7, 2018, https://bit.ly/2FPINSJ. Charles C. W. Cooke, "The New York Times Overstates the Case for Stricter Gun Laws," *National Review*, December 22, 2015, accessed May 7, 2018, https:// bit.ly/2IjvLlX. Robert VerBruggen, "Do Guns Cause Violence?" RealClear Policy, August 26, 2015, accessed May 7, 2018, https://bit.ly/2wkP1uz. Robert VerBruggen, "Another Iffy Gun Study," RealClear Policy, September 2, 2015, accessed May 7, 2018, https://bit .ly/2HVJikb. Christen Smith, "Gun Violence Study Results 'Should Be Interpreted with Caution,'" Guns.com, October 21, 2016, accessed May 7, 2018, https://bit.ly/2JWXOor. Brian Doherty, "5 Problems with the New Study 'Proving' That More Background Checks Lowered Connecticut's Gun Murder Rate by 40 Percent," Reason.com, June 24, 2015, accessed May 7, 2018, https://bit.ly/1Mbidod.

11. Meghan Rosen, "Gun Research Faces Roadblocks and a Dearth of Data," *Science News*, May 3, 2016, accessed May 7, 2018, https://bit.ly/2rrdbxD.

12. Crifasi et al., "Effects of Changes."

13. Webster et al., "Effects of the Repeal."

WHAT WAS THE RISK?

1. "Fatal Injury Data," Centers for Disease Control and Prevention, accessed May 7, 2018, https://bit.ly/2BTH6W5.

2. At the same time, we noted that none of the warnings about reliability directly applied to the categories we wished to study—namely, suicide via firearm.

3. "Why Doesn't the Census Include Hispanic As a Race?," Hispanic Research Inc., accessed May 7, 2018, https://bit.ly/2FQfjEz. "Chapter 7: The Many Dimensions of Hispanic Racial Identity," Pew Research Center, June 11, 2015, accessed May 7, 2018, https://pewrsr.ch/1FLoJul.

4. Michael D. Anestis, Joye C. Anestis, and Sarah E. Butterworth, "Handgun Legislation and Changes in Statewide Overall Suicide Rates," *American Journal of Public Health* 107, no. 4 (2017): 579–581, doi:10.2105/ajph.2016.303650.

5. For an example of this type of logic, see, for instance, Leah Libresco, "I Used to Think Gun Control Was the Answer. My Research Told Me Otherwise," *Washington Post*, October 3, 2017, accessed May 7, 2018, http://wapo.st/2xP99Vd?tid=ss_tw&utm_term= .f8ce7dad89b6.

6. "Past Summary Ledgers," Gun Violence Archive, accessed May 7, 2018, https:// bit.ly/1NZKAlS. "Mass Shootings," Gun Violence Archive, accessed May 7, 2018, https:// bit.ly/2wkwbDD. "Officer Shot or Killed," Gun Violence Archive, 2014, accessed on January 15, 1016, www.gunviolencearchive.org/reports/mass-shooting?year=2014. "Part IV.

What Is the Threat to the United States Today?," New America, accessed May 7, 2018, https://bit.ly/2jK2tzK. Linda Qiu, "Fact-Checking a Comparison of Gun Deaths and Terrorism Deaths," *Politifact*, 2015, https://www.politifact.com/truth-o-meter/statements/2015 /oct/05/viral-image/fact-checking-comparison-gun-deaths-and-terrorism-/.

7. Politics, for instance, that recognized that some forms of "limitation [to the right to bear arms are fairly supported by the historical tradition of prohibiting the carrying of 'dangerous and unusual weapons,'" as US Supreme Court justice Antonin Scalia described it in the infamous *District of Columbia v. Dick Anthony Heller* decision. See Andrew Rosenthal, "Justice Scalia's Gun-Control Argument," *New York Times*, December 11, 2015, accessed May 7, 2018, https://nyti.ms/2FSNVFD. Scalia thus sought to find reasonable balance between "prefatory clause" and "protected right." See Antonin Scalia, "DISTRICT OF COLUMBIA v. HELLER," Legal Information Institute, March 18, 2008, accessed May 7, 2018, https://bit.ly/22kPqTo. Tomas Witkowski, "After Half a Century of Research, Psychology Can't Predict Suicidal Behaviours Better Than by Coin Flip," *British Psychological Society Research Digest*, January 25, 2017, accessed May 7, 2018, https://bit.ly/2kjEWXh.

8. J. W. Gardner and J. S. Sanborn, "10 Calculating Potential Years of Life Lost (PYLL)," Association of Public Health Epidemiologists in Ontario, June 1, 2006, accessed May 7, 2018, https://bit.ly/2KDSQ0R.

9. By way of comparison, this amount nearly doubled the $146 million that Missouri governor Eric Greitens cut from Missouri universities, schools, and transportation programs on taking office in January 2017. See Kurt Erickson, "Gov. Greitens Cuts $146 Million from Missouri Budget, with Higher Education Taking Brunt," *St. Louis Post-Dispatch*, January 17, 2017, accessed May 7, 2018, https://bit.ly/2rqJL2G.

10. Noam Cohen, "Tornado Hits Missouri City, Killing Many," *New York Times*, May 23, 2011, accessed May 7, 2018, https://nyti.ms/2wku2If.

11. "Questions About Removing Firearms," Maine Suicide Prevention Program, accessed May 7, 2018, https://bit.ly/2rrjli9.

12. "Missouri Suicide Prevention Project (MSPP)," Missouri Institute of Mental Health, accessed May 7, 2018, https://bit.ly/2wkB3Zr.

UNAFFORDABLE

1. "Donald Trump ROCKS Anderson, SC Rally HQ Version (10-19-15)," YouTube video, 58:03, posted by "Presidential Election 2016," October 27, 2015, https://youtu.be /PJ66dV-dGuk. Josh Israel, "Trumpcare Breaks Every Promise Trump Made About Health Care," *ThinkProgress*, March 7, 2017, accessed April 24, 2018, https://thinkprogress.org /trump-obamacare-replacement-breaks-more-promises-42b2fda950f.

2. Editorial Board, "Trumpcare Is Already Hurting Trump Country," *New York Times*, May 19, 2017, accessed April 24, 2018, https://www.nytimes.com/2017/05/19/opinion /trumpcare-health-care-bill.html.

3. Holly Fletcher, "Tennessee's Insurance Chief Seeks Elusive Answers in Washington," *Tennessean*, May 12, 2017, accessed April 24, 2018, https://tnne.ws/2rnsHvl. Also see Reed Abelson, "Iowa's Largest Insurer Says It Will Withdraw from Obamacare Exchanges," *New York Times*, April 3, 2017, accessed April 24, 2018, https://nyti.ms/2nVkBZA. Robert Pear, "Trump, Shouting 'Death Spiral,' Has Nudged Affordable Care Act Downward," *New York Times*, May 20, 2017, accessed April 24, 2018, https://nyti.ms/2qEr3W6.

4. Patrick Caldwell, "Here's Exactly How Many People Will Be Uninsured Under Each Republican Health Care Bill," *Mother Jones*, July 21, 2017, accessed April 24, 2018, https://bit.ly/2eCSQTm. Jeffrey Young, "Trump Says He Should Let Obamacare 'Collapse.' That's Cruel And Irresponsible," *Huffington Post*, March 24, 2017, accessed April 24, 2018, https://bit.ly/2F5We4O. Benjamin Hart, "New Trump Executive Order Could Gut Obamacare Markets," *New York Magazine*, October 8, 2017, accessed April 24, 2018, https://nym.ag/2ySB1EK. Louise Radnofsky, Stephanie Armour, and Anna Wilde Mathews, "Trump to Sign Order Easing Health Plan Rules, Official Says," *Wall Street Journal*, October 17, 2017, accessed April 24, 2018, https://on.wsj.com/2wDY0CL. Jordan Fabian, "Trump: GOP Tax Bill 'Essentially' Repeals ObamaCare," *Hill*, December 20, 2017, accessed April 24, 2018, https://bit.ly/2HNLLNn.

5. Editorial Board, "Trumpcare Is Already Hurting Trump Country."

6. Dees Stribling, "The Five Largest Public Healthcare Companies Based in Nashville," Bisnow, October 20, 2016, accessed April 24, 2018, https://bit.ly/2JPyIaX. Alex Tolbert, "TN Health Insurance: Hope for Best, Prepare for Worst," *Tennessean*, February 26, 2017, accessed April 24, 2018, https://tnne.ws/2JWR2PE.

7. Moon-Kie Jung, *Beneath the Surface of White Supremacy: Denaturalizing US Racisms Past and Present* (Palo Alto, CA: Stanford University Press, 2015), 3–54. James Baldwin, *The Fire Next Time* (New York: Dell, 1962), 19, 127.

Cost

1. Abby Goodnough, "Governor of Tennessee Joins Peers Refusing Medicaid Plan," *New York Times*, March 27, 2013, accessed April 24, 2018, https://nyti.ms/2ju1Nxr.

2. According to the 2010 census, the racial makeup of the city was 84.53 percent Caucasian and 10.35 percent African American. Data obtained from American FactFinder, which is maintained by the US Census Bureau, at https://factfinder.census.gov. Joey Garrison, "Tennessee Denies Request to Block Confederate Statue," *USA Today*, July 20, 2015, accessed April 24, 2018, https://usat.ly/2wdL3Un.

3. "Eating Fried Foods Tied to Increased Risk of Diabetes, Heart Disease," Harvard School of Public Health, accessed April 24, 2018, https://bit.ly/2JPO0fG. "Know the Facts About High Blood Pressure," Centers for Disease Control and Prevention, accessed April 24, 2018, https://bit.ly/2HPl2jH.

4. Community Currencies in Action, *People Powered Money: Designing, Developing & Delivering Community Currencies* (London: New Economics Foundation, 2015).

In the Name of Affordable Care

1. "About the Affordable Care Act," US Department of Health & Human Services, December 7, 2017, accessed April 24, 2018, https://bit.ly/2oHr3kh.

2. "Patient Protection and Affordable Care Act," *Wikipedia*, accessed April 24, 2018, https://bit.ly/1tPf8MG. At the time of this writing, President Obama's comments remained on the White House website, at https://www.whitehouse.gov/the-press-office/remarks-president-affordable-care-act-and-new-patients-bill-rights.

3. And that as such, at least prior to 2016, people who could afford to should be required to invest in the system, and people who could not at the least maintained their

health while they nursed illnesses, injuries, or embodied injustices, or took care of their families, or looked for work.

4. Jim Patterson, "Vanderbilt Law Professor Influences SCOTUS Health Care Decision," *Vanderbilt News*, July 3, 2012, accessed April 24, 2018, https://news.vanderbilt .edu/2012/07/03/aca-scotus. "The Supreme Court Decision on Obama's Health Care Law," *New York Times*, accessed April 24, 2018, https://nyti.ms/2rlIJG9. "A Guide to the Supreme Court's Decision on the ACA's Medicaid Expansion," Henry J. Kaiser Family Foundation, August 1, 2012, accessed April 24, 2018, https://kaiserf.am/2rlwZCI.

5. Joe Hall, "McWherter Slays Big 'Bear' with Model TennCare Plan," *Nashville Business Journal*, May 31, 1993, 1. "TennCare Boosts Health Coverage to 94 Percent in State," *News Sentinel* (Knoxville, TN), August 28, 1994, A1. Bill Lewis, "TennCare Captures Strong Interest from Other States," *Nashville Business Journal*, October 4, 1993, 20. "TennCare: Problems May Show Way to Go," *Commercial Appeal* (Memphis, TN), January 23, 1995, A4.

6. See, for instance, "Lessons from Tennessee's Failed Health Care Reform," Heritage Foundation, April 7, 2000, accessed April 24, 2018, https://bit.ly/2HPUwXB. "Achieving a Critical Mission in Difficult Times—TennCare's Financial Viability," McKinsey & Company, December 11, 2003, accessed April 24, 2018, https://bit.ly/2jwhQe3. "Managed Care and Low-Income Populations: A Case Study of Managed Care in Tennessee," Henry J. Kaiser Family Foundation, December 30, 1996, accessed April 24, 2018, https://kaiserf .am/2rlr6oZ. Richard Locker, "Gov. Bill Haslam Signs Hall Income Tax Cut, Repeal into Law," *Tennesseean*, May 20, 2016, accessed April 24, 2018, https://tnne.ws/2KCdcrr.

7. Tara Culp-Ressler, "Tennessee's GOP Governor Rejects Medicaid Expansion, Leaves Residents to 'Health Care Lottery,'" *ThinkProgress*, March 27, 2013, accessed April 24, 2018, https://bit.ly/2rkD4iw. Abby Goodnough, "Tennessee Race for Medicaid: Dial Fast and Try, Try Again," *New York Times*, March 25, 2013, accessed April 24, 2018, https://nyti.ms/2jwzrCR.

8. "About Healthier Tennessee," Healthier Tennessee, accessed April 24, 2018, http://healthiertn.com/about. Jim Patterson, "Legislators, Stakeholders Briefed on Health Care Status of Tennessee," *VUMC Reporter*, January 15, 2015, accessed April 24, 2018, https://bit.ly/2jviKaX.

9. Christina Bennett, *TennCare: One State's Experiment with Medicaid Expansion* (Nashville: Vanderbilt University Press, 2014), 133.

10. "'Lamar Was Right' Television Advertisement," Lamar Alexander's website, video, 0:30, 2014, www.alexanderforsenate.com/repeal-obamacare-tn. Chas Sisk and Blake Farmer, "Ron Ramsey, Powerful Figure in Tennessee Politics for Two Decades, Ready to Just Be Granddad," Nashville Public Radio, March 16, 2016, accessed April 24, 2018, https://bit.ly/2IltTca. TN Press Release Center, "Ramsey: Fight Against 'Obamacare' Doesn't End Here," *TN Report*, June 28, 2012, accessed April 24, 2018, https://bit .ly/2wcNmam.

11. Tony Messenger, "Prop C Passes Overwhelmingly," *St. Louis Post-Dispatch*, August 4, 2010, accessed April 24, 2018, https://bit.ly/2FLCW0S. Also see Josie Wales, "What Missouri's Law Against ObamaCare Does and Doesn't Do," *Breitbart*, August 7, 2010, accessed April 24, 2018, https://bit.ly/2HURqxa. House Bill No. 1764, Ninety-Fifth Missouri General Assembly (2010), accessed April 24, 2018, https://bit.ly/2wcAX69http. "Report: Total Cost of Obamacare Website to Exceed $1 Billion," *Breitbart*, October 24,

2013, accessed April 24, 2018, https://bit.ly/2wg0MSY. See also Elizabeth Sheld, "Californians Experience Obamacare Sticker Shock," *Breitbart*, October 28, 2018, accessed April 24, 2018, https://bit.ly/2jtikSq. John Nolte, "ObamaCare Forces Woman into Welfare Program," *Breitbart*, November 21, 2013, accessed April 24, 2018, https://bit.ly/2HRUBWA. Kate Scanlon, "Marco Rubio Marks Fifth Anniversary by Rolling Out Alternative Plan," *Daily Signal*, March 24, 2015, accessed April 24, 2018, https://bit.ly/1MSmlEW.

12. Jeffrey Dorfman, "The High Costs of Obamacare Hit Home for the Middle Class," *Forbes*, October 31, 2013, accessed April 24, 2018, https://bit.ly/2juIIv6. Reed Abelson and Margot Sanger-Katz, "Yes, Obamacare Premiums Are Going Up," *New York Times*, June 15, 2016, accessed April 24, 2018, https://nyti.ms/1UwN69Y. J. Baumgardner, L. T. Bilheimer, M. B. Booth, W. J. Carrington, N. J. Duchovny, and E.C. Werble, "Cigarette Taxes and the Federal Budget—Report from the CBO," *New England Journal of Medicine* 367 (2012): 2068–2070. Aaron E. Carroll, "Preventive Care Saves Money? Sorry, It's Too Good to Be True," *New York Times*, January 29, 2018, accessed April 24, 2018, https://nyti.ms/2EjkEVF. Joseph L. Dieleman, Ellen Squires, Anthony L. Bui, Madeline Campbell, Abigail Chapin, Hannah Hamavid, Cody Horst, Zhiyin Li, Taylor Matyasz, Alex Reynolds, Nafis Sadat, Matthew T. Schneider, and Christopher J. L. Murray, "Factors Associated with Increases in US Health Care Spending, 1996–2013," *Journal of the American Medical Association* 318, no. 17 (2017): 1668–1678.

13. Gregory Krieg, "New Report Shows Obamacare Is Working, Especially for the Poor," *Mic*, August 12, 2015, accessed April 24, 2018, https://bit.ly/2HRWYIV. Stacey McMorrow and John Holahan, "The Widespread Slowdown in Health Spending Growth Implications for Future Spending Projections and the Cost of the Affordable Care Act: An Update," Robert Wood Johnson Foundation, June 2016, accessed April 24, 2018, https://rwjf.ws/2jwCRpg. Sarah Kliff, "The US Is Spending Trillions Less Than Expected on Health Care—and Uninsured Rates Are at an All-Time Low," *Vox*, June 21, 2016, accessed April 24, 2018, https://bit.ly/2Ii8HDW. Sabrina Tavernise and Robert Gebeloff, "Immigrants, the Poor and Minorities Gain Sharply Under Affordable Care Act," *New York Times*, April 18, 2016, accessed April 24, 2018, https://nyti.ms/2EexAhS.

FOCUS

1. Lynne Ames, "The View from Peekskill; Tending the Flame of a Motivator," *New York Times*, August 2, 1998, accessed April 24, 2018, https://nyti.ms/2HPvnMx. Also see Michael T. Kaufman, "Robert K. Merton, Versatile Sociologist and Father of the Focus Group, Dies at 92," *New York Times*, February 24, 2003, accessed April 24, 2018, https://nyti.ms/2HQUVZO.

2. Carol Vlassof, "Gender Differences in Determinants and Consequences of Health and Illness," *Journal of Health, Population, and Nutrition* 25, no. 1 (2007): 47–61. "The Top 10 Reasons Men Put Off Doctor Visits," American Heart Association, February 6, 2018, accessed April 24, 2018, https://bit.ly/2FMWkue.

3. J. Wardle and A. Steptoe, "Socioeconomic Differences in Attitudes and Beliefs About Healthy Lifestyles," *Journal of Epidemiology and Community Health* 57 (2003): 440–443.

4. "Frontiers (Anniversary Edition 2006)—Celebrating 50 Years," *Frontiers Magazine*, accessed April 24, 2018, https://bit.ly/2rrgWEf. Stanley J. Folmsbee, "The Origin of

the First 'Jim Crow' Law," *Journal of Southern History* 15, no. 2 (1949): 235–247. "Early History," Meharry Medical College, accessed April 24, 2018, www.mmc.edu/education /som/aboutus/somhistory.html. "The History of Nashville's Health Care Industry," Nashville Health Care Council, accessed April 24, 2018, https://bit.ly/2wcX2BI.

5. Michael Ralph, "'Life . . . in the Midst of Death': Notes on the Relationship Between Slave Insurance, Life Insurance, and Disability," *Disability Studies Quarterly* 32, no. 3 (2012), accessed April 24, 2018, https://bit.ly/2K7DQHL. Virginia Groark, "Slave Policies," *New York Times*, May 5, 2002, accessed April 24, 2018, https://nyti.ms/2HUcaoR. This history of slavery itself conveyed complex tensions in twenty-first-century Tennessee. For instance, in 2012, Tea Party activists in the state made national news when they fought to remove references to slavery and mentions of the country's founders being slave owners from school textbooks. See Trymaine Lee, "Tea Party Groups in Tennessee Demand Textbooks Overlook US Founder's Slave-Owning History," *Huffington Post*, January 23, 2012, accessed April 24, 2018, https://bit.ly/2HRGfcI.

6. Nadine Cohodas, *Strom Thurmond & the Politics of Southern Change* (Macon, GA: Mercer University Press, 1994), 355. Robert D. Schremmer and Jane F. Knapp, "Harry Truman and Health Care Reform: The Debate Started Here," *Pediatrics* 127, no. 3 (2011): 399–401, https://bit.ly/2rvZSw4. Paul Starr, "The Health Care Legacy of the Great Society," in Norman J. Glickman, Laurence E. Lynn, and Robert H. Wilson, eds., *LBJ's Neglected Legacy: The Policy and Management Legacies of the Johnson Years* (University of Texas Press, 2015), 235–258. Also see Atul Gawande, "Now What?," *New Yorker*, January 23, 2012, accessed April 24, 2018, https://stanford.io/2JUK79s.

7. Alondra Nelson, *Body and Soul: The Black Panther Party and the Fight Against Medical Discrimination* (Minneapolis: University of Minnesota Press, 2013). Bobby Seale, "Interviews: Black Panthers Today," interview by *POV*, PBS, September 21, 2004, accessed April 24, 2018, https://to.pbs.org/2Ijd2ah.

8. Michael Tesler, "The Spillover of Racialization into Health Care: How President Obama Polarized Public Opinion by Racial Attitudes and Race," *American Journal of Political Science* 56, no. 3 (2012): 690–704. "As Health Care Law Proceeds, Opposition and Uncertainty Persist," Pew Research Center, September 16, 2013, accessed April 24, 2018, https://pewrsr.ch/2KBHj20. Also see Maxwell Strachan, "Obamacare 3 Times More Popular Among Blacks Than Whites: Study," *Huffington Post*, September 16, 2013, accessed April 24, 2018, https://bit.ly/2rmgoyp.

9. Tim Brown, "Obama Ignores Nullification, Says Federal Agents Will Enforce Obamacare," *Freedom Post*, March 25, 2013, accessed April 24, 2018, https://bit .ly/2KBGRkA.

10. Lenny Bernstein and Joel Achenbach, "A Group of Middle-Aged Whites in the US Is Dying at a Startling Rate," *Washington Post*, November 2, 2015, https://wapo.st /2rjrNQG.

11. Michael Kimmel and Amy Aronson, eds., "Muscular Christianity," in *Men & Masculinities: A Social, Cultural, and Historical Encyclopedia*, vol. 1 (Santa Barbara, CA: ABC Clio, 2004). Richard Gray, *South to a New Place: Region, Literature, Culture* (Baton Rouge: Louisiana State University Press, 2002.) Also see C. V. Woodward, *The Burden of Southern History* (Baton Rouge: Louisiana State University Press, 1960) and Paul M. Gaston, *The New South Creed: A Study in Southern Mythmaking* (New York: Alfred A. Knopf, 1970).

SOCIALISM

1. Ted Tunnell, "Creating 'The Propaganda of History': Southern Editors and the Origins of "Carpetbagger and Scalawag," *Journal of Southern History* 72, no. 4 (2006): 789–822. Eric Foner, *A Short History of Reconstruction: 1863–1877* (New York: Harper & Row, 1990). Jason Sokol, *There Goes My Everything: White Southerners in the Age of Civil Rights, 1945–1975* (New York: Vintage Books, 2007).

2. Daniel Greenfield, "O'Reilly: Obamacare Is Pure Socialism," *Truth Revolt*, July 24, 2017, accessed April 24, 2018, https://bit.ly/2K7lq9O.

3. Edith Mitchell, "50 Years Ago, Medicare Helped to Desegregate Hospitals," interview with Renee Montagne, *Morning Edition*, July 30, 2015, https://n.pr/2rkRujx. Marilyn Elias, "Tennessee Pastor Rails Against Interracial Marriage," Southern Poverty Law Center, February 19, 2014, accessed April 24, 2018, https://bit.ly/2jwEzHc.

EVERYBODY

1. W. E. B. Du Bois, *The Souls of Black Folk* (New York: Dover, 1994), 2.

2. "Newspapers: The Chicago Defender," PBS, accessed April 24, 2018, https://to.pbs.org/1yz70ru. Roi Ottley, *The Lonely Warrior* (Chicago: Henry Regnery, 1955).

3. Issac J. Bailey, "How Bernie Sanders Exposed the Democrats' Racial Rift," *Politico*, June 8, 2016, accessed April 24, 2018, https://politi.co/2Ia29HJ. Also see Issac J. Bailey, *Proud. Black. Southern. (But I Still Don't Eat Watermelon in Front of White People)* (New York: Star Books, 2008).

4. David M. Cutler, *The Quality Cure: How Focusing on Health Care Quality Can Save Your Life and Lower Spending Too* (Oakland: University of California Press, 2014).

DE-PROGRESSIVE

1. At this writing, President Obama's comments appeared at https://www.whitehouse.gov/the-press-office/remarks-president-affordable-care-act-and-new-patients-bill-rights.

2. Jeff Woods, "Governor Says No to ObamaCare—at Least for Now," *Nashville Scene*, March 27, 2013, accessed April 24, 2018, https://bit.ly/2HS7h3O. For *Jackson Sun*, see Jeff Woods, "Haslam's Day of Reckoning Draws Nigh: Time to Decide ObamaCare Question," *Nashville Scene*, March 25, 2013, accessed April 24, 2018, https://bit.ly/2FLa09k.

3. "Ramsey: Fight Against 'Obamacare' Doesn't End Here," *TN Report*, June 28, 2012, accessed April 26, 2018, http://tnreport.com/2012/06/28/ramsey-fight-against-obamacare-doesnt-end-here/.

4. Dave Boucher, "Tennessee's GOP Gov to Expand Medicaid Program," *USA Today*, December 15, 2014, accessed April 24, 2018, https://usat.ly/2rmBFbj. Andrea Zelinski, "Vandy Poll: 2-to-1 Support for Insure Tennessee, Even More Want a Vote," *Nashville Post*, accessed April 24, 2018, https://bit.ly/2rm4QMJ. "Martha Ingram Backs Insure Tennessee Push," *Nashville Post*, accessed April 24, 2018, https://bit.ly/2waDmOR.

5. Hank Hayes, "Ramsey: Insure Tennessee Doesn't Have a Chance," *Times-News* (Kingsport, TN), January 16, 2016, accessed April 24, 2018, https://bit.ly/2JWhucb. Jeff Woods, "Ramsey Tells Insure TN Supporters to Shove It," *Nashville Scene*, January 18, 2016, accessed April 24, 2018, https://bit.ly/2KAEheu. Tom Humphrey, "Insure TN DOA in House Committee?," *Tom Humphrey's Humphrey on the Hill*, January 29, 2015,

accessed April 24, 2018, https://bit.ly/2HVnf9e. Dave Boucher, "Haslam Medicaid Plan Faces Long Odds in House Committee," *Tennessean*, January 28, 2015, accessed April 24, 2018, https://tnne.ws/2JWDYcZ. Paul Demko, "Tennessee Becomes Exhibit A in GOP's Obamacare Repeal Push," *Politico*, March 5, 2017, accessed April 24, 2018, https://politi .co/2FKhz02.

6. January Angeles, "How Health Reform's Medicaid Expansion Will Impact State Budgets," Center on Budget and Policy Priorities, July 25, 2012, accessed April 24, 2018, https://bit.ly/2fZYCzr. Also see Woods, "Governor Says No."

7. George Lipsitz, *The Possessive Investment in Whiteness: How White People Profit from Identity Politics*, revised and expanded ed. (Philadelphia: Temple University Press, 2006).

8. Daniel Hayes, "Donald Trump Takes Aim," *New York Times*, August 21, 2016, accessed April 24, 2018, https://nyti.ms/2wmO19p.

9. Saidiya V. Hartman, *Scenes of Subjection: Terror, Slavery, and Self-Making in Nineteenth-Century America* (Oxford: Oxford University Press, 1997), 51–52. Barbara Baumgartner, "The Body as Evidence: Resistance, Collaboration, and Appropriation in 'The History of Mary Prince,'" *Callaloo* 24, no. 1 (2001): 253–275. Philosophers, too, talk of pain as resistance. Michel Foucault famously set resistance and power within the same provider networks and dared to suggest that pleasure emerged from the interaction of the two. Friedrich Nietzsche subtly suggested that pleasure emerged from the feeling of overcoming resistance as well as from controlling somebody else. See Michel Foucault, *The History of Sexuality, Volume 1: An Introduction* (London: Allen Lane, 1979). Also see Friedrich Nietzsche, *The Antichrist*, trans. R. J. Hollingdale (Middlesex, England: Penguin, 1968).

The Numbers Tell the Story

1. Benjamin D. Sommers, Katherine Baicker, and Arnold M. Epstein, "Mortality and Access to Care Among Adults After State Medicaid Expansions," *New England Journal of Medicine* 367 (2012): 1025–1034, https://www.nejm.org/doi/full/10.1056 /NEJMsa1202099#t=article.

2. Benjamin D. Sommers, Sharon K. Long, and Katherine Baicker, "Changes in Mortality After Massachusetts Health Care Reform: A Quasi-Experimental Study," *Annals of Internal Medicine* 160 (2014): 585–593, https://bit.ly/2FNWWQE.

3. "What Is CDC Wonder?," Centers for Disease Control and Prevention, https:// wonder.cdc.gov/wonder/help/faq.html#1.

4. CDC WONDER Database: Sort by year and gender; Tennessee; all categories of urbanization included; age groups 25 through 85+; all genders; non-Hispanic black; years 2011 through 2015; all weekdays, autopsy values, and places of death; all causes of death. The 11.36 percent comes from the fact that deaths dropped -41/100,000, and the baseline death rate was 361/100,000.

5. Joseph Antos, "The Medicaid Expansion Is Not Such a Good Deal for States or the Poor," *Journal of Health Politics, Policy, and Law* 38, no. 1 (2013): 179–186, https://bit .ly/2HUDYcP. Further broken down by Tennessee census demographics suggests that this would mean saving between 921 and 2,273 black female lives, and between 942 and 2,326 black male lives. Gender breakdown is provided by CDC WONDER, and the database also provides the population for each year.

6. CDC WONDER Database: Sort by year and gender; Tennessee; all categories of urbanization included; age groups 25 through 85+; all genders; non-Hispanic white; years 2011 through 2015; all weekdays, autopsy values, and places of death; all causes of death. The 4.53 percent comes from the fact white deaths declined -14/100,000, and there was a baseline of 309 deaths. Also see Anne Case and Angus Deaton, "Rising Morbidity and Mortality in Midlife Among White Non-Hispanic Americans in the 21st Century," *PNAS* 112, no. 49 (2015): 15078–15083, accessed April 24, 2018, www.pnas.org /content/112/49/15078.full.

7. Further broken down by census demographics suggests that this would mean saving between 3,177 and 5,995 white female lives and between 3,188 and 6,018 white male lives.

8. Using numbers from Fenggang Peng, *Life Expectancy in Tennessee* (Nashville: Tennessee Department of Health, Division of Policy, Planning, and Assessment, 2013): Weighted average to predict the average age of the deaths, which turns out to be 66.1 years. Black women in Tennessee have a life expectancy of 18.4 years once they reach the age of 65, so at 66.1 years, they will have 17.3 years of life remaining. Black men at 65 have a life expectancy of 14.9 years, so at 66.1 years, they will have 13.8 years of life remaining. As a result, a minimum of 21,565 and a maximum of 28,933 black life years would have been saved if Tennessee expanded Medicaid between 2011 and 2015. This translates to as much as 37.1 days of life per African American Tennessee resident. Weighted average used to predict the average age of the deaths, which turns out to be 71.7 years. White women in Tennessee have a life expectancy of 19.7 years once they reach the age of 65, so at 71.7 years, they will have 13 years of life remaining. White men at 65 have a life expectancy of 16.7 years, so at 71.7 years, they will have 10 years of life remaining. As a result, a minimum of 73,181 and a maximum of 138,115 white life years would have been saved if Tennessee expanded Medicaid between 2011 and 2015. This translates to as much as 14.1 days of life per white Tennessee resident.

9. "Medicaid Expansion Benefits Everyone," National Association of Public Hospitals and Health Systems, October 2012, accessed April 24, 2018, https://bit.ly/2FNEAis.

10. "Tennessee vs. Kentucky," IndexMundi, accessed April 24, 2018, https://bit .ly/2KRh1sG. Beth Musgrave and Jack Brammer, "Beshear Says Kentucky Will Join Obamacare Plan to Expand Medicaid," *Lexington (KY) Herald-Leader*, May 9, 2013, accessed April 24, 2018, https://bit.ly/2HXsg12. Rachana Pradhan, "Kentucky Begins Dismantling Obamacare Exchange," *Politico*, January 12, 2016, accessed April 24, 2018, https://politi.co/2FMHDr6. "Proposed Changes to Medicaid Expansion in Kentucky," Henry J. Kaiser Family Foundation, August 4, 2017, accessed April 24, 2018, https:// kaiserf.am/2HWFwTF. Abby Goodnough, "Kentucky, Beacon for Health Law, Now a Lab for Its Retreat," *New York Times*, November 28, 2015, accessed April 24, 2018, https:// nyti.ms/1Pi9Hpr. Benjamin D. Sommers, Robert J. Blendon, and E. John Orav, "Both the 'Private Option' and Traditional Medicaid Expansions Improved Access to Care for Low-Income Adults," *Health Affairs* 35 (2016): 1, accessed April 24, 2018, https://bit .ly/2KaFJ6b. "Proposed Changes," Kaiser Family Foundation.

11. Sommers et al., "'Private Option.'" "Proposed Changes," Kaiser Family Foundation. "Health, United States, 2015, with Special Feature on Racial and Ethnic Health Disparities," Centers for Disease Control and Prevention, June 22, 2017, accessed April 24, 2018, https://bit.ly/2lSQ5Ly.

12. "Health, United States, 2015," CDC.

13. Susan L. Hayes, Sara R. Collins, David Radley, Douglas McCarthy, and Sophie Beutel, "A Long Way in a Short Time: States' Progress on Health Care Coverage and Access, 2013–2015," Commonwealth Fund, December 21, 2016, accessed April 24, 2018, https://bit.ly/2hTBr6n.

14. "Current Population Survey (CPS) Table Creator," United States Census, accessed April 24, 2018, https://bit.ly/2FZOkXf.

15. A. P. Wilper, S. Woolhandler, K. E. Lasser, D. McCormick, D. H. Bor, and D. U. Himmelstein, "Health Insurance and Mortality in US Adults," *American Journal of Public Health* 99, no. 12 (2009): 2289–2295, doi:10.2105/AJPH.2008.157685, https://www.ncbi.nlm.nih.gov/pmc/articles/PMC2775760. Ross Douthat, "Is Obamacare a Lifesaver?," *New York Times*, March 29, 2017, accessed April 24, 2018, https://nyti.ms/2owZFFQ.

16. Hayes et al., "A Long Way."

17. Sara Collins, David Radley, Munira Gunja, and Sophie Beutel, "The Slowdown in Employer Insurance Cost Growth: Why Many Workers Still Feel the Pinch," Commonwealth Fund, October 26, 2016, accessed April 24, 2018, https://bit.ly/2eQUYlb.

18. Michael Hiltzik, "Donald Trump, Rand Paul and the Myth of a Cheap Obamacare Replacement," *Los Angeles Times*, January 17, 2017, accessed April 24, 2018, https://lat.ms/2iETMCR. Douthat, "Is Obamacare a Lifesaver?" Robert Pear, Maggie Haberman, and Reed Abelson, "Trump to Scrap Critical Health Care Subsidies, Hitting Obamacare Again," *New York Times*, October 12, 2017, accessed April 24, 2018, https://nyti.ms/2kKn0GP.

19. Hiltzik, "Donald Trump."

20. "Under #ACA, Medical Bankruptcy Continues," *American Journal of Medicine Blog*, January 12, 2016, accessed April 24, 2018, https://bit.ly/2K865px. Margot Sanger-Katz, "Even Insured Can Face Crushing Medical Debt, Study Finds," *New York Times*, January 5, 2016, accessed April 24, 2018, https://nyti.ms/2n23AJG. "How the Poll on Medical Bills Was Conducted," *New York Times*, January 5, 2016, accessed April 24, 2018, https://nyti.ms/2HXthWU.

21. Peter A. Muennig, Ryan Quan, Codruta Chiuzan, and Sherry Glied, "Considering Whether Medicaid Is Worth the Cost: Revisiting the Oregon Health Study," *American Journal of Public Health* 105, no. 5 (2015): 866–871. Sophia Duong, "Study: Medicaid Benefits Are Well-Worth Its Costs," Georgetown University Health Policy Institute, April 20, 2015, accessed April 24, 2018, https://bit.ly/2uoOnWV.

22. Dan Mangan, "Medical Bills Are the Biggest Cause of US Bankruptcies: Study," CNBC, July 24, 2013, accessed April 24, 2018, https://cnb.cx/2xaLEGC. David U. Himmelstein, Deborah Thorne, Elizabeth Warren, and Steffie Woolhandler, "Medical Bankruptcy in the United States, 2007: Results of a National Study," *American Journal of Medicine* 122, no. 8 (2009): 741–746, https://bit.ly/2Ik4IH9. L. Hamel, M. Norton, K. Pollitz, L. Levitt, and G. Claxton, "The Burden of Medical Debt: Results from the Kaiser Family Foundation / New York Times Medical Bills Survey," Henry J. Kaiser Family Foundation, January 2016, accessed April 24, 2018, https://bit.ly/1JVqyqN. Michael Karpman and Kyle J. Caswell, "Past-Due Medical Debt Among Nonelderly Adults, 2012–2015," Urban Institute, March 2017, accessed April 24, 2018, https://urbn.is/2lAKFtg.

23. Alvin Powell, "The Costs of Inequality: Money = Quality Health Care = Longer Life," *Harvard Gazette*, February 22, 2016, accessed April 24, 2018, https://bit.ly/2HUkm8F. Kendal Orgera and Samantha Artiga, "Disparities in Health and Health

Care: Five Key Questions and Answers," Henry J. Kaiser Family Foundation, August 12, 2016, accessed April 24, 2018, https://kaiserf.am/2zoBWh0.

24. "Health Impact Assessment (HIA)," World Health Organization, accessed April 24, 2018, www.who.int/hia/evidence/doh/en.

25. "32 Mike Huckabee Quotes," Christian Quotes, accessed April 24, 2018, https://bit.ly/2roosQ4.

26. Nicole Chavez, "Sen. Orrin Hatch Calls Obamacare Supporters 'Stupidest, Dumbass People,'" CNN, March 2, 2018, accessed April 24, 2018, http://cnn.it/2F9UMeg.

27. Tara McKay and Stefan Timmermans, "Beyond Health Effects?," *Journal of Health and Social Behavior* 58, no. 1 (2017): 4–22, https://bit.ly/2roS66T.

28. Ralph Ellison, *Invisible Man* (New York: Random House, 1952).

29. Mary Rechtoris, "Donald Trump Quotes on Healthcare—'Repeal It, Replace It, Get Something Great!," *Becker's Hospital Review*, August 16, 2016, accessed April 24, 2018, https://bit.ly/2IkPm5m. Also see Sarah Kliff, "Donald Trump Has No Idea What Health Insurance Costs," *Vox*, May 11, 2017, accessed April 24, 2018, https://bit.ly/2q9LwQW.

There's No Place Like Home

1. L. Frank Baum, *The Wonderful Wizard of Oz*, ed. Susan Wolstenholme (New York: Oxford University Press, 1997), 44. John Funchion, "When Dorothy Became History: L. Frank Baum's Enduring Fantasy of Cosmopolitan Nostalgia," *Modern Language Quarterly* 71, no. 4 (2010): 429–451.

2. Bob Dole, *One Soldier's Story: A Memoir* (New York: Harper Collins, 2005), 36–37. Thomas Frank, *What's the Matter with Kansas?: How Conservatives Won the Heart of America* (New York: Holt, 2004), 50.

3. Annie, "These 14 Vintage Kansas Tourism Ads Will Have You Longing for the Good Ol' Days," Only in Your State, January 17, 2016, accessed April 25, 2018, https://www.onlyinyourstate.com/kansas/vintage-ks-ads.

4. Paul Ciotti, "Money and School Performance: Lessons from the Kansas City Desegregation Experiment," Cato Institute, March 16, 1998, accessed April 25, 2018, https://bit.ly/2JWbQGM. Peter Moran, "Too Little, Too Late: The Illusive Goal of School Desegregation in Kansas City, Missouri, and the Role of the Federal Government," *Teachers College Record* 107, no. 9 (2005): 1933–1935. "St. Louis Students Bused to Suburbs," *New York Times*, August 25, 1983, accessed April 25, 2018, https://nyti.ms/2taVDKa.

5. For a useful overview of this type of data, see National Center for Education Statistics, *State Comparisons of Education Statistics: 1969–70 to 1996–97* (Washington, DC: US Department of Education, 1998), accessed April 25, 2018, https://nces.ed.gov/pubs98/98018.pdf. Also see "2015 Reading State Snapshot Report: Kansas, Grade 4, Public Schools," National Center for Education Statistics, 2016, https://bit.ly/2HTzLtT.

6. For the formative role of nostalgia to identity, see Jacques-Alain Miller, ed. *The Seminar of Jacques Lacan, Book 1: Freud's Papers on Technique*, trans. John Forrester (New York: Norton, 1988), accessed April 25, 2018, www.lacan.com/seminars1a.htm.

7. Suzanne Perez Tobias, "Wichita Schools' Demographics Shifting Towards Greater Racial, Ethnic Diversity," *Wichita Eagle*, September 20, 2004, accessed April 25, 2018, https://bit.ly/2wocBqq.

THE KANSAS EXPERIMENT

1. John B. Judis, "This Is What's the Matter with Kansas," *New Republic*, September 29, 2014, accessed April 25, 2018, https://bit.ly/2v0GgDv. For an even more critical perspective, see Paul Krugman, "Who Ate Republicans' Brains?," *New York Times*, July 31, 2017, accessed April 25, 2018, https://nyti.ms/2ub9cVx.

2. Judis, "This Is What's the Matter." Also see David Atkins, "Austerity Fever Breaks in Kansas, Rebuking the Conservative Cult," *Washington Monthly*, June 20, 2017, accessed April 25, 2018, https://bit.ly/2jBT9Nw.

3. Bruce Japsen, "Republican Kansas Governor Rejects Medicaid Expansion and His Own Party," *Forbes*, March 30, 2017, accessed April 25, 2018, https://bit.ly/2IjMhlG. Tim Carpenter, "Brownback: Send Back $31.5M Federal Grant," *Topeka Capital-Journal*, August 9, 2011, accessed April 25, 2018, https://bit.ly/2HS4zuV. "NRA Endorses Sam Brownback for Governor of Kansas," NRA Political Victory Fund, September 22, 2014, accessed April 25, 2018, https://bit.ly/1udn7YW. Joseph P. Williams, "Last Call: New Gun Law Means No Training, No Permit, No Problem," *US News & World Report*, April 3, 2015, accessed April 25, 2018, https://bit.ly/2KF52yt. "Concealed Carry On Kansas College Campuses Begins July 1," KWCH, June 26, 2017, accessed April 25, 2018, https://bit.ly/2tehFL9.

4. Sabrina Tavernise, "In Missouri, Fewer Gun Restrictions and More Gun Killings," *New York Times*, December 22, 2015, accessed April 25, 2018, https://nyti.ms/2nlp5cK. Avery Johnson, "Tennessee Experiment's High Cost Fuels Health-Care Debate," *Wall Street Journal*, August 17, 2009, accessed April 25, 2018, https://on.wsj.com/2FQ8TFd.

5. "Governor Signs Tax Cuts in Statehouse Ceremony," *Great Bend (KS) Tribune*, accessed April 25, 2018, https://bit.ly/2IhgXEd. "Growing the Kansas Economy," Sam Brownback for Kansas Governor, accessed April 25, 2018, http://brownback.com/growing-kansas-economy. Justin Fox, "Kansas Tried Tax Cuts. Its Neighbor Didn't. Guess Which Worked," *Bloomberg*, March 29, 2016, accessed April 25, 2018, https://bloom.bg/2dgUmIt.

6. Bryan Lowry, "Brownback Signs School Finance Bill," *Kansas City Star*, April 21, 2014, accessed April 25, 2018, https://bit.ly/2rnWp2s.

7. Sam Brownback, "A Midwest Renaissance Rooted in the Reagan Formula," *Wall Street Journal*, May 28, 2014, accessed April 25, 2018, https://on.wsj.com/2HVzVkD.

8. "What Everyone Should Know About Their State's Spending," *Urban Institute*, accessed April 25, 2018, http://urbn.is/spending. *2013 Report Card for Kansas's Infrastructure* (Reston, VA: American Society of Civil Engineers, 2013), accessed April 25, 2018, https://bit.ly/2rq2Odx.

9. Edward M. Eveld, "Kansas Will Pay the Price for Diverting Money from Highway Fund, Some Lawmakers Say," *Kansas City Star*, December 28, 2015, accessed April 25, 2018, https://bit.ly/2FNYKZT. Henry Grabar, "Kansas' Insane Right-Wing Experiment Is About to Destroy Its Roads," *Slate*, June 30, 2016, accessed April 25, 2018, https://slate.me/299aEl7. Tim Carpenter, "KDOT Issues Record $400 Million in Bonds, Exceeds Previous Debt Cap," *Topeka Capital-Journal*, December 15, 2015, accessed April 25, 2018, http://cjonline.com/news-legislature-state/2015-12-15/kdot-issues-record-400-million-bonds-exceeds-previous-debt-cap.

10. "UPDATE 1: S&P Downgrades Kansas in Another Blow to Brownback Tax Cuts," Reuters, August 6, 2014, accessed April 25, 2018, http://reut.rs/1orlWMS. Barry Ritholtz, "The Kansas Supply-Side Experiment Unravels," *Bloomberg*, June 19, 2017, accessed

April 25, 2018, https://bloom.bg/2FPoRQ1. Howard Gleckman, "The Great Kansas Tax Cut Experiment Crashes and Burns," *Forbes*, June 7, 2017, accessed April 25, 2018, https://bit.ly/2rnRMFu.

11. Mark Binelli, "The Great Kansas Tea Party Disaster," *Rolling Stone*, October 23, 2014, accessed April 25, 2018, http://rol.st/1nAmTcm. "Tax Cuts Taking Toll on Kansas Communities," Kansas Center for Economic Growth, April 2015, accessed April 25, 2018, https://bit.ly/2rpTCXi.

12. Trends that in any case coincided with job gains nationwide during the Obama economy. See Gleckman, "Great Kansas Tax Cut." Also see Bryan Lowry, "Do Kansas Law-makers Personally Benefit from Business-Tax Cuts?," *Wichita Eagle*, October 10, 2016, accessed April 25, 2018, https://bit.ly/2cXTl8Z. Business owners who lived out of state also became subject to tax on nonwage income in their home states. See Jerry Siebenmark, "Kansas Small-Business Owners Say Elimination of Income Tax is a Big Help," *Wichita Eagle*, May 24, 2012, accessed April 25, 2018, https://www.kansas.com/news/business /article1092681.html.

13. Alicia Parlapiano, "Pence Ranks Low in Approval, but Not as Low as Trump and Clinton," *New York Times*, July 14, 2016, accessed April 25, 2018, https://nyti.ms/2IjRtWI. Amanda Holpuch, "Kansas School Funding Cuts Mean Summer Comes Uncomfortably Early," *Guardian*, May 5, 2015, accessed April 25, 2018, https://bit.ly/2wgAq3l. Brooke Lennington (@BrookeKSNT), "Governor Brownback Got a Tip from a Waitress," Twitter, 9:41 a.m., May 3, 2015, https://bit.ly/2HTfvsg. Catherine Rampell, "Kansas Shows Us What Could Happen If Republicans Win in 2016," *Washington Post*, April 30, 2015, accessed April 25, 2018, http://wapo.st/1GKl3eO.

14. Richard Rubin and Will Connors, "Sam Brownback Calls on Donald Trump to Mimic His Kansas Tax Plan," *Wall Street Journal*, December 23, 2016, accessed April 25, 2018, https://on.wsj.com/2KF9jC1. Sophia Tesfaye, "Sam Brownback Urges Donald Trump to Replicate His Kansas Disaster on a National Scale," *Salon*, December 23, 2016, accessed April 25, 2018, https://bit.ly/2HZ1N3h. Dominic Rushe, "Kansas Abandons Massive Tax Cuts That Provided Model for Trump's Plan," *Guardian*, June 7, 2017, accessed April 25, 2018, https://bit.ly/2r2dEZZ. Julie Hirschfeld Davis and Alan Rappeport, "Trump Proposes the Most Sweeping Tax Overhaul in Decades," September 27, 2017, *New York Times*, accessed April 25, 2018, https://nyti.ms/2k0Iz5y. Also see Ritholtz, "Kansas Supply-Side Experiment," and Gleckman, "Great Kansas Tax Cut."

15. Paul Krugman, "Taxpayers, You've Been Scammed," *New York Times*, March 1, 2018, accessed April 25, 2018, https://nyti.ms/2t7VhEf.

16. Alan Finder, "Here's an Idea: Put 65% of the Money into Classrooms," *New York Times*, January 4, 2006, accessed April 25, 2018, https://nyti.ms/2twBLRK.

17. "Budget Brings Out Partisanship at His Best," Kansas National Education Association, May 13, 2011, accessed April 25, 2018, http://knea.org/home/998.htm. Tim Carpenter, "Study: Kansas Cuts K–12 Education Funding by Fourth-Most in Nation," *Topeka Capital-Journal*, September 12, 2013, accessed April 25, 2018, https://bit.ly/2wfUvXy. Mark Tallman, "New Study Finds Kansas Funding Falling Behind Highest Achieving States," Kansas Association of School Boards, October 21, 2016, accessed April 25, 2018, https://bit.ly/2roMr1N.

18. "What Trump's Education Secretary Could Mean for Kansas School Choice," Kansas Policy Institute, December 14, 2016, accessed April 25, 2018, https://bit.ly/2rkSu6y.

Joe Robertson, "No Truce in Kansas Education Battle as Block Grants Plan Keeps Many Districts on Edge," *Kansas City Star*, March 28, 2015, accessed April 25, 2018, https://bit .ly/2rzkwfH. Holpuch, "Kansas School Funding."

19. Dion Lefler, Bryan Lowry, and Suzanne Perez Tobias, "Kansas Supreme Court: School Funding Inequitable," *Wichita Eagle*, February 11, 2016, accessed April 25, 2018, https://bit.ly/1O4VLse. Mitch Smith and Julie Bosman, "Kansas Supreme Court Says State Education Spending Is Too Low," *New York Times*, March 2, 2017, accessed April 25, 2018, https://nyti.ms/2lEArUG.

20. Ted Carter, "Educational Funding and Student Outcomes: The Relationship as Evidenced by State-Level Data," Kansas Association of School Boards, September 2014, accessed April 25, 2018, https://bit.ly/2Kcdlkt.

21. *State Education Report Card: 2017 Update* (Topeka, KS: Kansas Association of School Boards, forthcoming).

AUSTERITY

1. Tim Carpenter, "Study: Kansas Cuts K–12 Education Funding by Fourth-Most in Nation," *Topeka Capital-Journal*, September 12, 2013, accessed April 25, 2018, https://bit.ly/2wfUvXy. Mark Tallman, "New Study Finds Kansas Funding Falling Behind Highest Achieving States," Kansas Association of School Boards, October 21, 2016, accessed April 25, 2018, https://bit.ly/2roMr1N. "American Recovery and Reinvestment Act of 2009," Wikisource, accessed April 25, 2018, https://bit.ly/2Ib6nja. "Estimated Impact of the American Recovery and Reinvestment Act on Employment and Economic Output from October 2011 through December 2011," Congressional Budget Office, February 2012, accessed April 25, 2018, https://bit.ly/11j9aNm.

2. Buttonwood, "What Is Austerity?," *Economist*, May 20, 2015, accessed April 25, 2018, https://econ.st/2KJ6UGi.

3. Isaac Martin, "How Republicans Learned to Sell Tax Cuts for the Rich," *New York Times*, December 18, 2017, accessed April 25, 2018, https://nyti.ms/2kFpbbE.

4. Paul Krugman, "How the Case for Austerity Has Crumbled," *New York Review of Books*, June 6, 2013, accessed April 25, 2018, https://bit.ly/1XOg0BW. Mark Blyth, *Austerity: The History of a Dangerous Idea* (New York: Oxford University Press, 2013). Paul Krugman, "The Austerity Agenda," *New York Times*, June 1, 2012, accessed April 25, 2018, https://nyti.ms/2u9I74V.

5. Paul Starr, "Nothing Neo," *New Republic*, December 4, 1995, accessed April 25, 2018, https://bit.ly/2rphCsO.

6. See, for instance, Randolph Hohle, *Race and the Origins of American Neoliberalism* (New York: Routledge, 2015.) Also see Maya Goodfellow, "A Toxic Concoction Means Women of Colour Are Hit Hardest by Austerity," *Guardian*, November 28, 2016, accessed April 25, 2018, https://bit.ly/2gCbOX8. "Intersecting Inequalities: The Impact of Austerity on Black and Minority Ethnic Women in the UK," Women's Budget Group, October 2017, accessed April 25, 2018, https://bit.ly/2HWVuB2. Binyamin Appelbaum, "Trump Tax Plan Benefits Wealthy, Including Trump," *New York Times*, September 27, 2017, accessed April 25, 2018, https://nyti.ms/2jADrlU. Anne Lowrey, "Trump Says His Tax Plan Won't Benefit the Rich—He's Exactly Wrong," *Atlantic*, September 2017, accessed April 25, 2018, https://theatln.tc/2HVkQ2w. Dylan Scott and Alvin Chang, "The Republican

Tax Bill Will Exacerbate Income Inequality in America," *Vox*, December 2, 2017, https://bit.ly/2i9nwdx.

7. Binyamin Appelbaum and Robert Gebeloff, "Even Critics of Safety Net Increasingly Depend on It," *New York Times*, February 12, 2012, accessed April 25, 2018, https://www.nytimes.com/2012/02/12/us/even-critics-of-safety-net-increasingly-depend-on-it.html. Gary Younge, "Working Class Voters: Why America's Poor Are Willing to Vote Republican," *Guardian*, October 29, 2012, accessed April 25, 2018, https://bit.ly/2rn3otk. J. D. Vance, "How Donald Trump Seduced America's White Working Class," *Guardian*, September 11, 2016, accessed April 25, 2018, https://bit.ly/2cdhVCv.

8. "Kansas' Tax Plan Makes Racial Economic Disparities Worse," Kansas Center for Economic Growth, October 14, 2016, accessed April 25, 2018, https://bit.ly/2jADG0g.

9. John Rawls, *A Theory of Justice* (Harvard, MA: Harvard University Press, 1971). "Tax Cuts Taking Toll on Kansas Communities," Kansas Center for Economic Growth, April 2015, accessed April 25, 2018, https://bit.ly/2rpTCXi.

10. Dion Lefler, Bryan Lowry, and Suzanne Perez Tobias, "Kansas Supreme Court: School Funding Inequitable," *Wichita Eagle*, February 11, 2016, accessed April 25, 2018, https://bit.ly/1O4VLse. Also see "Charter School Provision to Be Tossed from Kansas Funding Bill," *Kansas City Star*, March 21, 2014, accessed April 25, 2018, https://bit.ly/1rN61zO. Julie Bosman, "Kansas Parents Worry Schools Are Slipping Amid Budget Battles," *New York Times*, May 31, 2016, accessed April 25, 2018, https://nyti.ms/2HY6aPZ. Mitch Smith and Julie Bosman, "Kansas Supreme Court Says State Education Spending Is Too Low," *New York Times*, March 2, 2017, accessed April 25, 2018, https://nyti.ms/2lEArUG.

11. Smith and Bosman, "Kansas Supreme Court." Edwin Rios, "Kansas Court Orders Governor to Fund Public Schools," *Mother Jones*, March 3, 2017, accessed April 25, 2018, https://bit.ly/2Ijv0sR.

12. Bryan Lowry, "Do Kansas Lawmakers Personally Benefit from Business-Tax Cuts?," *Wichita Eagle*, October 10, 2016, accessed April 25, 2018, https://bit.ly/2cXTl8Z.

13. Bryan Lowry, "Block-Grant School Funding Bill Could Be Approved Quickly," *Wichita Eagle*, March 10, 2015, accessed April 25, 2018, https://bit.ly/2rpV7E3. For an excellent overview of Kansas school budget politics, see Michael Kranish, "Old Battle Lines Drawn Anew in Kansas," *Boston Globe*, April 25, 2015, accessed April 25, 2018, https://bit.ly/1EwUMRn.

14. "Saline County Commissioner's Racial Slur Featured on the *Daily Show*," *Salina (KS) Post*, April 12, 2013, accessed April 25, 2018, https://bit.ly/2rng8QI. Elspeth Reeve, "Kansas Politician Is the Latest Accidental Racist After Dropping the N-Word," *Atlantic*, April 2013, accessed April 25, 2018, https://theatln.tc/2HTFjVk. Jonathan Shorman and Hunter Woodall, "Kansas Lawmaker Makes Racist Comments About African-Americans, Marijuana," *Pittsburgh Post-Gazette*, January 8, 2018, accessed April 25, 2018, https://bit.ly/2roWdjv.

15. John Celock, "Jim Gile, Kansas County Official, Apologizes for Racist Comment," *Huffington Post*, April 9, 2013, accessed April 25, 2018, https://bit.ly/2KEOqXP. "Saline County Officials Sworn-In," KSAL, January 9, 2017, accessed April 25, 2018, https://bit.ly/2G8NuY0. Lisa Graves, "Like His Dad, Charles Koch Was a Bircher (New Documents)," *Progressive*, July 8, 2014, accessed April 25, 2018, https://bit.ly/2rpTAy2. "The Kochs' Anti–Civil Rights Roots: New Docs Expose Charles Koch's Ties to John Birch

Society," *Democracy Now!*, July 8, 2014, accessed April 25, 2018, https://bit.ly/2rpVL4r. "Sam Brownback, America's Worst Governor: He's Gutted Kansas with an Ultraconservative, Religious Agenda—and It's Getting Worse," *Salon*, March 21, 2016, accessed April 25, 2018, https://bit.ly/2l2gKkQ.

16. Nathan Lean, "The Islamophobia Industry Strikes in Kansas," *Huffington Post*, June 1, 2012, accessed April 25, 2018, https://bit.ly/2HV1j2a.

17. "Executive Order 16-01: Protecting Kansas from Terrorism," Office of the Governor of Kansas, January 8, 2016, accessed April 25, 2018, https://governor.kansas.gov /executive-order-16-01. "First 100 Days: Rules, Regulations, and Executive Orders to Examine, Revoke, and Issue," House Freedom Caucus, December 14, 2016, accessed April 25, 2018, https://bit.ly/2hQ8c7q. "Ryan Cuts Immigration Deal with House Freedom Caucus Members," NumbersUSA, October 27, 2015, accessed April 25, 2018, https://bit .ly/2FQBf26.

18. Mica Rosenberg and Julia Edwards Ainsley, "Immigration Hardliner says Trump Team Preparing Plans for Wall, Mulling Muslim Registry," Reuters, November 11, 2016, accessed April 25, 2018, https://reut.rs/2rpt4pg. Oliver Morrison, "Hispanic Kansans Increase Their Percentage of State's Population, Census Data Says," *Wichita Eagle*, June 25, 2015, accessed April 25, 2018, https://bit.ly/2jyNR5m. Gustavo López and Renee Stepler, "Latinos in the 2016 Election: Kansas," Pew Research Center, January 19, 2016, accessed April 25, 2018, http://pewrsr.ch/1ODXtT0. Heidi Beirich, "What's the Matter with Kansas's Kris Kobach?," Southern Poverty Law Center, November 2, 2015, accessed April 25, 2018, https://bit.ly/1kqg0d0.

19. "Kansas Survey Results," Public Policy Polling, accessed April 25, 2018, https:// bit.ly/2HUsIRV.

THE SCHOOLS

1. R. L. Lyman, "The Junior High Schools of Kansas City, Kansas," *School Review* 36, no. 3 (1928): 176–191.

2. B. F. White, "The Effect of Supervised Study in Kansas High Schools on Success in the University of Kansas," *School Review* 35, no. 1 (1927): 55–58. F. R. Aldrich, "The Distribution of High-School Graduates in Kansas," *School Review* 24, no. 8 (1916): 610–616. H. T. Steeper, "The Status of History Teaching in the High Schools of Kansas: Enrolment and Preparation of Teachers," *School Review* 22, no. 3 (1914): 189–191. J. W. Shideler, "The Junior-College Movement in Kansas," *School Review* 31, no. 6 (1923): 460–463.

3. Warren focuses her study on Kansas, thought by many to be the quintessential free state not only because it was home to sizable populations of Indian groups and former slaves but also because of its unique history of conflict over freedom during the antebellum period. See Kim Cary Warren, *The Quest for Citizenship: African American and Native American Education in Kansas, 1880–1935* (Durham: University of North Carolina Press, 2010).

4. Mary L. Dudziak, "The Limits of Good Faith: Desegregation in Topeka, Kansas, 1950–1956," *Law and History Review* 5, no. 2 (1987): 351–391. Bruce D. Baker and Preston C. Green III, "Tricks of the Trade: State Legislative Actions in School Finance Policy That Perpetuate Racial Disparities in the Post-Brown Era," *American Journal of Education* 111, no. 3 (2005): 372–413, accessed April 25, 2018, https://bit.ly/2I8SJwL. K. F. Gotham,

"Urban Space, Restrictive Covenants and the Origins of Racial Residential Segregation in a US City, 1900–50," *International Journal of Urban and Regional Research* 24 (2000): 616–633, doi:10.1111/1468-2427.00268.

5. Michael Kranish, "Old Battle Lines Drawn Anew in Kansas," *Boston Globe*, April 25, 2015, accessed April 25, 2018, https://bit.ly/1EwUMRn.

6. Robert Wuthnow, *Red State Religion: Faith and Politics in America's Heartland* (Princeton, NJ: Princeton University Press, 2011). "Annie on My Mind," *Wikipedia*, accessed April 25, 2018, https://bit.ly/2IxfH04.

7. *State Education Report Card: 2016 Update* (Topeka, KS: Kansas Association of School Boards, 2016), accessed April 25, 2018, https://kasb.org/wp-content/uploads/2016/12/ReportCard-Full.pdf. Also see *KASB State Education Report Card: 2017 Update* (Topeka, KS: Kansas Association of School Boards, forthcoming).

8. Dion Lefler, "Private-School Vouchers Next Round in School Funding Debate," *Wichita Eagle*, March 5, 2017, accessed April 25, 2018, https://bit.ly/2Ijo9Qk.

9. Julie Bosman, "Kansas Parents Worry Schools Are Slipping Amid Budget Battles," *New York Times*, May 31, 2016, accessed April 25, 2018, https://nyti.ms/2HY6aPZ.

10. Ibid.

11. "Melissa Rooker," Melissa Rooker for Kansas House, accessed April 25, 2018, http://melissarooker.com/about-me/bio.

12. "NY Times Commits Journalistic Malpractice," Kansas GOP Insider (Wannabe), June 1, 2016, accessed April 25, 2018, www.insideksgop.com/2016/06/ny-times-commits-journalistic.html. "Student Outcomes Not Improving Despite Huge Increases in Education Spending," Kansas Policy Institute, May 24, 2017, accessed April 25, 2018, https://bit.ly/2K0iETP. "2017 State of the State Address," Office of the Governor of Kansas, January 10, 2017, accessed April 25, 2018, https://bit.ly/2Ifwkx9. "Measurable Success from a Proven Leader," Sam Brownback for Governor, accessed April 25, 2018, http://brownback.com/record. "SFFF Lawyers Clean Up with $7M from Schools," *Sentinel*, September 27, 2017, accessed April 25, 2018, https://sentinelksmo.org/sfff-lawyers-clean-7m-schools. "Kansas Tax Experiment: Not a Cautionary Tale but Lessons to Be Learned," Kansas Policy Institute, March 1, 2018, accessed April 25, 2018, https://kansaspolicy.org/kansas-tax-experiment.

13. Howard Gleckman, "The Great Kansas Tax Cut Experiment Crashes and Burns," *Forbes*, June 7, 2017, accessed April 25, 2018, https://bit.ly/2rnRMFu. "Kansas Lawmakers Override Governor Veto," *US News & World Report*, June 6, 2017, accessed April 25, 2018, https://bit.ly/2FQ9Hd7.

14. Kansas City Star Editorial Board, "Kansas Is In Better Shape in 2018. Gov. Brownback's Impending Goodbye Is One Reason Why," *Kansas City Star*, January 7, 2018, accessed April 25, 2018, https://bit.ly/2rqpv1h.

15. "Senate Bill 30: The Legislature Sets Kansas on the Road to Recovery," Kansas Center for Economic Growth, accessed April 25, 2018, https://bit.ly/2K0EQ0d.

16. Bryan Lowry, "Kris Kobach Launches Campaign for Kansas Governor," *Kansas City Star*, June 8, 2017, accessed April 25, 2018, https://bit.ly/2r6ig18.

17. Peter Hancock, "Lawmakers Pass School Funding and Tax Package," *Lawrence (KS) Journal-World*, June 5, 2017, accessed April 25, 2018, https://bit.ly/2KIpoqG.

18. Mark Tallman, "Key Facts: How Much Does Kansas Provide Per Pupil for K–12 Education?," Kansas Association of School Boards, October 17, 2016, accessed April

25, 2018, https://bit.ly/2rpYI5g. Lyndsey Layton, "Connecting School Spending and Student Achievement," *Washington Post*, July 9, 2014, accessed April 25, 2018, http://wapo .st/1sv9PDa. Michael Leachman and Chris Mai, "Most States Still Funding Schools Less Than Before the Recession," Center on Budget and Policy Priorities, October 16, 2014, accessed April 25, 2018, https://bit.ly/2rojmU5. "New York School Districts," Center for American Progress, 2011, accessed April 25, 2018, https://ampr.gs/2wkdXlJ.

19. Ulrich Boser, *Return on Educational Investment: A District-by-District Evaluation of U.S. Educational Productivity* (Washington, DC: Center for American Progress, 2014), accessed April 25, 2018, http://files.eric.ed.gov/fulltext/ED561093.pdf.

Congestive Heart Failure

1. "One Nation, by Ben Carson: On Education," *On the Issues*, accessed April 25, 2018, https://bit.ly/2Ga8Jsm.htm. Quinn McNeill, "11 Quotes on Education from 2016 Presidential Candidates," MSNBC, October 5, 2015, accessed April 25, 2018, https:// on.msnbc.com/1VCVXDF. "An Excerpt from *Tough Choices: A Memoir*, Written by: Carly Fiorina," Penguin Random House, accessed April 25, 2018, https://bit.ly/2IuDQEm.

2. "Malcolm X's Speech at the Founding Rally of the Organization of Afro-American Unity (1964)," BlackPast.org, accessed April 25, 2018, https://shar.es/1SQCXU. In an address to the World Bank Conference, UN secretary-general Kofi Annan claimed that "knowledge is power. Information is liberating. Education is the premise of progress, in every society, in every family." See "'If Information and Knowledge Are Central to Democracy, They Are Conditions for Development,' Says Secretary-General," United Nations, June 23, 1997, accessed April 25, 2018, https://bit.ly/2jzb7Ab.

3. Emily B. Zimmerman, Steven H. Woolf, and Amber Haley, "Understanding the Relationship Between Education and Health: A Review of the Evidence and an Examination of Community Perspectives," Agency for Healthcare Research and Quality, September 2015, accessed April 25, 2018, https://bit.ly/2mKZYMi. Point three is, in essence, life remaining for individuals who are twenty-five years of age. This figure is a more accurate representation of remaining years because total life expectancy from infancy takes into account childhood deaths.

4. Zimmerman et al., "Understanding the Relationship."

5. J. K. Montez and L. F. Berkman, "Trends in the Educational Gradient of Mortality Among US Adults Aged 45 to 84 Years: Bringing Regional Context into the Explanation," *American Journal of Public Health* 104, no. 1 (2014): 82–90, doi:10.2105 /AJPH.2013.301526. Jacob S. Hacker and Paul Pierson, "The Path to Prosperity Is Blue," *New York Times*, July 30, 2016, accessed April 25, 2018, https://nyti.ms/2k2f8ve.

6. As but a few examples, see Ledyard King, "Superfund Cuts Would Lead to Delays in Toxic Cleanups, Experts Warn," *USA Today*, August 1, 2017, accessed April 25, 2018, https://usat.ly/2f7WzbW. Michelle Martin, "Budget Cuts Could Lead to More Radon Deaths," *Newsweek*, May 12, 2017, accessed April 25, 2018, https://bit.ly/2pVe1mQ. Barbara B. Brown, Ken R. Smith, Wyatt A. Jensen, and Doug Tharp, "Transit Rider Body Mass Index Before and After Completion of Street Light-Rail Line in Utah," *American Journal of Public Health* 107, no. 9 (2017): 1484–1486. K. M. Parker, J. Rice, J. Gustat, J. Ruley, A. Spriggs, and C. Johnson, "Effect of Bike Lane Infrastructure Improvements on Ridership in One New Orleans Neighborhood," *Annals of Behavioral Medicine* 45 (2013): 101–107.

7. Steve Benen, "What Kansans Don't Know Might Hurt Them," *MaddowBlog*, October 25, 2016, accessed April 25, 2018, https://on.msnbc.com/2eG9vCH. "Kansas Policy Institute," SourceWatch, accessed April 25, 2018, https://bit.ly/2rClXZH (also https://kansaspolicy.org). Steve Rose, "Phony Numbers Meant to Smear Superb Kansas Services," *Kansas City Star*, July 2, 2016, accessed April 25, 2018, https://bit.ly/2HTfAfE (also https://kac.org).

8. "KASB State-Level Database," Tableau Public, accessed April 25, 2018, https://tabsoft.co/2rpCn8G. *State Education Report Card: 2016 Update* (Topeka, KS: Kansas Association of School Boards, 2016), accessed April 25, 2018, https://kasb.org/wp-content/uploads/2016/12/ReportCard-Full.pdf. *State Education Report Card: 2017 Update* (Topeka, KS: Kansas Association of School Boards, forthcoming). *2016 State Education Report Card: Executive Summary: Overall Rankings and School Funding* (Topeka, KS: Kansas Association of School Boards, 2016), accessed April 25, 2018, https://bit.ly/2ImkYYc. *State Education Report Card: 2017 Update* advance copy, (Topeka, KS: Kansas Association of School Boards, forthcoming), 7–8, https://kasb.org.

9. In other words, we laid the NAEP results over the KASB report. The NAEP scores help rank students as basic or proficient, while the KASB report provided the differences in achievement levels by income. We pulled yearly data from 2008 to 2015 (i.e., the four years before the Brownback cuts and the four years after they began to take effect).

10. "State Performance Comparison," Nation's Report Card, 2017, accessed April 25, 2018, https://bit.ly/2IqdjVZ. "Kansas K–12 Report Generator," KSDE Data Central, 2016, accessed April 25, 2018, https://bit.ly/2I1IACc. "KASB State-Level Database," Tableau Public.

11. "State Performance Comparison," Nation's Report Card. Search criteria included NCES as the source, Kansas as the state, and 2009, 2011, 2013, and 2015 as the years for analysis. NAEP 4 Math All Score, NAEP 4 Math Black Score, NAEP 4 Math White Score, and NAEP 4 Hispanic Score were selected for analysis. Then search criteria, NCES, Kansas as the state, and 2009, 2011, and 2015 as the years for analysis (2013 did not report this score). NAEP 4 Math White Basic or Above, NAEP 4 Math Black Basic or Above, and NAEP 4 Math Hispanic Basic or Above were selected. Then search criteria included NCES as the source, Kansas as the state, and 2009, 2011, 2013, and 2015 as the years for analysis. NAEP 8 Math All Score, NAEP 8 Math Black Score, and NAEP 8 Math White Score, and NAEP 8 Math Hispanic Score were selected for analysis. For the comparison charts, Proficient and Above and Basic and Above were selected for these analyses.

12. *KASB State Education Report Card: 2017 Update*, advance copy, 12–13.

13. "Essential Tools: Increasing Rates of School Completion: Moving from Policy and Research to Practice: A Manual for Policymakers, Administrators, and Educators," National Center on Secondary Education and Transition, accessed April 25, 2018, https://bit.ly/2KHh6PZ. E. A. Houck and A. Kurtz, "Resource Distribution and Graduation Rates in SREB States: An Overview," *Peabody Journal of Education* 85, no. 1 (2010): 32–48. Liang Zhang, "Does State Funding Affect Graduation Rates at Public Four-Year Colleges and Universities?," *Educational Policy* 23, no. 5 (2009): 714–731, https://bit.ly/2wiFkMZ.

14. "Kansas K–12 Report Generator," KSDE Data Central. "Dropouts by grade, race, gender" for public schools only was selected as the variable for analysis. Each school year's data between 2006/2007 and 2015/2016 was downloaded individually to procure rates per year rather than totals.

15. Here I use the US census term, for consistency. See "Hispanic Origin," United States Census Bureau, accessed April 25, 2018, https://bit.ly/1TPcp5g.

16. As quoted in George Seldes, ed., *The Great Quotations* (New York: Pocket, 1971), 641.

17. Even before the Trump administration's threat of DACA repeal, which would take away the only opportunities that many had to go to college in the first place. Of the estimated 13,000 students eligible for DACA in Kansas, 34 percent enrolled in primary or middle schools while 32 percent enrolled in high schools. See "Deferred Action for Childhood Arrivals (DACA) Profile: Kansas," Migration Policy Institute, accessed April 25, 2018, https://bit.ly/2wghCRO.

18. "Kansas School District Demographic Characteristics," Proximity, accessed April 25, 2018, https://bit.ly/2IdJ43X.

19. In other words, had pre-budget-cut trends remained in place, the white dropout rate should have been 1.11 percent in 2016. Instead, after the cuts, the white dropout rate rose to 1.5 percent. Thus, 4,400.72 white students were projected to drop out of high school. But in reality, 5,069.11 students actually dropped out in the four years after the cuts began. Ultimately, 668.39 *more* white students dropped out than might have otherwise done so based on a continuation of previous education funding.

20. "Sharp Partisan Divisions in Views of National Institutions," Pew Research Center, July 10, 2017, accessed April 25, 2018, https://pewrsr.ch/2tAL2GP. Paul Fain, "Deep Partisan Divide on Higher Education," *Inside Higher Ed*, July 11, 2017, accessed April 25, 2018, https://bit.ly/2HXZCNe.

21. Scott Jaschik, "Losing the White Working Class, Too," *Inside Higher Ed*, July 31, 2017, accessed April 25, 2018, https://bit.ly/2I00j8I. "House Majority PAC White Working Class Voter Project (Continued)," Expedition Strategies, July 2017, accessed April 25, 2018, https://bit.ly/2FNU1a.D.

22. Kansas City Star Editorial Board, "What Kansas City Can Learn from Bidding for Amazon's HQ2," *Kansas City Star*, October 17, 2017, accessed April 25, 2018, https://bit.ly/2K0l2tZ.

MILLIONS OF MILLIONS

1. Editorial Board, "Kris Kobach Has It Wrong on Education," *Wichita Eagle*, May 15, 2018, https://www.kansas.com/opinion/editorials/article211201214.html. Sherman Smith, "In School Funding Fight, Kobach Uses 'Crystal Palaces' to Promote 75% Mandate," *Topeka Capital-Journal*, July 1, 2018, http://cjonline.com/news/20180701/in-school-funding-fight-kobach-uses-crystal-palaces-to-promote-75-mandate.

2. Mr. Kobach argued that while there had been a relatively small number of noncitizens in Kansas who had tried to vote, he believed that they were only "the tip of the iceberg." In her ruling, Judge Robinson dismissed Mr. Kobach's claim: "Instead, the Court draws the more obvious conclusion that there is no iceberg; only an icicle, largely created by confusion and administrative error." Julie Bosman, "Judge Rejects Kansas Law Requiring Voters to Show Proof of Citizenship," *New York Times*, June 18, 2018, https://nyti.ms/2ljRq0d. Allyson Chiu, "'I Will Not Back Down': Kansas Republican Defends Displaying Replica Machine Gun in Parade," *Washington Post*, June 4, 2018, https://wapo.st/2xEPacN?tid=ss_tw&utm_term=.08856f2493c0. Ella Nilsen, "Kris

Kobach's Campaign Is Accused of Hiring White Nationalists. Trump Just Endorsed Him," *Vox*, August 6, 2018, https://www.vox.com/policy-and-politics/2018/8/6/17656700 /kris-kobach-kansas-governor-trump-endorsement-primary.

CONCLUSION: THE CASTLE DOCTRINE

1. Joel Currier, "Mother of Florissant Woman Who Protested in Ferguson Believes Daughter's Death Was Accident," *St. Louis Post-Dispatch*, November 28, 2014, accessed April 26, 2018, https://bit.ly/2KnuMOQ.

2. Robert Samuels, "Ferguson Police Chief Asks St. Louis County Police to Manage Protests," *Washington Post*, October 3, 2014, accessed April 26, 2018, https://www .washingtonpost.com/news/post-nation/wp/2014/10/03/ferguson-police-chief-asks-st-louis -county-police-to-manage-protests. Alison Vingiano, "Pro–Darren Wilson Cardinals Fans Clash with Pro–Michael Brown Ferguson Protesters in St. Louis," BuzzFeed, October 7, 2014, accessed April 26, 2018, https://bzfd.it/2IgHuTb. "Michael Brown Protesters Interrupt St. Louis Symphony Orchestra Concert," *St. Louis Post-Dispatch*, October 6, 2014, accessed April 26, 2018, https://bit.ly/2wGtaOg. Jon Swaine, "Missouri Governor Declares State of Emergency as National Guard Called in to Ferguson," *Guardian*, November 17, 2014, accessed April 26, 2018, https://www.theguardian.com/us-news/2014/nov/17 /missouri-governor-state-of-emergency-ferguson.

3. Among the multiple sources reporting on the Campbell incident, see, for instance, Currier, "Mother of Florissant Woman." Also see: Evan Perez and Shimon Prokupecz, "Police: Woman Allegedly Kills Herself with Gun Bought to Prepare for Ferguson Unrest," CNN, November 23, 2014, accessed April 26, 2018, https://www.cnn.com/2014/11/23 /us/ferguson-woman-kills-herself/index.html; Catherine Thompson, "Police: Woman Saying She's 'Ready for Ferguson' Shoots, Kills Self by Accident," *Talking Points Memo*, November 24, 2014, accessed April 26, 2018, https://talkingpointsmemo.com/livewire /ferguson-woman-kills-self-gun-accident.

4. Hilary Hanson, "Becca Campbell Dead After Gun Bought to Prepare for Ferguson Decision Discharges: Report," *Huffington Post*, November 24, 2014, accessed April 26, 2018, https://bit.ly/2KXZnUe. Also see Lisa Suhay, "Ferguson Spurs Rise of New Gun Owners in St. Louis: Another Safety Threat?," *Christian Science Monitor*, November 24, 2014, accessed May 10, 2016, https://www.csmonitor.com/USA/Society/2014/1124 /Ferguson-spurs-rise-of-new-gun-owners-in-St.-Louis-Another-safety-threat. Also see refs 1–3 above.

5. Mary Sanchez, "Fear of Immigrants Paved Kris Kobach's Path to Candidate for Kansas Governor," *Kansas City Star*, May 3, 2018, accessed May 8, 2018, https://www .kansascity.com/opinion/opn-columns-blogs/mary-sanchez/article210414974.html.

6. Hanson, "Becca Campbell." Nickarama, "#Ferguson Protester Becca Campbell Killed with Her Own Gun," Weaselzippers, November 24, 2014, accessed April 26, 2018, https://www.weaselzippers.us/206098-ferguson-protester-killed-with-her-own-gun. Currier, "Mother of Florissant Woman."

7. Currier, "Mother of Florissant Woman."

8. In 1968, the civil rights activist Stokely Carmichael famously assailed forms of racial bias that maintained the status quo through such structures as zoning laws, economics, welfare bureaucracies, schools, criminal law enforcement, and courts. Institutionalized

racism, he argued, "is less overt, far more subtle, less identifiable in terms of specific individuals committing the acts, but is no less destructive of human life." Stokely Carmichael, "Black Power, A Critique of the System of International White Supremacy & International Capitalism," in *The Dialectics of Liberation*, ed. David Cooper (New York: Penguin, 1968), 151. Also see E. Bonilla-Silva, "Rethinking Racism: Toward a Structural Interpretation," *American Sociological Review* 62 (2003): 465–480.

9. Brittaney Jewel Bethea, "Effects of Segregation Negatively Impact Health," *Source*, November 6, 2013, accessed April 26, 2018, https://source.wustl.edu/2013/11 /effects-of-segregation-negatively-impact-health. Also see Drew Margary, "The Most Racist City in America: St. Louis?," *Gawker*, September 26, 2013, accessed April 26, 2018, http://gawker.com/5946663/the-most-racist-city-in-america-st-louis. Michael B. Sauter and Thomas C. Frohlich, "America's Most Segregated Cities," *24/7 Wall Street*, September 8, 2016, accessed April 26, 2018, https://247wallst.com/special-report/2016/09/08 /americas-most-segregated-cities-2/5/. Govin Vatsan, "St. Louis: A Segregated City," *Washington University Political Review*, May 16, 2013, accessed April 26, 2018, www.wupr .org/2013/05/16/st-louis-a-segregated-city. Maggie Clark, "St. Louis Police Predict Dire Impact from Sequestration," *Governing*, October 15, 2012, accessed April 26, 2018, www .governing.com/news/state/sl-police-predict-dire-impact-from-sequestration.html.

10. "Investigation of the Ferguson Police Department," United States Department of Justice Civil Rights Division, March 4, 2015, accessed April 26, 2018, https://bit .ly/1lV31kb. Ryan J. Reilly, "Police Research Group Shocked by Predatory Ticketing Practices in St. Louis County," *Huffington Post*, May 4, 2015, accessed April 26, 2018, https:// www.huffingtonpost.com/2015/05/04/st-louis-county-predatory-policing_n_7201964.html. Kera Mashek, "Residents Voice Worries as Raytown Budget Cuts Could Lead to Loss of More Than a Dozen Police Officers," Fox 4 News, September 26, 2017, http://via.fox4kc .com/rJLFK. Kurt Erickson, "Nixon Cuts Another $51 Million from Budget amid Slow Revenue Growth," *St. Louis Post-Dispatch*, December 7, 2016, accessed April 26, 2018, https://bit.ly/2IC6i7t. Garrett Haake, "Feds Warn: Sequester Is 'Crime-Fighting Kryptonite,'" KSHB, July 30, 2013, accessed April 26, 2018, https://www.kshb.com/news/state /missouri/national-budget-cuts-could-impact-personal-safety. Christine Byers and Chuck Raasch, "Feds Stop Sharing Asset Forfeitures with Local Police After $1.2 Billion in Spending Cuts," *St. Louis Post-Dispatch*, December 23, 2015, accessed April 26, 2018, https://bit.ly/2rIYVRc. In May 2015, a report about Missouri policing produced by the Police Executive Research Forum found that "the crisis in many St. Louis County departments is driven by the need to generate more and more revenue . . . police departments are being pushed into the role of revenue generators for their cities and towns. They are being diverted away from their traditional roles of community guardians and protectors." See *Overcoming the Challenges and Creating a Regional Approach to Policing in St. Louis City and County* (Bethesda, MD: Police Executive Research Forum, 2015), 10, accessed April 26, 2018, www.bettertogetherstl.com/wp-content/uploads/2015/04/PERF-Report -Overcoming-the-Challenges.pdf.

11. *2013 Report Card for Missouri's Infrastructure* (Reston, VA: American Society of Civil Engineers, 2013), accessed April 26, 2018, https://bit.ly/2rH6FmL.

12. Denise Hollinshed, "Woman Fatally Shot Inside Vehicle in St. Louis," *St. Louis Post-Dispatch*, November 22, 2014, accessed April 26, 2018, https://bit.ly/1xiMQMb. Also see Ashton Edwards and CNN Wire, "Woman Says, 'We're Ready for Ferguson,' Accidentally

Shoots Self in Head," Fox 13 Salt Lake City, November 24, 2014, accessed April 26, 2018, http://fox13now.com/2014/11/24/woman-says-were-ready-for-ferguson-accidentally -shoots-self-in-head. "History of Barnes-Jewish Hospital," Barnes-Jewish Team, December 7, 2012, accessed April 26, 2018, http://barnesjewishblog.org/history-barnes-jewish -hospital. "Affordable Care Act, Sequestration Hit St. Louis Hospitals Hard," CBS St. Louis, November 12, 2013, accessed April 26, 2018, https://stlouis.cbslocal .com/2013/11/12/affordable-care-act-sequestration-hit-st-louis-hospitals-hard. Associated Press and Andrew Nichols, "Nixon: Tax Cut Bill Would Harm Education, Eliminate Funding for Fulton Hospital," KBIA, July 30, 2013, accessed April 26, 2018, http://kbia.org /post/nixon-tax-cut-bill-would-harm-education-eliminate-funding-new-fulton-hospital.

13. Sabrina Tavernise, "In Missouri, Fewer Gun Restrictions and More Gun Killings," *New York Times*, December 22, 2015, accessed April 26, 2018, https://www.nytimes .com/2015/12/22/health/in-missouri-fewer-gun-restrictions-and-more-gun-killings.html. Associated Press in Jefferson City, "Missouri Approves Concealed Gun at Schools and Open Carry in Public," *Guardian*, September 11, 2014, accessed April 26, 2018, https://www .theguardian.com/world/2014/sep/11/missouri-guns-schools-law-concealed-open -governor. "Missouri:Castle Doctrine and Training Bill Passes House," NRA Institute for Legislative Action, April 30, 2015, accessed April 26, 2018, https://www.nraila.org /articles/20150430/missouri-castle-doctrine-and-training-bill-passes-house. For the spike in gun sales in St. Louis during the Ferguson protests, see Suhay, "Ferguson Spurs Rise."

14. Chuck Raasch, "Missouri Had Highest Black Homicide Rate in 2012, Gun Control Group Says," *St. Louis Post-Dispatch*, January 14, 2015, https://bit.ly/2Ig8ySm. Selwyn Duke, "Misery in Missouri? Claim: Looser Gun Laws Leading to More Murder," *New American*, March 14, 2016, accessed April 26, 2018, https://www.thenewamerican.com/usnews /crime/item/22753-misery-in-missouri-claim-looser-gun-laws-leading-to-more-murder. Results of a search for "white:black unintentional firearm deaths, 2008–2013" at http:// webappa.cdc.gov/cgi-bin/broker.exe.

15. George Lipsitz, *The Possessive Investment in Whiteness: How White People Profit from Identity Politics* (Philadelphia: Temple University Press, 2006).

16. Editorial Board, "The Death of Michael Brown," *New York Times*, August 12, 2014, https://nyti.ms/1vF2jea. Adam D. Kiš, *The Development Trap: How Big Thinking Fails the Poor* (New Jersey: Routledge, 2018).

17. "Why Traffic-Choked Nashville Said 'No Thanks' to Public Transit," *Wired*, May 19, 2018, accessed May 20, 2018, https://www.wired.com/story/nashville-transit -referendum-vote-plan/?mbid=email_onsiteshare.

18. Kansas City Star Editorial Board, "Kansas Is In Better Shape in 2018. Gov. Brownback's Impending Goodbye Is One Reason Why," *Kansas City Star*, January 7, 2018, accessed April 26, 2018, https://www.kansascity.com/opinion/editorials/article193296389 .html.

19. Linda Tirado, "Dear Dana Loesch: How Do You Sleep at Night?," *Daily Beast*, March 9, 2018, accessed April 26, 2018, https://www.thedailybeast.com/dear-dana-loesch -how-do-you-sleep-at-night.

20. Lena H. Sun and Juliet Eilperin, "CDC Gets List of Forbidden Words: Fetus, Transgender, Diversity," *Washington Post*, December 15, 2017, http://wapo.st/2j7DbdS?tid=ss _tw&utm_term=.270f056ef431. Thomas B. Edsall, "Trump Has Got Democrats Right Where He Wants Them," *New York Times*, February 1, 2018, accessed April 26, 2018,

https://www.nytimes.com/2018/02/01/opinion/trump-democrats-immigration.html. Katherine W. Phillips, "How Diversity Makes Us Smarter," *Scientific American*, October 1, 2014, accessed April 26, 2018, https://www.scientificamerican.com/article/how-diversity-makes-us-smarter. S. E. Page, *The Difference: How the Power of Diversity Creates Better Groups, Firms, Schools, and Societies* (Princeton, NJ: Princeton University Press, 2008).

21. Mike Spies, "When Kids Pull the Trigger, Who Is Responsible? Not Gun Owners, the NRA Says," *Newsweek*, October 10, 2016, accessed April 26, 2018, https://www.newsweek.com/2016/10/21/when-kids-pull-trigger-who-responsible-507656.html.

22. Shelby Black, "Trump's Tweet About the Super Bowl Was So, So Underwhelming," *Elite Daily*, February 5, 2018, accessed April 26, 2018, https://www.elitedaily.com/p/trumps-tweet-about-the-super-bowl-was-so-so-underwhelming-8095741.

23. James P. McClure and J. Jefferson Looney, eds., *The Papers of Thomas Jefferson*, digital edition (Charlottesville: University of Virginia Press, 2008), accessed April 26, 2018, http://rotunda.upress.virginia.edu/founders/TSJN.html.

24. Javion Simmons, "'Evil Doesn't Care About Laws': Ky. Governor Responds to Shooting, Gun Violence," WKRN, January 25, 2018, accessed April 26, 2018, https://bit.ly/2IhavOB. Daniel Desrochers, "'You Can't Regulate Evil,' Bevin Says of Vegas Shooting. Here's How Twitter Reacted," *Lexington (KY) Herald-Leader*, October 2, 2017, accessed April 26, 2018, https://www.kentucky.com/news/politics-government/article176616521.html. Bryan Lowry, "'It's a Pit.' As He Leaves Kansas, Brownback Decries Underfunding of State Facilities," *Kansas City Star*, January 30, 2018, accessed April 26, 2018, https://www.kansascity.com/news/politics-government/article197379284.html. "Brownback Calls for $600 Million More in Education Funding, but Offers No Way to Pay," *Kansas City Star*, January 28, 2018, accessed May 15, 2018, https://www.kansascity.com/news/politics-government/article193831104.html. Also see Sherman Smith, "Report Refutes Brownback Claim That 'Rural Recession' Caused Budget Woes," *Topeka Capital-Journal*, March 24, 2018, accessed March 20, 2018, http://cjonline.com/news/20180324/report-refutes-brownback-claim-that-rural-recession-caused-budget-woes.

25. Linley Sanders, "Kentucky School Shooting: Doctor Who Treated Students Says Politicians 'Will Do Nothing' to Stop Next Attack," *Newsweek*, January 24, 2018, accessed April 26, 2018, https://www.newsweek.com/doctor-kentucky-school-shooting-victims-politicians-will-do-nothing-789899.

26. "Former CNN Anchor's Husband Shoots, Kills Motel Robber," *Kansas City Star*, July 2, 2015, accessed April 26, 2018, https://www.kansascity.com/news/nation-world/national/article26038183.html. Jason Kravarik and Stephanie Elam, "Good Samaritan with a Gun Saves Wounded Cop," CNN, April 6, 2017, accessed May 1, 2018, https://www.cnn.com/2017/03/17/us/beyond-the-call-of-duty-arizona/index.html.

27. Richard Clark, "Man Accidentally Shoots Self While Guarding 'Muslim-Free' Oktaha Gun Store," NewsOn6.com, August 18, 2015, accessed May 1, 2018, www.newson6.com/story/29826547/man-accidentally-shoots-self-while-guarding-muslim-free-oktaha-gun-store. David Moye, "NRA Employee Accidentally Shoots Himself on the Job," *Huffington Post*, April 7, 2017, accessed May 1, 2018, https://www.huffingtonpost.com/entry/nra-employee-shoots-himself_us_58e7f971e4b00de1410384e7#. "Man Shoots Himself in the Head During NRA 500 at Texas," *USA Today*, April 14, 2013, accessed May 1, 2018, https://www.usatoday.com/story/sports/nascar/2013/04/14/fan-death-investigation-texas-motor-speedway/2081395.

28. Jonathan M. Metzl and Kenneth T. Macleish, "Mental Illness, Mass Shootings, and the Politics of American Firearms," *American Journal of Public Health* 105, no. 2 (2015): 240–249, doi:10.2105/ajph.2014.302242. "More than 80 percent of Americans believe illegal gun dealers and poor access to mental health care are to blame for mass shootings." See Jeremy Lin, "Poll: Americans Are Split on Who's to Blame for 2018's School Shootings," *Politico*, May 25, 2018, accessed May 28, 2018, https://www.politico.com/interactives/2018/school-shooting-poll.

29. Dimitrios Pagourtzis, the Sante Fe shooter, "did not appear to have a history of mental health or legal issues." Evan Perez, Jason Morris, and Ralph Ellis, "What We Know About Dimitrios Pagourtzis, the Alleged Santa Fe High School Shooter," CNN, May 21, 2018, accessed May 22, 2018, https://www.cnn.com/2018/05/18/us/dimitrios-pagourtzis-santa-fe-suspect/index.html.

INDEX

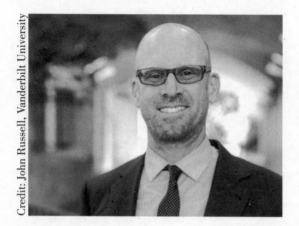

Jonathan M. Metzl is the Frederick B. Rentschler II Professor of Sociology and Psychiatry and Director of the Center for Medicine, Health, and Society at Vanderbilt University. A leading national voice on gun violence and mental illness, Metzl writes extensively for medical, psychiatric, and popular publications. His books include *The Protest Psychosis*, *Prozac on the Couch*, and *Against Health*. He hails from Kansas City, Missouri, and lives in Nashville, Tennessee.